# Paediatric Endocrinology and Diabetes

# Oxford Specialist Handbooks published and forthcoming

# Paediatric Endocrinology and Diabetes

**Second edition**

## Gary Butler

Consultant in Paediatric and Adolescent Medicine and
Endocrinology, University College London Hospital;
Clinical Professor in Child and Adolescent Health, UCL
Great Ormond Street Institute of Child Health; and
Honorary Consultant in Paediatric and Adolescent
Endocrinology, Gender Identity Development Service,
Tavistock and Portman Trust

## Jeremy Kirk

Consultant Paediatric Endocrinologist, Birmingham
and Research and Innovation Director, Women's and
Children's Hospital NHS Foundation Trust; Honorary
Professor, University of Birmingham and also University
of Wolverhampton; and Clinical Director, NIHR Clinical
Research Network (CRN), West Midlands

OXFORD
UNIVERSITY PRESS

## OXFORD
UNIVERSITY PRESS

Great Clarendon Street, Oxford, OX2 6DP,
United Kingdom

Oxford University Press is a department of the University of Oxford.
It furthers the University's objective of excellence in research, scholarship,
and education by publishing worldwide. Oxford is a registered trade mark of
Oxford University Press in the UK and in certain other countries

© Oxford University Press 2020

The moral rights of the authors have been asserted

First Edition published in 2011
Second Edition published in 2020

Published in the United States of America by Oxford University Press
198 Madison Avenue, New York, NY 10016, United States of America

British Library Cataloguing in Publication Data
Data available

Library of Congress Control Number: 2019950488

ISBN 978–0–19–878633–7

Printed and bound by CPI Group (UK) Ltd, Croydon, CR0 4YY

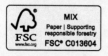

MIX
Paper | Supporting
responsible forestry
FSC® C013604

The manufacturer's authorised representative in the EU for product safety is
Oxford University Press España S.A. of el Parque Empresarial San Fernando de
Henares, Avenida de Castilla, 2 – 28830 Madrid (www.oup.es/en).

To my wife Lizzie, and children Jules, Chris and Mariana.
GB

To my wife Katie, and children Olivia and Lucinda.
JK

# Contents

# Contents

# Preface to second edition

We were astounded at how popular the first edition was, having sold out completely. Listening to the positive feedback, we have kept the format unchanged, with an easily accessible emergencies section. All chapters have now been fully revised, taking into account new developments in classification, diagnosis, and management. We are grateful to Dr Billy White UCLH for help with revising the diabetes chapter. Other chapters have taken into account new diagnostic classifications based on newly identified genes, and changes in treatment schedules based on evidence-based studies, newer therapies, and revised product availabilities. There is now also a new chapter on endocrine support for young people with gender incongruence.

We hope that this second edition will be as helpful in guiding safe and effective care of children and adolescents with endocrine conditions. Whereas we have taken every care in checking investigation protocols, normal laboratory ranges and drug dosages, we advise the reader to consult with the local laboratory and pharmacy as well.

Gary Butler and Jeremy Kirk

# Symbols and abbreviations

| | |
|---|---|
| ➔ | cross-reference |
| ▶ | important |
| 🔊 | website |
| ~ | approximately |
| 1° | primary |
| 2° | secondary |
| 3° | tertiary |
| 17OHP | 17-hydroxyprogesterone |
| 21OHD | 21-hydroxylase deficiency |
| ACDC | Association of Children's Diabetes Clinicians |
| ACE | angiotensin-converting enzyme |
| ACR | albumin:creatinine ratio |
| ACTH | adrenocorticotropic hormone |
| AD | autosomal dominant |
| ADA | American Diabetes Association |
| ADH | antidiuretic hormone |
| AFP | alpha fetoprotein |
| AHO | Albright's hereditary osteodystrophy |
| ALL | acute lymphoblastic leukaemia |
| ALS | acid-labile subunit |
| AMH | anti-Müllerian hormone |
| APS | autoimmune polyglandular syndrome |
| AR | autosomal recessive |
| AVP | arginine vasopressin |
| BBS | Bardet–Biedl syndrome |
| bd | twice daily |
| BMC | bone mineral content |
| BMD | bone mineral density |
| BMI | body mass index |
| BMT | bone marrow transplantation |
| BSPED | British Society for Paediatric Endocrinology and Diabetes |
| BWS | Beckwith–Wiedemann syndrome |
| CAH | congenital adrenal hyperplasia |
| CAIS | complete androgen insensitivity syndrome |
| CDGP | constitutional delay of growth and puberty |
| CDI | cranial diabetes insipidus |
| CFRD | cystic fibrosis-related diabetes |

| | |
|---|---|
| CGM | continuous glucose monitoring |
| CGMS | continuous glucose monitoring system |
| CH | congenital hypothyroidism |
| CNS | central nervous system |
| CPHD | combined pituitary hormone deficiency |
| CPP | central precocious puberty |
| CRH | corticotropin-releasing hormone |
| CRI | chronic renal insufficiency |
| CSI | craniospinal irradiation |
| CSII | continuous subcutaneous insulin infusion |
| DCCT | Diabetes Control and Complications Trials |
| DDAVP | 1-deamino-8-D-arginine vasopressin |
| DHEA | dehydroepiandrosterone |
| DHEA-S | dehydroepiandrosterone sulphate |
| DHT | dihydrotestosterone |
| DI | diabetes insipidus |
| DIDMOAD | diabetes insipidus, diabetes mellitus, optic atrophy, and deafness |
| DKA | diabetic ketoacidosis |
| DSD | disorder of sex development |
| DXA | dual-energy X-ray absorptiometry |
| EDTA | ethylenediaminetetraacetic acid |
| ESPE | European Society for Paediatric Endocrinology |
| ESR | erythrocyte sedimentation rate |
| FBC | full blood count |
| FDA | Food and Drug Administration |
| FGD | familial glucocorticoid deficiency |
| FSH | follicle-stimulating hormone |
| FSS | familial short stature |
| GAD | glutamic acid decarboxylase |
| GH | growth hormone |
| GHD | growth hormone deficiency |
| GHIS | growth hormone insensitivity syndrome |
| GHR | growth hormone receptor |
| GHRH | growth-hormone releasing hormone |
| GI | gastrointestinal |
| GIPP | gonadotropin-independent precocious puberty |
| GnRH | gonadotropin-releasing hormone |
| GnRHa | gonadotropin-releasing hormone analogue |
| GSD | glycogen synthase deficiency |
| GTT | glucose tolerance test |

| | |
|---|---|
| HbA1c | glycated haemoglobin |
| hCG | human chorionic gonadotropin |
| HDL | high-density lipoprotein |
| HH | hypogonadotropic hypogonadism *or* hyperinsulinaemic hypoglycaemia |
| HHS | hyperosmolar hyperglycaemic state |
| HPA | hypothalamic–pituitary–adrenal |
| HSD | hydroxysteroid dehydrogenase |
| HV | height velocity |
| IAA | insulin autoantibodies |
| ICA | islet cell antibodies |
| IFG | impaired fasting glycaemia |
| IGF-1 | insulin-like growth factor 1 |
| IGFBP3 | insulin-like growth factor binding protein 3 |
| IGT | impaired glucose tolerance |
| IHH | idiopathic hypogonadotropic hypogonadism |
| IM | intramuscular |
| ISPAD | International Society for Pediatric and Adolescent Diabetes |
| ISS | idiopathic short stature |
| ITT | insulin tolerance test |
| IU | international unit(s) |
| IUGR | intrauterine growth retardation |
| KS | Kallmann syndrome |
| LCH | Langerhans cell histiocytosis |
| LFT | liver function test |
| LH | luteinizing hormone |
| LHRH | luteinizing hormone-releasing hormone |
| MAS | McCune–Albright syndrome |
| mcg | microgram(s) |
| MDI | multiple daily injection |
| MEN | multiple endocrine neoplasia |
| MODY | maturity-onset diabetes of the young |
| MPH | mid-parental height |
| MPHD | multiple pituitary hormone deficiency |
| MRI | magnetic resonance imaging |
| MTC | medullary thyroid cancer |
| NHS | National Health Service |
| NICE | National Institute for Health and Care Excellence |
| NS | Noonan syndrome |
| OGTT | oral glucose tolerance test |
| OHD | hydroxylase deficiency |

| OI | osteogenesis imperfecta |
| OSA | obstructive sleep apnoea |
| PAIS | partial androgen insensitivity syndrome |
| PCOS | polycystic ovary syndrome |
| PTH | parathyroid hormone |
| PWS | Prader–Willi syndrome |
| QoL | quality of life |
| RCPCH | Royal College of Paediatrics and Child Health |
| SAPT | sensor augmented pump therapy |
| SC | subcutaneous |
| SD | standard deviation |
| SDS | standard deviation score |
| SGA | small for gestational age |
| SHBG | sex hormone-binding globulin |
| SIADH | syndrome of inappropriate antidiuretic syndrome secretion |
| SMBG | self-monitoring of blood glucose |
| SOD | septo-optic dysplasia |
| SST | short Synacthen test |
| StAR | steroidogenic acute regulatory protein |
| T1DM | type 1 diabetes mellitus |
| T2DM | type 2 diabetes mellitus |
| $T_3$ | triiodothyronine |
| $T_4$ | thyroxine |
| TBG | thyroid-binding globulin |
| TBI | total body irradiation |
| TFT | thyroid function test |
| TPO | thyroid peroxidase |
| TRAb | thyrotropin receptor antibody |
| TRH | thyrotropin-releasing hormone |
| TS | Turner syndrome |
| TSH | thyroid-stimulating hormone |
| TSI | thyroid-stimulating immunoglobulin |
| U | units(s) |
| U&E | urea and electrolytes |
| WFH | weight for height |
| WHO | World Health Organization |

# Growth (including short stature and tall stature)

# Introduction

## Introduction

Failure to grow normally may be:
- due to a 1° growth disorder
- 2° to chronic illness.

## Normal growth

Fig. 1.1 shows the earliest known growth chart, that of the son of the Comte Philibert de Montbeillard (1759–1777). Growth data can be shown in terms of either height achieved (Fig. 1.1a) or increase in height over a period of time—the height velocity (Fig. 1.1b).

## Physiology

Growth consists of three phases superimposed upon each other, each of which is under different controls, nutritional and hormonal (Fig. 1.2):

### Infantile phase

This is predominantly under nutritional control, as children with congenital hormone deficiencies usually have relatively normal birthweights/lengths.

It is both a rapid and rapidly decelerating growth curve, lasting from birth until around 3 years of age, and is a continuation of the intrauterine growth curve. During the first year of life, an infant grows more rapidly than at any other period of their (extrauterine) life, at up to 2.5 cm a month. By 2 years of age, a child is roughly half its adult height, indicating that ~50% of growth has already occurred.

### Childhood phase

This is under hormonal control, predominantly growth hormone (GH) and thyroid hormone, although nutritional factors also play a role.

It is a steady and slowly decelerating growth curve which starts at around 2–3 years of age and continues until puberty. By their 8th birthday most children will have achieved around three-quarters of their final height.

### Puberty phase

This is under the control of GH and sex hormones acting synergistically.

It lasts from adolescence onwards, and has different timing and strength in the two sexes. It is this phase of growth which accounts for the sex differences in final height of around 14 cm between males and females. While girls enter their growth spurt earlier, the peak height velocity is not as great as that in boys (Fig. 1.3 and Fig. 1.4, p. 6).

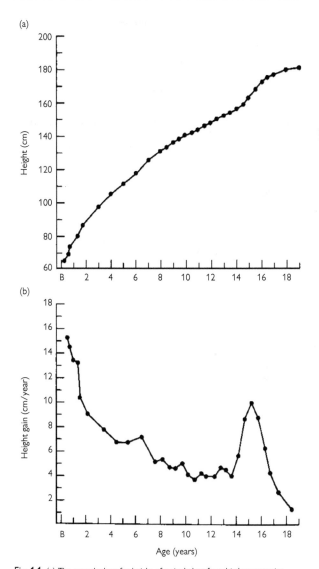

**Fig. 1.1** (a) The growth chart for height of a single boy from birth to maturity. (b) The same data as in (a), but expressed as height gain or velocity.

Reproduced with permission from Wass JAH, Shalet SM (eds) (2002). *Oxford Textbook of Endocrinology and Diabetes*, Oxford University Press, Oxford. Copyright © 2002 OUP.

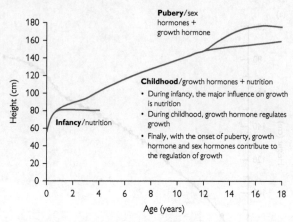

**Fig. 1.2** The infancy–childhood–puberty (ICP) model of growth.

Reproduced with permission from Karlberg JA (1989). Biologically-oriented mathematical model (ICP) for human growth. *Acta Paediatr Scand Suppl* (ACTA PAEDIATRICA: NURTURING THE CHILD) 350: 70–94. Copyright © 1989 John Wiley and Sons.

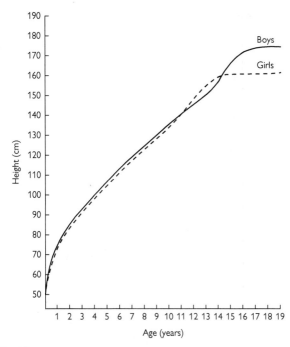

**Fig. 1.3** Typical individual height-attained curves for boys and girls (supine length to the age of 2 years; integrated curves of Fig. 1.2).

Reproduced with permission from Turner HE, Wass JAH (2002). *Oxford Handbook of Endocrinology and Diabetes*, Oxford University Press, Oxford. Copyright © 2002 OUP.

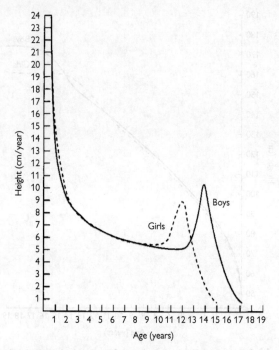

**Fig. 1.4** Mean growth velocity curves of British girls and boys whose peak growth spurt is reached at an average age (12 years and 14 years respectively).

Reproduced from Tanner JM, Whitehouse RH, Takaishi M (1966). Standards from birth to maturity for height, weight, height velocity, and weight velocity: British children, 1965. I. *Arch Dis Child* 41: 454–71. Copyright © 1966 BMJ Publishing Group Ltd.

# Measurement techniques

- When measuring children ≤2 years, all clothes and nappies should be removed.
- In those >2 years, only minimal clothing should be worn, and shoes must be removed.

Measurers should be appropriately trained, especially in height/length measurements. Measure height/length recorded to the last millimetre.

## Standing height

This is performed from 2 years onwards, producing measurements ~1 cm less than supine length. Measurement should be performed without shoes and with only thin socks being worn.

Measurement should be made with the feet together, heels on the floor and against the backboard, with the head held in the Frankfurt plane (an imaginary line drawn from the centre of the auditory meatus to the lower border of the eye). Ideally, repeat height measurements should be carried out at the same time of day and by the same measurer.

## Supine length

This is performed before 2 years of age or if unable to stand: appropriate equipment is a length board or mat. This measurement requires two people: one to hold the head vertically against the headboard in the Frankfurt plane, and the other to straighten the knees and hold the feet flat against the footboard.

Measuring equipment varies in cost but, if properly set up and maintained, all produce consistent and accurate measurements in trained hands. Height measurements should be accurate to the nearest 1 mm; significantly better than that seen in many biochemical investigations.

## Weight

This is performed using class III electronic scales in metric setting, which do not require regular calibration. Children <2 years of age are usually measured naked, and after that in light clothing only, with nappies and shoes removed. If minimal clothing is used, its estimated weight (about 100 g) should be subtracted before weight is recorded. Scales are usually graduated to 10 g.

Typically an infant doubles their birthweight in the first 4 months of life (gaining 150–190 g per week), and trebles it by 1 year. A child is approximately half the adult weight by 9–11 years.

## Body mass index (BMI)

This is a way of assessing weight for height, and calculated by dividing the weight $W$ (in kilograms) by the square of height $H$ (in metres): $W/H^2$. It is most easily calculated on a smartphone by entering weight (in kilograms) then dividing twice by height (in metres).

BMI varies throughout childhood:
- rises steeply in infancy
- falls during the preschool years
- rises progressively into adulthood.

An alternative, the ponderal index (cube root of weight/height), is often used in babies.

## Head circumference

This is the measurement to the nearest millimetre (using a non-stretchable plastic or paper tape) of the maximum head circumference (from the mid-point of the forehead to the occipital prominence). It is routinely measured up to 2 years of age, but is usually only measured subsequently if there are any clinical concerns.

At birth, head circumference is ~75% of its adult size, and subsequent growth phases are:
1. the first years of life, when most postnatal growth occurs
2. a relative plateau period of growth in mid-childhood
3. a further increase from puberty onwards.

## Other measurements

### Sitting height

This is not routinely measured, although it is important to assess short stature with disproportion. For example:
- skeletal dysplasias, where limb length is usually reduced
- spinal irradiation in the treatment of malignant disease, where spinal growth is retarded.

Subtraction of sitting height from standing height produces subischial leg length, and these measurements are then plotted onto special charts to assess any discrepancy. Discrepancies between measurements of >2 standard deviations (SD) prepubertally and >2.5 SD during puberty indicate significant disproportion.

Alternatives are:
- standing height vs arm span
- upper and lower segment measurements (taken from the pubis).

## Growth charts

NB: website links to various growth charts are listed in ➔ 'Further reading', p. 12.

The original UK growth charts, based on growth data from the 1950s to the 1960s,[1] were updated in the early 1990s and subsequently in 2013 because:
- there was a secular trend towards increased height and earlier maturation
- the data were not representative of the UK as a whole.

Compared with the earlier charts, the secular trend is 1.2 cm in total, with most of this being due to increased leg length.

The normal distribution of organic variables such as height and weight can be shown as either:
- centiles
- SD from the mean.

The nine centile lines (0.4th, 2nd, 9th, 25th, 50th, 75th, 91st, 98th, 99.6th), are each set two-thirds of a SD away from each other; therefore the 2nd and 98th centiles are −2 and +2 SD from the mean. Outer lying lines for very tall +4 SD or small −4 and −5 SD are given in SD scores (SDS). As with any normally distributed measure, the further from the mean, the more likely there is to be pathology, and it is estimated that ~25% of children with heights below −3 SD from the mean have growth hormone deficiency (GHD).

Along with the World Health Organization (WHO), the Royal College of Paediatrics and Child Health (RCPCH) has produced a number of growth charts:

- 0–4 years
- Neonatal and Infant Close Monitoring (NICM)
- 2–18 years
- Childhood and Puberty Close Monitoring (CPCM).

### 0–4 years growth chart

This second edition (2013) combines WHO standards with UK preterm and birth data. The data from 2 weeks to 4 years of age are based on WHO data of healthy, non-deprived, breastfed children of non-smoking mothers. It can be used for all children regardless of whether they were breastfed or formula fed, and also for infants born moderately preterm (32–36 weeks' gestation).

The chart also includes a BMI centile lookup and an adult height predictor.

### Neonatal and Infant Close Monitoring (NICM) growth chart

Formerly called the Low Birth Weight chart, this is designed for plotting:
- very preterm infants, and
- those with significant early health problems in the first 2 years of life.

It features low lines for very short or underweight children, and aids for gestational correction. It consists of three different charts:

1. *23–42 weeks' gestation.* This is based on reanalysis of the UK 1990 data and illustrates the size measurements of infants born at different gestational ages.
2. *2 weeks' to 6 months' corrected age.*
3. *6 months' to 2 years' corrected age.* These charts are derived from the UK-WHO 0–4 years growth charts, and don't reflect usual growth of preterm infants. However, individual infants who have remained well should follow the trajectory indicated by the centile lines at their corrected age.

For children born preterm (i.e. <37 weeks gestational age), plotting should involve a correction for gestational age which should continue until at least 1 year of age.

### 2–18 years growth chart

This combines data from the UK 1990 growth charts at birth and 4–18 years with the WHO growth standards from 2–4 years, and is aimed at assessment of school-age children.[2] The chart also includes guidance on:
- onset and progression of puberty
- BMI centile lookup

- adult height predictor
- mid-parental height (MPH) comparator.

### Childhood and Puberty Close Monitoring (CPCM) growth chart

Published in 2013, this is a modification of the 2–18 years growth chart, aimed at children with growth and/or nutritional problems.

It is intended for use in specialist clinics and special schools. The chart extends to age 20 years and also features:

- a BMI chart
- low and high lines for very short, thin, or overweight children
- puberty-phase specific thresholds for assessment of short children with late puberty, and tall children with early puberty.

### Weight

If weight is above the 75th centile or if weight and height centiles differ, the BMI centile should be calculated, as the BMI centile is the best indicator of thinness and fatness. The BMI lookup allows you to read off the BMI centile, accurate to a quarter of a centile space. There is a BMI centile grid at the top of the growth chart where the centiles for children with high or low values can be plotted.

### Height velocity

Growth is not a continuous process, but has a number of superimposed phases.

1. Weeks: growth spurts with intervening growth arrest ('saltation and stasis').
2. Months: seasonal variation in growth (usually faster in spring and summer compared with autumn and winter).
3. Years: longer-term variation over a number of years.

Height velocity standards have been devised over a 12-month period (Fig. 1.4), and shorter intervals will tend to emphasize measurement errors.

Given the inherent challenges of growth measurement accuracy and the knowledge about the variable pattern of childhood growth, what then is the best method for recognizing abnormal growth? In a review of practice from the Netherlands, Finland, and the UK, the most accurate parameters are deflection in height and distance from mid-parental target height.[3] There is a significantly greater chance of pathology in a child who is tall or short for their family, whose height increases or decreases by 0.5 SD over 1 year or >0.7 SD over 2 years. On the UK RCPCH growth charts, this equates to a shift of over half a centile bandwidth in 1 year and across greater than one intercentile space (0.67 SD) over 2 years.

### Weight velocity

The term 'centile crossing' rather than 'weight velocity' is usually used, especially in infants. The phenomenon of regression to the mean means that children born large for dates tend to catch down, while those born small for dates catch up.

- ~50% of children cross at least one centile line between 6 weeks and 12–18 months.
- 5% cross two centile lines.

Abnormal centile crossing downwards, 'faltering growth', may need investigation.

*Pubertal assessment*

→ This is included in Chapter 2.

## References

1. Tanner JM, Whitehouse RH, Takaishi M. Standards from birth to maturity for height, weight, height velocity, and weight velocity: British children, 1965. I. *Arch Dis Child* 1966;41:454–471.
2. Royal College of Paediatrics and Child Health. Growth charts for children aged 2–18 years. http://www.rcpch.ac.uk/growthcharts/
3. Stalman SE, Hellinga I, Dommelen P, et al. Application of the Dutch, Finnish and British screening guidelines in a cohort of children with growth failure. *Horm Res Paediatr* 2015;84:376–382.

# Physiology

After the initial infantile period, GH is the main factor involved in growth. The factors involved in GH secretion are shown in ➲ Fig. 3.3 p. 94.

At the hypothalamic level, GH is secreted under the influence of the peptides somatostatin (inhibitory) and growth-hormone releasing hormone (GHRH; stimulatory). There are a number of other factors which also act at the hypothalamic level, including exercise, sleep, and drugs, which are used diagnostically to stimulate GH secretion. Ghrelin, a peptide secreted from the stomach, may also be involved in secretion of GH.

GH is secreted in a pulsatile fashion, with pulses approximately every 180 minutes. The largest pulses are at night-time with low trough levels in between.

GH itself is a 191-amino acid polypeptide which circulates bound in the blood to its binding protein (GHBP). Most (~75%) is a 22 kDa protein, but other isoforms (such as the 20 kDa protein) are also found which may have differing biological activities.

GH binds to the transmembrane growth hormone receptor (GHR), which then dimerizes to produce intracellular signalling via the Janus kinase/signal transducers and activators of transcription (JAK/STAT pathway).

The metabolic effects of GH are predominantly direct, whereas the growth-promoting effects are indirectly mediated via growth factors such as insulin-like growth factor 1 (IGF-1).

## Indirect GH effects

These are mediated via IGF-1, a 79-amino acid polypeptide which is produced by the liver in an endocrine fashion, and by other tissues in a paracrine/autocrine fashion.

## Direct GH effects

### Carbohydrate metabolism

Maintenance of normal blood glucose via an anti-insulin activity, through suppression of insulin-stimulated glucose uptake in peripheral tissues, and enhanced glucose synthesis within the liver.

### Protein metabolism

Anabolism via increased amino acid uptake, increased protein synthesis, and decreased protein oxidation.

### Fat metabolism

Fat utilization through triglyceride breakdown and adipocyte oxidation. In addition to indirect effects of GH mediated via IGF-1, there is also some evidence of a direct effect of GH on the growth plate; the 'dual effector hypothesis'.

# Growth disorders

It is estimated that:
- ~20% of children with a height <−2 SD below the mean (2nd centile), and
- ~50% of children with a height <−3 SD below the mean have an underlying pathological cause for their short stature.

## Familial

Familial height:
- familial short stature (FSS).

Familial growth patterns:
- constitutional delay of growth and puberty (CDGP).

Within a population, ~80% of height variation is explained by genetic factors. A number of other factors affect growth.

## Genetic disorders

Examples include:
- Turner syndrome (TS)
- Noonan syndrome (NS)
- Russell–Silver syndrome (RSS).

## Skeletal

Skeletal dysplasias.

## Birth size

- Small for gestational age (SGA)
- Intrauterine growth retardation (IUGR).

## Chronic illness

- Respiratory: asthma, cystic fibrosis
- Cardiovascular: chronic heart failure
- Gastrointestinal: coeliac disease, inflammatory bowel disease
- Renal: chronic renal insufficiency
- Hepatic: biliary atresia, post transplantation, chronic hepatitis
- Haematology: chronic anaemia
- Rheumatological: SLE, rheumatoid arthritis.

## Psychological factors

- Psychosocial deprivation.

## Environmental

- Nutritional
- Malnutrition
- Socioeconomic
- Poverty.

## Endocrine disorders

- GH: GH deficiency
- Thyroid hormone: hypothyroidism
- Corticosteroids: Cushing syndrome
- Sex steroids: precocious puberty
- Pseudo(pseudo)hypoparathyroidism.

# Causes of short stature

## Genetic

Two major sets of genes determine a child's height: one set determines how tall they will be, and the other determines the tempo of growth. These are assessed using MPHs and bone age, respectively.

### Mid-parental height

From 2 years of age there is a strong correlation between:
- a child's centile position for height, and their final height centile
- a child's centile position, and their parents' height centiles.

As adult males are on average 14 cm taller than adult females, MPH for a boy is calculated as follows.
1. Father's height and mother's height are measured in centimetres and added together.
2. This total is divided by 2.
3. 7 cm is added to the result.
4. This is the MPH.
For a girl, 7 cm is deducted rather than added in step 3.

The new RCPCH/WHO growth charts also have a chart to plot the parents' heights and assess MPH.
- Plot the mother's and father's heights on their respective scales and join the two points with a line. The mid-parental centile is where this line crosses the centile line in the middle.
- Compare the mid-parental centile to the child's current height centile, plotted on the adult height predictor centile scale.
- 80% of both boys and girls have an adult height <±7 cm of the MPH target height.
- 90% of children's height centiles are <±2 centile spaces of the MPH.
- Only 1% are >3 centile spaces below.

### Predictive adult height calculator

The child's adult height centile can be predicted from the child's current height centile with a given accuracy of ±6cm in 80% of cases. There is usually a reasonably close correlation at most ages except at the time of puberty on account of the wide variation in the timing and magnitude of the adolescent growth spurt.

### When is further assessment required?

If any of the following are present:
- Where weight, height, or BMI is <0.4th centile, unless previously fully investigated.
- If the height centile is >3 centile spaces below the mid-parental centile.
- A drop in height centile position of >2 centiles.
- Smaller centile falls or discrepancies between child's and mid-parental centile, if seen in combination, or if associated with possible underlying disease.
- When the predictive adult height varies significantly from the MPH then pathology is more likely.
- If there are any other concerns about the child's growth.

*Bone age*

Although GH secretion continues throughout life, final height is achieved in the mid to late teens when the bony epiphyses fuse under the influence of oestrogen. As the hand and wrist contain numerous epiphyses, a radiograph of the non-dominant hand enables a 'bone age' to be calculated, which is an estimate of the 'biological' rather than the 'chronological' age. By quantifying the years of remaining growth, it also enables an estimation of final height to be made (⊙ see also 'Introduction to tall stature', p. 34). The most common method used in routine clinical practice is that of Greulich and Pyle, where the child's radiograph is compared with standards from an atlas. The Tanner Whitehouse-3 (TW3) method is a different system which assesses the development of the radius, ulna, and the short bones (metacarpals and phalanges) separately and maturity scores are given to each of these bones. A computerized method, BoneXpert, has been derived which actually calculates the bone maturity in a three-phase process, analysing the size, shape, and density of the long and short bones. This has the advantage of significantly reduced inter-observer variability.

Bone age is less useful for children under the age of 5 years due to the lack of epiphyses.

As tall and obese children mature faster than short children, it is usual for the bone age to be advanced in these children and delayed in short children.

It is also:
- advanced in or precocious puberty (adrenarche)
- delayed in GH deficiency, delayed puberty, or chronic illness.

## Familial short stature

In this condition:
- birthweight is normal
- height is short but appropriate for parental heights (as is final height)
- height velocity is normal
- bone age is not substantially delayed
- there is an absence of any other clinical features which might suggest an underlying disease
- endocrine and other baseline testing is normal.

## Idiopathic short stature (ISS)

Children with ISS are a heterogeneous group; there are some unidentified causes but causes include CDGP and FSS.

ISS is defined as follows:
- height <−2 SDS (2nd centile) for sex and age
- poor adult height prediction (<162.5 cm (5ft 4in) for males and <150 cm (4ft 11in) for females), may or may not fall within target range
- normal birthweight and no dysmorphism
- no detectable cause (systemic, endocrine, nutritional, or chromosomal abnormalities) for the short stature (including no GH deficiency)
- height velocity can be either normal or reduced
- short stature homeobox (*SHOX*) gene mutations have been described in 2–5% of children with ISS

- heterozygous gene mutations of natriuretic peptide receptor-B (*NPR2*) (homozygous mutations cause acromesomelic dysplasia) are also described in ISS
- ~60–80% of all children with heights <−2 SDS can be diagnosed with ISS.

## Constitutional delay of growth and puberty

This is also dealt with in → Chapter 2. It is one of the most common causes of (relative) short stature, and is often a diagnosis of exclusion. It is more common in boys than girls (male:female ratio 7:1). Features include:

- short stature during childhood when assessed by chronological age, but not bone age
- poor growth from ~9–11 years of age onwards, as peers enter the pubertal growth spurt
- delayed bone age (>2 SD)
- delayed puberty (from 13 years onwards in girls and 14 years onwards in boys)
- no evidence of any other underlying disorder which might produce delayed puberty
- often a history of CDGP in immediate relatives.

## Turner syndrome

This occurs in ~1 in 2500 live female births, although it is estimated that ~98% of affected fetuses miscarry spontaneously.

It is the most common gonadal dysgenesis in females. Approximately 50% have a missing complete X chromosome (45,X); the remainder have other abnormalities involving the X chromosome, including:

- deletions of the short and long arms of the X chromosome
- duplications (isochromosomes)
- ring chromosomes
- mosaicism.

Short stature is due to a combination of:

- IUGR
- poor growth in childhood; characteristically from 4–5 years onwards
- mild skeletal dysplasia
- absent pubertal growth spurt.

As a result, final height is reduced by ~20 cm from MPH, with mean final height being 136–147 cm. Taller patients with TS (~>91st centile) may have final heights within the normal adult female range.

### Biochemical features

- Abnormal GH secretion, with other GH isoforms
- GH insensitivity
- Deficient oestrogen secretion.

Short stature is due to *SHOX* gene haploinsufficiency.

### Diagnosis

Diagnosis be made at a number of stages.

- *At any age*—dysmorphic features:

- skeletal—short neck, webbed neck, wide carrying angle (cubitus valgus), shield chest, short 4th metacarpal and metatarsal, broad feet, hyperconvex nails
- facial—low-set ears, high-arched palate
- other—horseshoe kidneys, streak ovaries, increased naevi, chronic serous otitis media (glue ear), hearing loss, coarctation of aorta.
- *In utero*: on amniocentesis, either as an incidental finding or following a finding of increased nuchal folds.
- *Neonatal*: puffy hands and feet, cardiac lesions (especially coarctation of the aorta).
- *Childhood*: short stature, dysmorphic features, educational problems.
- *Adolescence*: delayed/absent/arrested puberty, amenorrhoea.

## Noonan syndrome

NS is an autosomal dominant condition occurring in ~1 in 1000–2500 children.

### Dysmorphic features

- *Facial*: high forehead, low hairline, curly hair, webbed neck, wide epicanthic folds, hypertelorism, down-slanting palpebral fissures, ptosis, low-set and posteriorly rotated ears, deep philtrum, small upturned nose, high-arched palate.
- *Cardiac (in 80%)*: pulmonary stenosis (~50%), hypertrophic cardiomyopathy (~20%), atrial and ventricular septal defects (aortic coarctation).
- *Gonadal*: cryptorchidism and delayed puberty.
- *Feeding problems*: leading to failure to thrive. Usually resolve by 18 months of age.
- *Intellectual*: mean full-scale IQ is 85, with mild motor delay in >70%.
- *Other*: pectus excavatum or carinatum, cubitus valgus, winged scapula, scoliosis, ophthalmological and hearing abnormalities, haematological problems; juvenile myelomonocytic and acute lymphocytic leukaemia.

A number of clinical scoring systems exist, although there are now a number of genes within the mitogen-activated protein kinase (MAPK) system implicated in NS.

At least nine genes have now been implicated in NS and NS-like conditions. All are involved in the RAS–MAPK signal transduction pathway, involved in growth factor-mediated cell differentiation, proliferation, and death (Table 1.1).

### Growth

Disease-specific growth charts are available. Mean final height is ~162 cm in males and 152 cm in females, i.e. ~2nd centile on UK 1990 charts. On this basis ~50% of patients will have short stature, especially those with *PTPN11* and *RAF1* gene mutations, while those with *SOS1* and *BRAF* gene mutations are associated with better height preservation.

### Biochemical features

- Low mean GH concentrations, with irregular wide pulses, and high trough concentrations.
- Low IGF-1 levels.

Table 1.1 Genes implicated in Noonan syndrome

| Gene | Location | % of NS patients | Mutated in other conditions |
|---|---|---|---|
| PTPN11 | 12q24 | ~50 | LEOPARD syndrome |
| SOS1 | 2p22 | 11 | |
| RAF1 | 3p25 | 5 | LEOPARD syndrome |
| KRAS | 12p12 | ~1.5 | Cardiofaciocutaneous syndrome |
| NRAS | 1p13 | 0.2 | |
| RIT1 | 1q22 | ? 3–5 | |
| MEK1 and MEK2 (MAP2K1) | 15q22 | ? | Cardiofaciocutaneous syndrome |
| SHOC2 | 10q25 | ~2 | NS-like syndrome |
| CBL | 11q23 | ? | NS-like syndrome |

## 3-M syndrome

This is named after the three authors Miller, McKusick, and Malvaux who first described it. Characterized by:
- dysmorphic facial features
- severe postnatal growth failure
- radiological abnormalities (tall vertebral bodies and slender long bones)
- fleshy prominent heels.

It is due to mutations in (currently) three genes involved in IGF-2 signalling:
- CUL7 (70%)
- OBSL1 (25%)
- CCDC8 (5%).

Patients with CUL7 gene mutations tend to have the shortest stature.

## Down syndrome

This is due to trisomy (whole or part) of chromosome 21, with an incidence of ~1 in 800–1000 births.

Disease-specific growth charts are available, with a mean final height of 157 cm in males and 146 cm in females (➡ see also ➡ 'Further reading', p. 9).

These are useful as in addition to height reduction due to the trisomy, children may also have additional medical conditions which may further jeopardize growth including:
- congenital heart disease
- feeding problems
- sleep-related upper airway obstruction
- autoimmune disorders: coeliac disease and thyroid hormone deficiency.

## Russell–Silver syndrome

RSS is also known (outside the UK) as Silver–Russell syndrome (SRS). Occurs in 1 in 30,000–100,000 births. Most cases are sporadic, although RSS can be transmitted in an autosomal dominant, autosomal recessive, and/or X-linked dominant fashion.

### Clinical features

- Pre- and postnatal growth failure
- Dysmorphism: relatively large head with prominent forehead, triangular face, micrognathia, thin upper lip, clinodactyly (short incurved little fingers)
- Body/limb asymmetry
- Hypospadias and undescended testes in males
- Hypoglycaemia and sweating
- Poor feeding, especially for solids.

Several different clinical scoring systems exist; in the most commonly used at least four of the following six criteria should be present to make a diagnosis of RSS:

1. SGA (see later in this topic)
2. postnatal growth failure
3. relatively normal head circumference
4. prominent forehead
5. body asymmetry
6. feeding problems and/or low BMI.

Although the diagnosis is predominantly clinical, two genetic abnormalities have now been identified.

1. Maternal uniparental disomy of chromosome 7 (MUPD7) occurs in 5–10% of patients.
2. Methylation defects in the Beckwith–Wiedemann syndrome gene (BWS on 11p15), resulting in reduced expression of the gene coding for IGF-2, and reducing fetal growth, have been shown to account for 30–60% of cases of RSS.

NB: characteristically patients with genetic abnormality (1) have fewer clinical features of SRS than those with genetic abnormality (2), but more neurocognitive issues.

## Small for gestation age and intrauterine growth retardation

Although these terms are often used interchangeably, they are not the same.

### Small for gestational age

This is a statistical auxological term, and defines those babies who have birthweights/birth lengths below a specific level for sex and gestational age (some definitions also include maternal height). Current consensus is that this is below −2.0 SDS (~2nd centile). In the UK, birth length is rarely measured accurately, so usually birthweight alone is used.

### Intrauterine growth retardation

- This implies that a pathological process is at work, and that serial intrauterine measurements have been performed (at least two serial measurements performed at least 2 weeks apart). Usually also includes a birthweight < 10th centile.

• It is not synonymous with SGA, as a child can be SGA and not have IUGR, and vice versa.

The recognition that low-birthweight children are more likely to develop diabetes mellitus and cardiovascular and respiratory disease, suggesting that factors acting in fetal life and infancy may be important in programming abnormal physiology ('the Barker hypothesis'), has stimulated interest in prevention and early treatment of IUGR.

• Fetal factors account for ~1/3 of children born SGA; the remainder are 2° to maternal and placental factors.
• In 40% no abnormality is found.

Broadly, the differential diagnosis of IUGR/SGA involves a number of categories: maternal, placental, and fetal.

*Maternal*

• Ethnicity, socioeconomic status, primiparity, reduced/increased maternal age, and short stature.
• Nutrition: protein–calorie malnutrition (both before and during pregnancy).
• Medical: hypertension, cardiac, respiratory, renal, haematological, and autoimmune disorders including collagen vascular disease and diabetes mellitus.
• Infection.
• Substance use/abuse: smoking, alcohol, and drugs (illicit and therapeutic).
• Uterine malformations.

*Placental*

• Placental insufficiency, pregnancy-induced hypertension (PIH), placenta praevia, chronic placental abruption, cord anomalies, or abnormal insertion.

*Fetal*

• Congenital infection, congenital malformations, chromosomal anomalies, genetic syndromes
• Multiple gestation.

NB: genetic causes account for 5–20% of babies with IUGR, especially if growth restriction has an early onset.

Most children born SGA show postnatal catch-up growth, with ~90% achieving normal heights (above −2 SDS) by 2 years of age, with the best predictors of catch-up growth being longer birth length and taller MPH. Little catch-up growth occurs subsequent to this, and by 18 years of age ~8% of infants born SGA remain short.

SGA infants born prematurely have a different pattern of catch-up growth; and can take up to 4 years or more to achieve a height in the normal range.

## Chronic illness

Any chronic disorder commonly causes varying impairment of growth. There are two major ways in which growth may be affected:
- growth delay
- absolute stunting of growth.

The former is seen in chronic disorders and indicates a degree of reversibility, i.e. growth is put 'on hold', whereas the latter suggests that the process is irreversible. It is possible that the disease process initially produces the former, and that the latter only occurs when the disease process has been continuing for some time or is severe.

### Organ system: disease
- Respiratory: asthma, cystic fibrosis
- Cardiovascular: congenital heart disease
- Gastrointestinal: coeliac disease, inflammatory bowel disease
- Urogenital: chronic renal insufficiency (CRI)
- Musculoskeletal: rheumatoid arthritis
- Other: sickle cell disease, thalassaemia major, diabetes mellitus, glycogen storage disease, and cerebral palsy
- Almost any chronic illness can produce short stature, dependent on chronicity and severity.

The aetiology of the short stature is probably multifactorial, but includes:
- nutritional factors:
  - malabsorption
  - intake limited by volume or content
  - anorexia
- protein loss
- chronic inflammation
- tissue anoxia or acid–base balance.

### Chronic renal insufficiency
Growth failure in CRI is thought to be multifactorial, with one of the factors believed to be reduced sensitivity to GH rather than decreased GH levels.

### Skeletal dysplasias
There are >400 different skeletal dysplasias currently described within >40 different groupings. Over 350 different genes have now been described.
   Where there is significant disproportion, a skeletal survey should be performed.

### Achondroplasia
- The most common non-lethal skeletal dysplasia, occurring in 1 in 16,000–26,000 live births.
- Autosomal dominant mutation; homozygous mutations are lethal.
- Nearly all show a specific point mutation in the fibroblast growth factor receptor gene 3 (FGFR3) gene (G1138A).
- Associated with increased paternal age.

Diagnosis can be made antenatally using an ultrasound scan (USS), which shows shortened femora. Postnatally, a skeletal survey may show:
- large skull with narrow foramen magnum

- short, flattened vertebral bodies with increased intervertebral disc width
- iliac wings squared and small, with a narrow sciatic notch
- trident hand with short metacarpals and phalanges
- thick and short tubular bones with cupping of metaphyses.

Disease-specific growth charts are available, with mean final heights of 131 cm in males and 126 cm in females.

### Hypochondroplasia

As with achondroplasia, this is due to mutations in the *FGFR3* gene, with two different mutations accounting for ~70% of cases. The incidence is unknown as clinical features are mild and heterogeneous, but probably similar to achondroplasia:

- short stature
- mesomelic limb shortening
- brachydactyly (short fingers)
- relative macrocephaly
- limited elbow extension
- generalized joint laxity.

A skeletal survey may show:

- failure of widening of lumbar interpedicular distances in the spine
- anteroposterior shortening of lumbar pedicles, with dorsal concavity of lumbar vertebral bodies
- long fibulae
- J-shaped sella turcica.

### Leri–Weill dyschondrosteosis

A rare skeletal dysplasia with:

- short forearms and legs (mesomelic dwarfism)
- characteristic deformity of the forearms (Madelung deformity).

This has been shown to be due to *SHOX* gene haploinsufficiency.

## Psychosocial deprivation (psychosocial short stature (PSS))

This is poor growth arising from adverse social conditions, abuse, and/or neglect/deprivation (both social and also psychological). The condition is heterogeneous, and a number of subtypes have been described, based on both age at presentation and clinical/biochemical findings.

- *Type 1 PSS*: onset in infancy. Presents with weight faltering. Depressed affect can occur. GH secretion is normal.
- *Type II PSS*: onset at 3 years or older. Bizarre behaviours involving eating and drinking, such as hyperphagia, food hoarding, and polydipsia, are usually observed. Patients are often depressed. Decreased or absent GH secretion is found which reverses on hospitalization. There is a poor response to GH therapy.
- *Type III PSS*: onset in infancy or older. Weight faltering is not usually present, nor are bizarre behaviours. GH secretion is normal, with a good response to GH therapy.

## Nutritional

Worldwide, this is the most common cause of poor growth. Growth of children with severe nutritional deprivation such as kwashiorkor (protein–energy-deficient malnutrition associated with loss of appetite and oedema) or marasmus (energy-deficient malnutrition associated with emaciation and preservation of appetite) is significantly disturbed, although less severe deficiencies may also cause growth problems.

GH levels, both spontaneous and stimulated, tend to be high, with low IGF-1 levels, indicating a degree of GH resistance.

### Endocrine disorders

These are also dealt with in other chapters.

#### Hypothyroidism

This can be associated with extreme short stature. Bone age is characteristically very delayed. GHD is also found, with reduced GH pulsatility which returns to normal on treatment with thyroxine.

#### Cushing syndrome

The most common cause in children is iatrogenic, as a result of exogenous steroid administration. Poor growth is very commonly noted, and is due to a direct effect of glucocorticoids on the growth plate.

#### Precocious puberty

Although these patients characteristically present with tall stature, early fusion of epiphyses results in long-term short stature.

#### Abnormalities of GH–IGF-1 axis

This is also dealt with in ➲ Chapter 3, 'Hypopituitarism', p. 83.

- GH receptor defects
- Extracellular/transmembrane/intracellular mutations
- GH signal transduction defects (e.g. STAT 3, STAT 5b)
- SHP-2 (encoded by PTPN11), K-RAS, H-RAS mutations
- IGF-1 gene mutations or deletions
- Bio-inactive IGF-1
- Acid-labile subunit (ALS) defect
- IGF-1 receptor mutations.

Understanding of the axis has led to elucidation of the various growth disorders associated with defects within the axis.

2° defects of the GH–IGF-1 axis:
- GH deficiency of hypothalamic or pituitary origin
- GH-neutralizing antibodies in patients with GH gene deletion
- bio-inactive GH.

Birthweight is characteristically:
- normal in defects involving the upper part of the axis (e.g. GH1 gene deletions)
- low in defects involving the lower half of the axis (e.g. IGF-1, IGF-1R mutations).

Isolated GH deficiency due to defects in the GHRH receptor or GH1 gene is at one extreme of a spectrum of genetic and associated biochemical and clinical phenotypes. At the other end of the spectrum, short stature may not be marked in heterozygous mutations of GHR, ALS, and the IGF-1R.

## GH insensitivity syndrome (GHIS; Laron syndrome)

This rare, autosomal recessive condition is usually due to mutations within the gene encoding the GHR. In addition, post-receptor abnormalities involving the JAK–STAT transcription pathway and the *IGF1* gene may produce a similar phenotype. Clinical features are similar to GHD, and in addition a micropenis is commonly found in males. Hypoglycaemia is also common and may produce seizures.

GH levels (both basal and stimulated) are characteristically raised, with very low levels of IGF-1 and the GH-dependent binding protein insulin-like growth factor binding protein 3 (IGFBP3). Those with GHR abnormalities also characteristically show reduced serum levels of growth-hormone binding protein (GHBP), which represents the extracellular portion of the GH receptor.

## Acquired disorders causing IGF-1 deficiency

* Malnutrition, parenchymal liver disease, and type 1 diabetes catabolic states (e.g. intensive care, postoperative)
* Chronic inflammatory and nutritional disorders (e.g. juvenile chronic arthritis, Crohn's disease).

### *Acid-labile subunit deficiency*

IGF-1 ALS is a GH-dependent glycoprotein which binds IGF-1 and extends its half-life in the circulation.

Short stature due to 1° ALS deficiency is characterized by:

* moderate postnatal short stature
* very low circulating levels of IGF-1 and IGF-B3, and also ALS
* no evidence of GHD or GHR
* insulin resistance in some patients.

# Investigation of short stature

Short stature is a considerable concern to children, parents, and healthcare professionals, and represents a significant number of referrals to paediatric endocrine clinics.

Although short stature is defined arbitrarily as those children whose heights lie (dependent on definition) below the 0.4th, 2nd, or 3rd centiles for age, it is important to recognize that this represents a vast number of children, most of whom are normal. Therefore the clinician must distinguish between those children who are normal and consequently require no therapy but merely reassurance, and those who have significant pathology requiring treatment (Table 1.2).

The purpose of investigation is to:
- determine whether there is a 1° growth disorder
- identify an underlying chronic disorder which needs treating.

Currently, height is routinely measured at primary school entry at 4–5 years and exit at 10–11 years, although it should also be measured at other opportunistic occasions. Suggested guidelines for specialist referral are as follows (based on the UK 1990 centile charts):
- Single height measurement:
  - refer any child whose height falls either below the 0.4th or above the 99.6th centile.
- Repeated height measurements:
  - the most accurate parameters are deflection in height and distance from mid-parental target height. There is a significantly greater chance of pathology in a child who is tall or short for their family, whose height increases or decreases by 0.5 SD over 1 year or >0.7 SD over 2 years. On the UK RCPCH growth charts, this equates to a shift of *over half a centile bandwidth* in 1 year and *across greater than one intercentile space (0.67 SD)* over 2 years.

The following steps should be taken initially.

**Table 1.2** Findings in different causes of short stature

| Aetiology | Weight for height | Height velocity | Bone age delay | Family history | Disproportion |
|---|---|---|---|---|---|
| FSS | Normal | Normal | No | Yes | No |
| CDGP | ↑ | ↓ | Yes | Yes | No |
| Endocrine disorders | ↑ | ↓ | Yes | Not usually | No[a] |
| Chronic disease | ↓ | ↓ | Yes | Possibly | No |
| Syndromic | Normal, ↑ or ↓ | Normal/↓ | Usually normal | Possibly | No[b] |

[a] Unless hypothyroidism. [b] Unless skeletal dysplasia.

- Accurate measurement of height, weight, and any other appropriate growth parameters. Measurement of heights of both parents. Obtain previous height measurements if available.
- Careful history, including:
  - details of pregnancy, delivery, birthweight, perinatal history, any significant past medical history
  - pattern of growth, systematic enquiry (including any symptoms of underlying disorder or chronic disease).
- Examination including evidence of disproportion, dysmorphic features, signs of underlying disorder, or chronic disease. Pubertal assessment.
- Plot data on appropriate growth charts to allow comparison with the population and also with parental target range.
- Estimation of skeletal maturity using bone age.
- A skeletal survey should be performed if there is unexplained disproportion.
- If appropriate, further investigations may be required at this stage, including screening bloods for underlying disorders. This process may enable a diagnosis to be made, even at initial consultation.

Screening bloods may include:

- chronic illness, e.g. full blood count (FBC), erythrocyte sedimentation rate (ESR), urea and electrolytes (U&E), liver function tests (LFTs), bone profile, coeliac antibodies
- endocrine, e.g. IGF-1, IGFBP3, thyroid function tests (TFTs), cortisol (9 am), prolactin, luteinizing hormone (LH), follicle-stimulating hormone (FSH), testosterone/oestradiol
- parathyroid hormone (PTH) if pseudohypoparathyroidism is being considered
- karyotype: probably mandatory in girls as (1) dysmorphism in TS may be minimal and (2) a proportion of girls with even 45,X may show spontaneous puberty, and in boys when a chromosomal anomaly is suspected. Further specific genetic testing may be indicated. This has usually been superseded by microarrays.

In the UK, familial patterns of growth are the most common cause of short stature, with endocrine problems being (relatively) uncommon. However, a diagnosis may not be apparent on initial assessment, and further growth data are required. Subsequent height measurements allow assessment of height velocity, but even if this is normal significant pathology may be indicated by:

- extreme short stature (even allowing for skeletal maturation)
- inappropriately short stature relative to parents.

GH stimulation tests are described in the section on hypopituitarism.

- They are usually performed to diagnose GHD (including in children born SGA who show clinical evidence of GHD)
- They are not routinely performed in other GH-treated groups.

NB: in IGF-1 deficiency, a low IGF-1 level in the presence of high baseline GH levels with a classic clinical phenotype is often sufficient to make the diagnosis.

# Therapy for short stature

Often, reassurance alone may be all that is required. Depending on the condition, various treatments are available. For chronic illnesses, treatment of the underlying disorder alone may often result in an improvement in growth.

## Sex steroid therapy

Treatment of delayed puberty with sex hormones (oestrogen in females and testosterone in males) is dealt with in ➲ Chapter 2. In CGDP, either sex steroids or anabolic steroids are given, although these do not produce increases in final height, and if given in excess will decrease final height through premature epiphyseal fusion.

## Growth hormone

GH therapy has been available for over 60 years, although until the availability of biosynthetic GH in the late 1980s supplies were highly restricted and reserved only for the most severely GH-deficient patients.

GH currently has a product licence in Europe and the UK for the following paediatric conditions (Table 1.3), with the approximate percentage of new patients in parentheses:

- GHD: (~55%)
- TS (~10%)
- CRI (2.5–4%)
- Prader–Willi syndrome (PWS) (5–6%)
- SGA (15–20%)
- SHOX deficiency (1–2%).

NB: unlicensed conditions account for 6–10% of new patients.

There is also a licence for adult GHD.

Approximately 1000 new patients are started on GH within the UK each year; with ~55–60% being male.

The Food and Drug Administration (FDA) in the USA has also approved all the previously listed indications plus ISS and also NS.

There is also a product licence for chondrodysplasias in Japan.

**Table 1.3** Recommended doses of growth hormone

| Diagnosis | Dose (mcg/kg/day) | Dose (mg/m²/day) |
|---|---|---|
| GHD | 23–39 | 0.7–1.0 |
| TS | 45–50 | 1.4 |
| CRI | 45–50 | 1.4 |
| PWS | 35[a] | 1.0[a] |
| SGA | 35–66 | 1.0–2.0 |
| SHOX deficiency | 45–50 | 1.4 |

[a] Daily maximum 2.7 mg/day.

*Turner syndrome*

In addition to GH therapy, sex hormones (anabolic steroids and oestrogen) also impact growth.

A recent UK randomized trial has shown benefit in terms of final height of:
1. addition of the mild anabolic steroid oxandrolone (0.05 mg/kg/day) from 9 years of age onwards
2. delaying starting oestrogen replacement therapy until 14 rather than 12 years of age.

There was not an additive effect of benefits (1) and (2), and so addition of oxandrolone might enable oestrogen to be started at 12 rather than 14 years of age.

*Chronic renal insufficiency*

GH is recommended for prepubertal children with CRI, provided that:
- nutritional status has been optimized
- metabolic abnormalities have been optimized
- steroid therapy has been reduced to a minimum.

*Prader–Willi syndrome*

(⊖ See also Chapter 6, p. 234.)

It is unclear whether these patients are truly GH deficient or not, although GH therapy results in improvement in height (~1 SD in the first year), body composition, and muscle strength/tone.

However, there have been a number of reports of sudden death in PWS patients treated with GH, especially if the patient is severely obese. In obese patients, sleep studies should be performed before GH therapy is commenced.

*Small for gestational age*

GH is licensed for children born SGA (birthweight and/or length below −2 SD (2nd centile) who fail to show catch-up growth (height velocity SDS <0 during the last year) by 4 years of age or later, and who are short compared with both their peers (height below −2.5 SD) and their parents (parental adjusted height <−1 SD).

## GH therapy

(⊖ See also Chapter 3, p. 98.)

All GH therapy is now biosynthetic, currently administered by subcutaneous injection, and usually given nightly to mimic physiological secretion. A number of different GH devices are available, which broadly fall into two groups:
- needled devices (pen, needle and syringe, electronic device)
- needle-free devices.

*Side effects of GH therapy*
- Local discomfort.
- Transient headache in some patients, especially those on higher-dosage regimens. Benign intracranial hypertension has been reported and usually responds to briefly stopping GH and then restarting, initially at a lower dose.
- Oedema may be exacerbated in TS but is rare in other patients.

- Malignancy: recurrence of brain tumours does not appear to be increased. Longer-term studies have not suggested an increased cancer risk when recommended GH doses are used.
- Hypothyroidism has been reported in 5–10% of patients undergoing treatment with GH.

GH should be stopped if there is:
- poor response to therapy (i.e. <50% increase in height velocity in the first year of GH)
- poor adherence to treatment
- achievement of final height (fusion of epiphyses on bone age and/or height velocity <2 cm over a whole year).

NB: in PWS, evaluation of response should also include body composition.

In addition, in children with CRI, GH should be stopped at the time of renal transplantation, and not restarted until at least 1 year post-transplantation to see if catch-up growth has occurred.

## Alternative therapies

### Medical

#### Depot forms of GH

A number of depots of GH are currently in development, using implants, hydrogels, implants, pegylation, conjugation with albumin or amino acid sequences, and fusion to immunoglobulin.[1]

They only need to be given weekly, fortnightly, or even monthly.

#### IGF-1 therapy

This has been used in patients with GHIS, and is now licensed for 1° IGF-1 deficiency, the diagnostic criteria for which are:
- height below −3.0 SDS
- IGF SDS <2.5th centile
- GH 'sufficiency' on provocative testing.

Because of the risk of hypoglycaemia, initiation of therapy may require admission, especially in younger children.
- Starting dose is 0.04 mg/kg bd, gradually increased over 3 months to maintenance dose of 0.12 mg/kg bd.
- After dose increase, capillary blood glucose should be checked before breakfast and evening meal for at least 2 days.
- Recombinant human IGF-1 (rhIGF-1) should be administered shortly after a meal or snack. If hypoglycaemia despite adequate food intake, dose should be reduced. If the patient cannot eat, rhIGF-1 should be omitted.

NB: despite therapy final height remains very short (usually <−5 SDS).

#### Others

The following have been shown in some studies to have an additive effect with GH in increasing final height.
1. Anabolic steroids: oral oxandrolone (0.05 mg/kg/day) plus GH in TS increased final height by a mean of 4.6 cm.

2. Gonadotropin-releasing hormone (GnRH) analogues: in GH-deficient children, and possibly children born SGA or with SHOX deficiency, who remain short at the onset of puberty.

Aromatase inhibitors (AIs) have been shown to improve predicted adult height in several conditions, but only one study (in CDGP) has shown an increase in near-final height.

A trial with a C-natriuretic peptide analogue in achondroplasia has shown an increase in height velocity over 6 months without serious adverse effects.

### Surgical
Surgical limb lengthening in skeletal dysplasias, with distraction of the bones at ~1 mm/day, can not only produce meaningful increases in height (up to 30 cm) but also improve disproportion.

### Reference
1. Cai Y, Xu M, Yuan M, et al. Developments in human growth hormone preparations: sustained-release, prolonged half-life, novel injection devices, and alternative delivery routes. *Int J Nanomed* 2014;9:3527–3538.

# Introduction to tall stature

As stature is a normally distributed variable, tall stature is (theoretically) as likely to occur as short stature. However, in clinical practice, both referrals to the paediatric endocrine service and the need to treat present much less commonly, and may reflect the fact that tall stature is more socially acceptable than short stature.

Assessment by a paediatric endocrinologist is important for a number of reasons:
- prediction of final height
- exclusion of an underlying disorder, especially if this has implications for both the patient and their family
- therapy to restrict final height if this is likely to be excessive.

While tall stature is usually arbitrarily defined as a height above a certain centile (i.e. >97th, 98th, or 99.6th centile) or alternatively >2 SD above the target height, the most important factor in deciding whether to treat is an estimate of final height. If this is likely to be excessive, then it may be appropriate to attempt to limit it (Box 1.1).

Broadly, tall stature is due to a number of different causes:
1. *normal variant*: familial/constitutional tall stature
2. *excess of growth factors*: IGF-1 and insulin (e.g. obesity), IGF-2 (e.g. BWS)
3. *excess sex steroid production*: precocious puberty
4. *deficiency of oestrogen/oestrogen action*: hypogonadotropic hypogonadism (HH), aromatase deficiency, oestrogen receptor deficiency
5. *deficiency of factors needed to prevent bone elongation*: Marfan syndrome, homocystinuria
6. *excess of growth genes*: SHOX (e.g. Klinefelter syndrome, 47,XYYX), Y-specific control gene
7. *excess GH secretion*: GH-secreting tumour (isolated or as part of multiple endocrine neoplasia (MEN) type 1).

Box 1.1 Causes of tall stature

*Normal variants*
- Constitutional tall stature
- 'Simple' obesity.

*Syndromic*

*Chromosomal*
- Klinefelter (47,XXY) syndrome and variants, 47,XYY.

*Genetic overgrowth syndromes*
- Marfan syndrome
- Homocystinuria
- Sotos syndrome
- Weaver syndrome
- BWS
- Marshall–Smith syndrome
- Simpson–Golabi–Behmel syndrome.

*Endocrine*
- GH excess
- Thyrotoxicosis
- Sex hormone related: precocious puberty (central and peripheral: testotoxicosis and McCune–Albright syndrome (MAS), HH, androgen insensitivity syndrome (AIS), defects of oestrogen production and action
- Adrenal related: adrenarche, congenital adrenal hyperplasia, adrenal tumours, isolated adrenocorticotropic hormone (ACTH) deficiency.

# Constitutional tall stature

Given the range of normal stature, there will inevitably be people whose height falls within the normal range, albeit at the extreme ends. According to the RCPCH centile charts,[1] in the UK the 98th and 99.6th centiles are 191 and 197 cm for adult males and 176 and 180 cm for adult females, respectively.

Features of constitutional tall stature are:
- height >98th or 99.6th centile (depending on cut-off)
- predicted adult height within mid-parental range
- normal height velocity 75th centile
- normal IGF-1 level (although often at the upper end of normal).

Mean birth length in these patients is on the 75th centile, and tall stature usually becomes apparent from 3–4 years of age. Height velocity may be increased at this stage, but it is usually normal from 4–5 years of age, when it parallels the normal growth lines.

## Management

In the case of constitutional tall stature, all that may be required is reassurance. As tall stature is perceived as more of a problem in females, they are more likely to seek attention than males.

## Reference

1. Royal College of Paediatrics and Child Health. Growth charts for children aged 2–18 years. ℳ http://www.rcpch.ac.uk/growthcharts/

# Exogenous obesity

Unlike most syndromic or endocrine obesity, where affected patients are characteristically short, classical exogenous obesity (so-called simple obesity) is associated with tall stature and with nutritionally derived growth factors such as IGF-1. Although patients may be tall, final height does not appear to be increased.

# Syndromic tall stature

A number of syndromes, chromosomal and otherwise, are associated with tall stature.

## Klinefelter syndrome

This is caused by an extra sex chromosome 47,XXY due to non-disjunction during meiosis. It is thought to occur in ~1 in 500–600 males.

Patients present with:
- tall stature
- eunuchoid proportions (increased arm span-to-height ratio)
- hypogonadism with characteristically small testes (2° to tubular hyalinization)
- increased incidence of gynaecomastia
- some degree of language learning difficulty may occur in some patients.

Diagnosis is made on karyotype.
- Biochemical evidence of gonadal failure presents in adolescence.
- Patients are subfertile with sperm usually only obtainable on surgical testicular extraction (TESE).
- Exogenous testosterone supplementation may be required from the onset of puberty.
- Testosterone therapy or surgery for gynaecomastia may be required.

## Other sex chromosomal variants associated with tall stature

- 47,XYY
- 47,XXX
- 48,XXXY
- 48,XXYY
- 49,XXXXY.

## Marfan syndrome

This is an autosomal dominant condition of connective tissue. It is said to have a prevalence of 1 in 5000–10,000.

Marfan syndrome is caused by mutations in the fibrillin gene *FBN1*, located on chromosome 15. Approximately 15–30% of all cases are due to *de novo* mutations, and mutations are found in a minority of sporadic cases (~20%) but in the majority (~80%) of familial cases. Clinically, Marfan syndrome is diagnosed using the Ghent criteria, which were modified in 2010 to recognize similar conditions which don't carry similar risk factors for aortic dissection/aneurysm seen with Marfan syndrome.

The clinical features involve a number of systems.

### Skeletal system
- Tall stature—in one study, mean final height was 191.3 ± 9 cm for males and 175.4 ± 8.2 cm for females
- Increased arm span-to-height ratio
- Long, slender fingers and toes (arachnodactyly)
- Scoliosis
- Pectus excavatum or carinatum.

*Cardiac*
- Prolapse of aortic or mitral valve
- Aortic aneurysm with dissection.

*Eyes*
- Subluxation of lens (ectopia lentis): superotemporal dislocation.

*Others*
- Spontaneous pneumothorax
- Dural ectasia.

## Homocystinuria

This is an autosomal recessive disorder. There is defective metabolism of methionine, often involving cystathionine beta synthase, and consequently the disease is also known as cystathionine beta synthase deficiency. As a result, homocysteine accumulates in the serum and there is increased urinary homocysteine excretion.

Features are similar to Marfan syndrome:
- tall stature
- increased arm span-to-height ratio
- arachnodactyly
- pectus excavatum and carinatum
- scoliosis
- ectopia lentis (although dislocation is inferonasal).

Other specific features:
- mental retardation
- psychiatric disorders
- accelerated atheroma.

Treatment consists of a diet low in certain amino acids such as methionine. High-dose vitamin B$_6$ (pyridoxine) may also be beneficial.

## Sotos syndrome

Also known as cerebral gigantism. The incidence is ~1 in 14,000 births.

*Features*
- Commonly large for gestational age (LGA).
- Tall stature with excessive growth, often from the first few years of life.
- Dysmorphism: large head and long head, with prominent forehead, and long chin. Down-slanting eyes. Large hands and feet.
- Dyspraxia.
- Hypotonia.

Patients may have a degree of intellectual impairment and also have behavioural problems.

The vast majority (~95%) of cases are sporadic. The gene *NSD1* has been found to be mutated in patients with Sotos syndrome (and also in Weaver syndrome, another overgrowth condition).

Life expectancy is normal. Although growth during childhood may be excessive, final height is usually normal.

## Weaver syndrome

Often mistaken for Sotos syndrome, with which it shares many phenotypic features including early overgrowth, advanced bone age, macrocephaly, and developmental delay. Clinical features include:

- prenatal and postnatal overgrowth
- facial dysmorphism (hypertelorism, large ears, depressed nasal bridge, down-slanting palpebral fissures, broad forehead and face, dimpled chin, prominent wide philtrum, micrognathia)
- hypotonia (but also hypertonia)
- advanced skeletal maturation
- permanent bending of fingers (camptodactyly).

Many have developmental delay and learning difficulties.

Characteristically associated with mutations in the *EZH2* (Enhancer of Zeste, *Drosophila* homolog 2) gene, although mutations in *NSD1* (as in Sotos syndrome) are also described.

Autosomal dominant transmission may occur.

## Tatton–Brown–Rahman syndrome (TBRS)

Also known as DNMT3A overgrowth syndrome.

### Features

- Tall stature with macrocephaly
- Joint hypermobility
- Hypotonia
- Characteristic facial dysmorphism: round face, thick horizontal eyebrows, narrowed palpebral fissures
- Cognitive disability (varying from mild to severe) and autism spectrum disorder.

First described in 2014. All cases occur due to new mutations in the *DNMT3A* gene.

## Beckwith–Wiedemann syndrome

This is a rare overgrowth syndrome with an incidence of ~1 in 15,000.

### Features

- Macrosomia and tall stature, with characteristic slowing of growth around 7–8 years of life
- Macroglossia (in ~80%)
- Hemihypertrophy
- Anterior abdominal wall defects (omphalocele)
- Neonatal hypoglycaemia.

BWS is caused by mutations in the gene *CDKN1C*, a growth-regulating gene adjacent to the Wilms tumour gene *WT1*. BWS usually occurs sporadically, but familial cases (e.g. autosomal dominant with incomplete penetrance) may occur in ~15%. Mutations in *CDKN1C* are found in 40% of familial cases and 5–10% of isolated cases. Consequently, patients with BWS are at increased risk of developing embryonal tumours (e.g. Wilms tumour, hepatoblastoma, adrenal carcinoma, neuroblastoma, and rhabdomyosarcoma).

# Endocrine causes of tall stature

## GH excess

Gigantism is caused by excessive production of GH prior to fusion of the epiphyses. GH excess in children is a very rare disorder, with only a few hundred cases reported in the literature. The most common cause is a pituitary secreting adenoma, although other underlying medical conditions include MEN-1, McCune–Albright syndrome (MAS), Carney complex, and neurofibromatosis.

- May be either GH-adenoma (somatotropinoma) or somatotrope hyperplasia.
- ~½ of somatotropinomas also co-secrete prolactin.

### Features

In addition to excessive growth, features of acromegaly may also be present:
- frontal bossing
- prominent jaw
- thickened facial features
- large hands and feet with thick fingers and toes.

### Tumour-size related

- Headache
- Double vision or visual field defect.

### Abnormal secretion (over/underproduction of other hormones)

- Breast milk secretion (galactorrhoea)
- Irregular menstruation (oligomenorrhoea)
- Delayed puberty
- Other pituitary hormone deficiencies.

NB: characteristically, adolescent girls present with menstrual abnormalities, while boys present with mass effects arising from the tumour.

### Other endocrine causes of tall stature

- *Hyperthyroidism*: growth is rapid, but advancement of the bone age means that final height is not increased.
- *Precocious puberty*:, both gonadotropin-dependent central precocious puberty (CPP) and gonadotropin-independent precocious puberty (GIPP): testotoxicosis, and MAS. In this condition, premature fusion of the epiphyses, if untreated, results in reduced final height. In MAS, other hormonal excesses producing tall stature may coexist, including thyrotoxicosis along with GH excess.
- *Pseudo-precocious puberty*: i.e. adrenarche, adrenal tumours, and congenital adrenal hyperplasia (CAH).

Rarer problems
- *Oestrogen abnormalities*: untreated HH, aromatase deficiency, oestrogen receptor abnormalities. These patients are characteristically of normal height during childhood, but have a very delayed bone age and continue to grow into their 30s.
- *Androgen insensitivity syndrome*.
- *Isolated glucocorticoid deficiency*: due to inactivating mutations of the adrenocorticotropic hormone (ACTH) receptor.

# Investigation of tall stature

The diagnosis may be apparent, but the following important points should be remembered.

## History

- Birthweight and length, neonatal problems (including hypoglycaemia)
- Postnatal growth (look at parent-held record—the 'Red Book')
- Parental heights (and also sibling heights)
- Family history of inherited disorders
- Evidence of developmental delay or behavioural problems.

## Examination

- Dysmorphic features
- Height, weight, BMI
- Head circumference
- Body proportions: sitting height, upper:lower body segments, arm span
- Pubertal rating
- Evidence of hypogonadism
- Height velocity (based on repeated measurements).

## Investigations

- Karyotype
- TFTs
- Androgens
- IGF-1
- Bone age.

### Investigation of suspected GH excess

- Serum IGF-1, IGFBP3
- Serum prolactin
- Assessment of other pituitary hormone defects (baseline and stimulated levels)
- Oral glucose tolerance test (to suppress GH levels)
- Visual fields
- Computed tomography (CT)/magnetic resonance imaging (MRI) scan of head and pituitary.

### Other conditions

- Precocious puberty: luteinizing hormone-releasing hormone (LHRH), consider tumour markers (alpha fetoprotein (AFP), human chorionic gonadotropin (hCG)).
- Marfanoid features: consider plasma homocysteine, mutation screening of *FBN1*.
- Store DNA if tall stature syndrome suspected.

## Height prediction

Several different techniques exist such as Tanner–Whitehouse (most commonly used in the UK) and Bayley–Pinneau. These use bone age estimation (Tanner–Whitehouse or Greulich–Pyle, respectively) as well as height to estimate final height.

Problems with bone age are:
- subjective assessment of bone age produces considerable inter- and intra-observer errors
- all systems are based on 'normal' children, and may not be as applicable to those with heights outside the normal range.

In various studies the bone age determined by the Greulich–Pyle method overestimates and the Tanner–Whitehouse method underestimates final height, more so in boys than girls. Automated bone age systems are now available (BoneXpert).

# Treatment of tall stature

Even in the absence of an underlying medical cause treatment may be warranted if predicted final height is felt to be excessive. There are no absolute rules, but treatment may be appropriate if final height will exceed +2.5 SDS, i.e. >180 cm in girls or >196 cm in males.

Although the basis for treatment of tall stature is for psychological reasons, there is little published data to support this. It is recognized that tall children feel different from their peers and are teased about their height, and coping mechanisms such as kyphotic (hunched) posture, social withdrawal, and even depression have been observed. There are also practical problems in obtaining suitable clothes and shoes.

Two main modalities are used to restrict final height, although there have been few controlled trials.

## Sex steroid therapy (to promote early epiphyseal fusion)

Large doses of oestrogen are not now were used in females, with height reduction inversely proportional to the bone age at which treatment was commenced, currently, in females, it is advised to use lower-dose physiological oestrogen is to promote normal but early pubertal development. As the pubertal growth spurt can add up to 30 cm to height, if it is wished to restrict final height to <185 cm, oestrogen needs to be added at ~155 cm (5ft 1in) if a girl shows no signs of spontaneous pubertal development.

In males, long-acting testosterone esters can be used at ~500 mg/m²/month. This is very supraphysiological, corresponding to ~4 times the normal testosterone production rate of adult men, *or* ~8–10 times that in early adolescence. Usually, IM injections of 500 mg fortnightly or 250 mg weekly are given, although studies indicate that testosterone 250 mg IM every 2 weeks is as effective in reducing final height as 500 mg every 2 weeks.

NB: male fertility does not appear to be affected by high-dose testosterone therapy.

In males, there is no evidence to support administration of both testosterone and oestrogen.

Girls treated with high-dose oestrogen in the past have reduced adult fertility with a depleted follicular pool and increased 1° ovarian insufficiency, which appears to be dose dependent.

Although there may be possible increases in various malignancies (breast, gynaecological, and melanoma) study numbers are too small to show a statistical increase.

## Epiphysiodesis

• This is a surgical procedure to destroy growth plates around the knee.
• Can be performed percutaneously.
• Recommended that this should not be performed if:
  • bone age is >12.5 years in girls and >14 years in boys
  • height in girls is >170 cm and boys >185 cm.
Remaining limb growth is reduced by approximately one-third, but as spinal growth is unaffected then disproportion may occur.

In one large retrospective study there was a mean reduction in final height in boys of 7 cm and in girls of 4.1 cm.

In some countries this has now become the treatment of choice for tall stature.

### Therapies to reduce the secretion/action of GH

Alternatively, somatostatin analogue (octreotide) has been shown to reduce growth velocity in the short term, although the (very) limited data do not support a significant reduction in final height.

Although there are anecdotal case reports it is unclear whether the GH receptor blocker pegylated GH (pegvisomant) is of therapeutic benefit in these patients.

### Treatment of GH excess

#### Surgical

Treatment is surgical in well-defined pituitary tumours, and is curative in ~80%. Radiotherapy is also effective, but may take up to 10 years. As an effect of the tumour or of its therapy, there may be other pituitary hormone deficits which need treating.

#### Medical

Dopamine agonists and somatostatin analogues (octreotide) have been used. Pegvisomant is also used in adults, although data for children are lacking. Sex steroid therapy to produce premature epiphyseal fusion.

# Further reading

Butler MG, Lee J, Manzardo AN, et al. Growth charts for non-growth hormone treated Prader-Willi syndrome. *Pediatrics* 2015;135:e126–e135.

Colao A, Pivonello R, Di Somma C, et al. Growth hormone excess with onset in adolescence: clinical appearance and long-term treatment outcome. *Clin Endocrinol (Oxf)* 2007;66:714–722.

Cole TJ. Conditional reference charts to assess weight gain in British infants. *Arch Dis Child* 1995;73:8–16.

Cole TJ, Freeman JV, Preece MA. Body mass index reference curves for the UK, 1990. *Arch Dis Child* 1995;73:25–29.

Dauber A, Rosenfeld RG, Hirschhorn JN. Genetic evaluation of short stature. *J Clin Endocrinol Metab* 2014;99:3080–3092.

Davies JH, Cheetham T. Investigation and management of short stature. *Arch Dis Child* 2014;99:767–771.

Davies JH, Cheetham T. Investigation and management of tall stature. *Arch Dis Child* 2014;99:772–777.

Down Syndrome Medical Interest Group. Growth charts. ♪ https://www.dsmig.org.uk/information-resources/growth-charts/

Freeman JV, Cole TJ, Chirin S, et al. Cross sectional stature and weight reference curves for the UK 1990. *Arch Dis Child* 1995;73:17–24.

Hannema SE, Savendahl L. The evaluation and management of tall stature *Horm Res* 2016;85:347–352.

Harlow Healthcare. Turner syndrome growth charts. ♪ http://www.healthforallchildren.com/shop-base/shop/growth-charts/turner-syndrome-growth-charts-100-pack/

Horton WA, Rotter JI, Rimoin DL, et al. Standard growth curves for achondroplasia. *J Pediatr* 1978;93:435–438.

Kant SG, Wit JM, Breuning MH. Genetic analysis of tall stature. *Horm Res* 2005;64:149–156.

Lee JM, Howell JD. Tall girls: the social shaping of a medical therapy. *Arch Pediatr Adolesc Med* 2006;160:1035–1034.

National Institute for Health and Care Excellence (NICE) (2010). Human growth hormone (somatropin) for the treatment of growth failure in children. TA 188. ♪ https://www.nice.org.uk/guidance/ta188

NHS Executive. *Child Health in the Community: A Guide to Good Practice.* London: Department of Health, 1996.

NHS. Healthy child programme. ♪ http://www.healthychildprogramme.com/

Noordam C, van Daalen S, Otten BJ. Treatment of tall stature in boys with somatostatin analogue 201-995: effect on final height. *Eur J Endocrinol* 2006;154:253–257.

Royal College of Paediatrics and Child Health. Growth charts. ♪ https://www.rcpch.ac.uk/resources/growth-charts

Royal College of Paediatrics and Child Health. UK-WHO growth charts—guidance for health professionals. ♪ https://www.rcpch.ac.uk/resources/uk-world-health-organisation-growth-charts-guidance-health-professionals

Savage MO, Burren CP, Rosenfeld RG. The continuum of growth hormone-IGF-I axis defects causing short stature: diagnostic and therapeutic challenges. *Clin Endocrinol (Oxf)* 2010;72:721–728.

Schilg S, Hulse T. *Growth Monitoring and Assessment in the Community: A Guide to Good Practice.* London: Child Growth Foundation, 1997.

Tanner JM, Whitehouse RH, Takaishi M. Standards from birth to maturity for height, weight, height velocity, and weight velocity: British children, 1965. I. *Arch Dis Child* 1966;41:454–471.

Venn A, Hosmer T, Hosmer D, et al. Oestrogen treatment for tall stature in girls: estimating the effect on height and the error in height prediction. *Clin Endocrinol (Oxf)* 2008;68:926–929.

Williams Syndrome Association. Growth charts. ♪ https://williams-syndrome.org/growth-charts/growth-charts

Wit JM, Oostdijk W. Novel approaches to short stature therapy. *Best Pract Res Clin Endocrinol Metab* 2015;29:353–366.

World Health Organization. The WHO child growth standards. ♪ http://www.who.int/childgrowth/standards/en/

# Puberty and its disorders

# Definition

Puberty is defined as the acquisition of 2° sexual characteristics, with a view to reproductive capability. These characteristics are:

- Females:
  - development of breasts (may also occur in males—gynaecomastia)
  - enlargement of the internal female organs, with achievement of menstruation (menarche).
- Males:
  - enlargement of genitalia (penis and scrotum) and increase in testicular volume
  - lowering of the voice frequency (also occurs to lesser extent in girls).
- Both sexes:
  - development of pubic and axillary hair
  - growth spurt
  - attainment of reproductive function.

Although the terms 'puberty' and 'adolescence' are commonly used interchangeably, puberty tends to be used for physical changes and adolescence for psychological changes.

# Physiology of normal puberty

The hypothalamic–pituitary (HP)–gonadal axis is shown in Fig. 2.1.

Although the precise mechanism is unclear, the onset of puberty is heralded by an increase in pulsatile gonadotropin-releasing hormone (GnRH) from the hypothalamus. In turn, pulsatile release of luteinizing hormone (LH) from the pituitary results from both increased secretion of GnRH and increased pituitary responsiveness. Follicle-stimulating hormone (FSH) secretion from the pituitary in response to GnRH also increases progressively from prepuberty to mid-puberty.

LH releases sex hormones from the gonads (testes and ovaries). In males it acts on the Leydig cells of the testis to produce androgens, including testosterone. In females it triggers ovulation, with formation of the corpus luteum which in turn secretes progesterone. It also supports ovarian thecal cells which produce androgens and oestrogen.

FSH stimulates germ cell maturation in the gonad in both sexes. In males it acts on the Sertoli cells to promote spermatogenesis. In females it initiates growth of the follicle.

The sex hormones (androgens and oestrogens) are produced in both sexes, although the levels differ.

- *Androgens* are produced by both gonads and adrenals, and are responsible for virilization, including development of pubic and axillary hair, as well as adult body odour, greasiness of skin and hair, and acne. The predominant androgen is testosterone, although the weaker dehydroepiandrosterone (DHEA) and dehydroepiandrosterone sulphate (DHEA-S) are produced in micromolar rather than the nanomolar amounts of most other androgens.
- *Oestrogens* are also produced in both sexes, through ovarian secretion in girls and by peripheral conversion of androgens in fat tissue in both sexes, and are responsible for breast development. They are also the hormones responsible for epiphyseal fusion in both sexes.

The different sensitivity of the HP–gonadal axis probably accounts for the earlier onset of puberty of girls, with precocious puberty more commonly seen in girls and delayed puberty in boys.

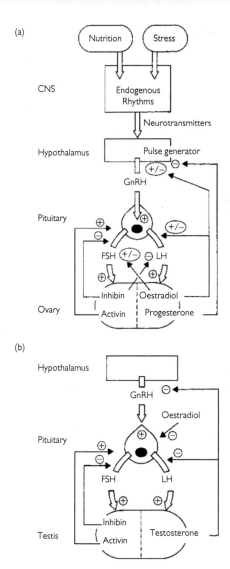

**Fig. 2.1** Hypothalamic–pituitary–gonadal axis for (a) females and (b) males.

# Pubertal staging

Pubertal assessment is typically done using the Tanner stages (Figs 2.2, 2.3 and 2.4). However correct use of this system requires training and a formal clinical examination.

For those not familiar with this system, or when a clinical examination is not possible or appropriate, then the RCPCH *puberty phases* system can be used (and can be used just by the history alone) (Table 2.1).

The 2–18- and 2–20-year RCPCH growth charts contain puberty lines, vertical black lines with legends, demarcating the earliest (99.6th) and latest (0.4th) centile ages for starting puberty and the latest age for the completing puberty phase (0.4th).

- Boys: genital development Tanner stages.
  - Stage 1: prepubertal
  - Stage 2: enlargement of scrotum and testes
  - Stage 3: enlargement of penis, initially in length; further growth of testes and scrotum
  - Stage 4: increased size of penis with growth in breadth
  - Stage 5: genitalia adult in size and shape.

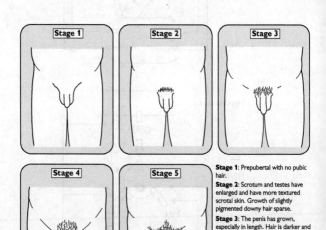

**Stage 1**: Prepubertal with no pubic hair.

**Stage 2**: Scrotum and testes have enlarged and have more textured scrotal skin. Growth of slightly pigmented downy hair sparse.

**Stage 3**: The penis has grown, especially in length. Hair is darker and curlier.

**Stage 4**: Further penile growth, in length and breadth, has occured. Glans is larger and broader, and hair is adult in type.

**Stage 5**: The testes and scrotum are adult in size. Pubic hair is adult in quantity and pattern, and presents along the inner borders of the thighs.

**Fig. 2.2** Male genital and pubic hair development by Tanner stage.

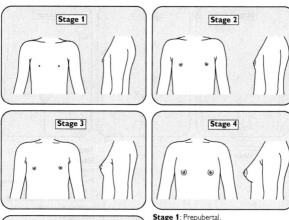

**Stage 1**: Prepubertal.

**Stage 2**: Breast bud beneath the areolar enlargement.

**Stage 3**: Enlargement of the entire breast with no protrusion of papilla or of secondary mound.

**Stage 4**: Enlargement of the areola and papilla as a secondary mound.

**Stage 5**: Adult configuration of the breast with protrusion of the nipple.

**Fig. 2.3** Female breast development by Tanner stage.

- *Girls: breast development Tanner stages.*
  - Stage 1: prepubertal
  - Stage 2: breast bud stage, with elevation of breast and papilla
  - Stage 3: further enlargement of breast and areola, with no separation of their contours
  - Stage 4: projection of areola and papilla to form a mound above the level of the breast
  - Stage 5: mature stage, with projection of papilla only.
- *Both sexes: pubic hair Tanner stages.*
  - Stage 1: prepubertal
  - Stage 2: sparse growth of long downy hair, chiefly along the base of the penis or labia
  - Stage 3: hair considerably darker, coarser, and curlier, spreading sparsely over the junction of the pubes
  - Stage 4: hair now adult in type, but area covered is still considerably smaller than in the adult
  - Stage 5: adult in quantity and quality, with spread to medial surface of the thighs
  - Stage 6: spread of hair to linea alba.

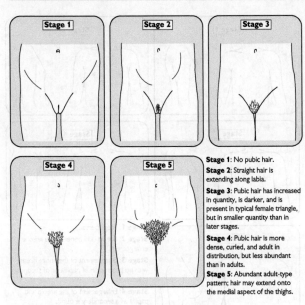

**Stage 1**: No pubic hair.

**Stage 2**: Straight hair is extending along labia.

**Stage 3**: Pubic hair has increased in quantity, is darker, and is present in typical female triangle, but in smaller quantity than in later stages.

**Stage 4**: Pubic hair is more dense, curled, and adult in distribution, but less abundant than in adults.

**Stage 5**: Abundant adult-type pattern; hair may extend onto the medial aspect of the thighs.

**Fig. 2.4** Female pubic hair development by Tanner stage.

Testicular volume is assessed using the orchidometer, a series of graduated beads from 1 to 25 mL. By definition, testicular volumes <3 mL are assessed as prepubertal, and those ≥3 mL as pubertal. Most of the testicular enlargement is due to seminiferous tubular development under the influence of FSH.

**Table 2.1** The three phases of puberty as assessed by history

|  | Pre-puberty (Tanner stage 1) if all of the following: | In puberty (Tanner stage 2–3) if any of the following: | Completing puberty (Tanner stage 4–5) |
|---|---|---|---|
| Girls | • No signs of nipple of breast development <br> • No pubic hair | • Any breast enlargement so long as nipples also enlarged <br> • Any pubic or axillary (armpit) hair growth | *If all of the following:* <br> Started periods (menarche) with breast, pubic, and axillary hair development |
| Boys | • High voice <br> • No growth of testes or penis <br> • No pubic hair | • Slight voice deepening <br> • Reddening of scrotum with growth of the testes <br> • Early testicular of penile enlargement <br> • Early pubic or axillary hair growth | *If any of the following:* <br> • Voice fully changed (broken) <br> • Adult size of penis with pubic and axillary hair growth |

Source: data from Royal College of Paediatrics and Child Health.

# Timing of puberty

Puberty is an ordered process with a specific consonance.

- *Girls.*
  - Puberty presents with breast budding or thelarche (Tanner stage 2 breast development, assessed by inspection and palpation), followed by pubic and axillary hair development.
  - Onset of the growth spurt occurs with breast budding, with peak height velocity at mid-puberty.
  - Commencement of periods (menarche) 2–3 years after the onset is the completion of puberty, with a mean height gain of ~6 cm post menarche.
- *Boys.*
  - Pubertal onset is marked by testicular and genital enlargement (Tanner stage 2 genital development, testicular volume ≥3 mL) followed by pubic and axillary hair development.
  - Although initial onset of puberty is similar to that of girls, the growth spurt in boys begins during mid-puberty (around 2 years later; testicular volume ≥10 mL).
  - Peak height velocity is in late puberty (testicular volume ≥15 mL). There is no equivalent event to menarche in males, although first conscious ejaculation has been used.

In addition to variation in onset of pubertal stages, there is also variation in transit from one stage to another, although roughly one stage a year is the norm.

Puberty is described as consonant if it follows the normal sequence of pubertal changes, or inconsonant if this is abnormal (Table 2.2).

The wide range of normal pubertal development means that abnormalities in puberty (both delayed and precocious) are usually defined as those that lie outside the normal range (characteristically >2.5 SD from the mean).

**Table 2.2** Mean for pubertal stage transit times

| Girls | | Boys | |
|---|---|---|---|
| B2–menarche | 2.3 years | G2–G5 | 3.0 years |
| B2–B5 | 4.5 years | G2–G3 | 1.1 years |
| B2–B3 | 0.9 years | G3–G4 | 0.8 years |
| B2–B4 | 2.0 years | G4–G5 | 1.0 years |

# Premature sexual maturation

This is diagnosed as the onset of 2° sexual characteristics:
- before the age of 8 years in girls
- before the age of 9 years in boys

or
- if menarche occurs before 11 years of age.

In the USA, the cut-off has now been reduced to 7 years in Caucasian girls, and 6 years for African Americans (especially for true puberty).

Premature sexual maturation can be further categorized as:
- isosexual (i.e. 2° sexual characteristics that are appropriate for the child's sex)
- heterosexual/contrasexual (where 2° sexual characteristics are contrary to phenotypic sex, i.e. there is virilization in girls).

Central precocious puberty (CPP) is always isosexual, whereas peripheral precocious puberty can be isosexual or heterosexual.

Premature sexual maturation is further classified as follows.
- *CPP or gonadotropin-dependent precocious puberty*:
  - idiopathic
  - 2°: tumours, hydrocephalus, trauma, cranial irradiation, abuse.
- Abnormal patterns of gonadotropin secretion:
  - premature thelarche
  - thelarche variant
  - isolated premature menarche
  - hypothyroidism.
- *Gonadotropin-independent precocious puberty* (GIPP; i.e. the source of sex steroids is extra-gonadal or gonadal but not under gonadotropin control):
  - McCune–Albright syndrome (MAS)
  - testotoxicosis.
- Virilization:
  - adrenarche
  - congenital adrenal hyperplasia (CAH)
  - Cushing disease
  - adrenal tumours
  - gonadal tumours.

> ❶ Long-standing or aggressive gonadotropin-*independent* precocious puberty can progress to gonadotropin-*dependent* precocious puberty.

# Central precocious puberty (gonadotropin-dependent precocious puberty)

### Idiopathic and secondary central precocious puberty

- The pattern of puberty is the same as that seen in normal puberty (consonant), but occurs abnormally early because of premature activation of the HP axis, either 2° to an underlying disorder or of unknown cause (idiopathic).
- In addition to pubertal changes patients also show:
  - tall stature (especially in relation to parental heights)
  - rapid growth rate
  - advanced skeletal maturation (assessed using bone age)
  - evidence of excess sex steroid production (greasy skin and hair, acne, body odour, and mood swings).
- Overall incidence is estimated to be 1 in 5000–10,000.
- CPP is more frequent in girls, with a female:male ratio of 10:1.
- Also been observed in girls adopted from developing countries.
- *In girls*, breast development is followed by other features of normal puberty including a growth spurt, development of axillary and pubic hair, and vaginal discharge.
- *In boys*, testicular enlargement is also followed by a rapid growth rate, often behavioural disturbances, and deepening of the voice.
- The fixed amount of growth in puberty means that although the child may present with tall stature, growth will finish early and therefore final height is reduced.
- Growth acceleration may occur relatively early in boys, and this may result in a final height that is more than expected.
- Psychological problems may arise due to pubertal levels of sex steroids, resulting in 'adolescent behaviour'. There is altered self-image and the child is expected to behave appropriately to height age.

### Familial central precocious puberty

- Loss of function mutations in paternal allele *DLK1* gene
- *KISS-1* activating mutations
- Loss of function in paternal allele *MKRN3* gene on chromosome 15q11–q13 (PWS region).

May be principal cause of apparently idiopathic CPP in boys.

### Investigations

- Bone age is advanced, often by >2 years.
- TFTs to exclude hyperthyroidism, which advances bone age and may precipitate CPP. In addition, in 1° hypothyroidism high levels of TSH may also stimulate the FSH receptor (van Wyk Grumbach syndrome).

- Baseline oestradiol or testosterone, which are elevated above prepubertal values, although oestradiol is not as helpful in girls as testosterone is in boys.
- Baseline gonadotropins may be of use; a basal LH level:
  - ≥0.3 IU/L predicts subsequent pubertal progression
  - ≤0.2 IU/L—nearly all patients do not progress.
- A GnRH (LHRH) test shows a pubertal gonadotropin response with LH predominance over FSH and peak responses >5 IU/L.
- A pelvic USS in girls shows ovarian follicular activity and uterine growth and maturation, and may also show an endometrial stripe.

### Features of pelvic USS associated with progressive CPP

- A uterine volume >2 mL or length >34 mm
- A pear-shaped uterus, and
- Endometrial thickening (ultrasound).

### Brain MRI (CT if MRI unavailable)

- This is mandatory in boys.
- It is advised in girls <6 years of age especially if E2 elevated.
- Unsuspected cranial pathology is found in 8% of girls and 40% of boys—the percentage decreases with age (e.g. 2–7% of girls aged 6–8 years).

## Treatment

Goals of treatment are to:
1. halt or cause regression of 2° sexual characteristics
2. prevent early menarche in girls
3. retard skeletal maturation and improve final height
4. avoid psychosocial/behavioural sequelae.

GnRH analogues (GnRHa) are the mainstay of treatment:
- Leuprorelin (Prostap®), triptorelin (Decapeptyl®) SC/IM 8–12-weekly, Triptorelin (Gonapeptyl®) SC/IM 3–4 weekly.

Adverse effects of GnRHa (rare in younger ages):
- Short term: headaches, hot flushes, mood swings.
- Injection site reactions: rashes, bruising, and sterile abscess formation.
- Long-term use: ? linked to polycystic ovary syndrome (PCOS).
- As GnRH analogues produce an initial increase of pituitary gonadotropin secretion, followed by suppression, female patients, especially those well established in puberty, may develop initial vaginal bleeding, and need to be warned about this.

Monitoring response to treatment:
- Abolition/reduction of mood swings is indicative of success in gonadotropin suppression. If breakthrough occurs, it is worth reducing the time period between injections.
- Halting breast development or testicular enlargement, with regression in some cases.
- Halting/regression of pelvic USS changes.
- Baseline testosterone/oestradiol and dynamic GnRH testing should show a prepubertal response if unclear.

- Bone age and height velocity are slow to show changes, and are usually preceded by the previously listed features if not fully suppressed (especially mood changes).

NB: progression of pubic hair may occur and indicates normal adrenarche. If there is failure of response, options are as follows:
- Gradually increase the frequency of GnRHa to half the recommended dosage interval.
- Alternatively, or subsequently if no control attained (and compliance assured), a double dose of GnRHa can be considered.
- Add cyproterone acetate at low dose (25 mg bd) and titrate upwards. Adrenal suppression can occur, so patients require a steroid card and emergency advice.

Effect of GnRHa on final adult height is:
- undisputed only in girls <6 years old with early-onset CPP
- not improved in girls beyond 8 years old
- only modestly improved in girls aged 6–8 years
- not recommended routinely for early normal pubertal onset.

Combined use of growth hormone and GnRH agonists is controversial, but may allow more growth in particularly short children.

# Abnormal patterns of gonadotropin secretion

## Premature thelarche

- A (usually) self-limiting condition of unilateral or bilateral thelarche (breast development) in girls.
- May be present from birth or develop within first few months of life.
- Breast development rarely progresses beyond Tanner stage 3, is usually cyclical, and is generally 'burnt out' by 4 years of age.
- Growth velocity is usually normal, and bone age is not advanced.
- Puberty occurs at the usual time, and final height is normal, as is (probably) fertility.
- Premature thelarche is thought to be due to episodic formation of ovarian cysts and/or increased sensitivity of breast tissue to normal levels of circulating oestrogen.
- A small percentage of patients (14% in one study) develop CPP.

### Management

- Investigation may be unnecessary in mild cases.
- Girls show a characteristic pattern of pulsatile FSH secretion which is unlike that seen in normal puberty.
- Pelvic USS may demonstrate ovarian cysts.
- Follow-up should be maintained as it may be difficult to distinguish from early true precocious puberty.

## Thelarche variant

Some patients may demonstrate a clinical picture intermediate between thelarche and CPP, a partial activation of the HP–gonadal axis:

- evidence of slow clinical progress in puberty (usually girls) and no rapid growth acceleration
- GnRH testing shows peak LH/FSH responses <5 IU/L or FSH predominance
- low oestradiol secretion
- bone age not advanced
- probably quite common, and described as 'slowly progressive variant of precocious puberty in girls'
- final height is not affected
- a conservative initial approach is sensible.

## Isolated premature menarche

This is sporadic or cyclical vaginal bleeding in girls with no or few signs of pubertal development.

- It usually occurs between 4 and 8 years of age.
- It is important to exclude other causes of bleeding such as exogenous administration of oestrogen, vulvovaginitis, foreign body, trauma, or sexual abuse. Rectal bleeding and fabricated bleeding should also be considered.
- Normal pubertal development, including menarche, generally occurs at the same time as other girls.

*Investigation and management*
- Bone age is not advanced.
- Pelvic USS shows a prepubertal uterus.
- GnRH testing may be necessary in doubtful cases. Activation of the HP–gonadal axis results in FSH secretion and increased sensitivity of the endometrium to oestradiol levels, which are too low to produce breast development.

No treatment is usually necessary but the child should probably be kept under follow-up.

## Gonadotropin-independent precocious puberty

GIPP is very rare, although probably occurs more commonly in boys than in girls.

Testotoxicosis is an autosomal recessive condition with an activating mutation of the LH receptor affecting the Leydig cells, in which testes develop on their own without stimulation from the pituitary gland. Familial cases are described. The pattern of development of pubertal changes is identical to that of true CPP.

GIPP may also occur rarely in girls, almost always as MAS, which is characterized by abnormal bone cysts (polyostotic fibrous dysplasia) and skin pigmentation (*café au lait* patches in 'coast of Maine' distribution).

Other autonomous endocrine hypersecretions may also occur, such as hyperthyroidism, hyperparathyroidism, Cushing syndrome, and GH-secreting pituitary adenoma.

# Virilization

(● See also Chapter 8.)

## Adrenarche (premature adrenarche or pubarche)

At birth, there is involution of the fetal zone of the adrenal cortex, which usually remains quiescent in early childhood. From 6 years of age in boys and girls there is a marked increase (5–10×) in adrenal androgen secretion, especially DHEA, DHEA-S, and androstenedione. This is called *adrenarche*. There is also a concomitant rise in blood pressure but little alteration in height velocity in growth velocity.

This rise in DHEA is thought to arise from need to increase cortisol production as a child grows, and hence there is a greater pituitary ACTH drive to do this. The higher internal cortisol levels inhibit enzyme 3βHSD2 activity which consequently raises DHEA production. DHEA is sulphated to DHEA-S by enzyme SULT2A1 to become the most abundant hormone in the body.

## Isolated premature pubarche

This refers to development of pubic hair at <8 years in girls and <9 years in boys, without any other pubertal signs. The most common cause of this is exaggerated or premature adrenarche, which also includes the following clinical features.

### Clinical features

- Characteristic onset from 4–6 years
- Pubic hair; characteristically along the labiae in girls rather than pubic area
- Axillary hair
- Adult body odour
- Minimal acne if present
- No virilization
- Slow/little advance in clinical signs
- Height velocity may be increased, but pubertal timing and adult height usually unchanged
- Bone age in upper normal range (usually <2 years advanced).

### Points

- More common in:
  - children of Mediterranean, Indian, and African-Caribbean origin
  - girls
  - children born small for gestational age (SGA).
- Increasingly seen, possibly because of increased levels of obesity.
- Despite advanced bone age, final height is normal
- No evidence that spontaneous androgen secretion is abnormal, and children may represent those at the top end of the normal range for secretion or be more sensitive to normal levels of androgens
- Although initially thought to be a benign condition, long-term sequelae include early puberty and PCOS.

*Investigations and management*
- Minimum investigation should be bone age, which should not be advanced by >2 years. Many would also do additional investigations, especially if there are any other features of concern.
- Adrenal androgens (usually DHEA and DHEA-S but also testosterone and androstenedione) are raised for age but not stage of pubic hair. These and other adrenal steroids, e.g. 17-hydroxyprogesterone (17-OHP), are also raised in both CAH and adrenal tumours. A Synacthen stimulation test may be required to identify steroid synthesis defects ( ) see 'Short Synacthen test for investigation of possible congenital adrenal hyperplasia', p. 404).

Symptomatic treatment only is probably required.
- Adult body odour: regular bathing, deodorant. Antiperspirant is not recommended.
- Excess hair: depilatories, shaving, trimming. There is no evidence that these make hair grow back faster or thicker.

## Precocious pseudopuberty

This occurs when there are signs of sexual maturation due to sex steroid secretion with a different mechanism from normal puberty, such as from cysts, tumours, or metabolic abnormalities of the adrenals (CAH) or gonads.

The condition is usually recognized because there is a disordered sequence of pubertal events (inconsonant puberty). Clinical features depend on the aetiology but often include:
- early onset in preschool years
- tall stature with rapid growth
- very advanced bone age (>2 years)
- pubic and axillary hair development in both sexes
- acne (may be marked)
- increased penile length with prepubertal testes (<3 mL) in boys
- clitoromegaly in girls
- rapid progression of symptoms.

*Investigation and management*
- Measure androgens (testosterone, DHEA-S, androstenedione, 17OHP) in serum or urine.
- Measure oestrogen if female gonadal tumour/cyst suspected.
- Measure tumour markers: βhCG and AFP.
- GnRH and a Synacthen test may be done as indicated.
- Assess bone age.
- Pelvic USS and adrenal MRI should also be considered to look for a gonadal or adrenal tumour.

Treatment is usually directed to the underlying cause.

# Delayed puberty

Is puberty delayed or just late? If delayed, is it a delayed *onset* and/or *completion*?

## Late puberty

This is defined as pubertal events occurring within the later (lower) centiles but within the normal range (0.4th–99.6th centiles).

## Delayed onset of puberty

- Diagnosed when there is absence of 2° sexual characteristics:
  - by 13 years in a girl
  - by 14 years in a boy
- It affects ~2% of adolescents.
- While it may be a normal variant, it might also indicate an underlying disorder.

NB: the definition does not involve pubic hair as this may be part of adrenarche.

The 2–18- and 2–20-year growth charts have puberty lines which depict the normal ranges and latest ages for starting puberty.

## Delayed completing puberty

The final puberty line depicts the latest age of the *completing puberty* phase (0.4th centile).

- In girls, this is if the first period does not occur by 15 years of age.
- In boys, this is if genital development is not complete, the voice fully lowered and facial hair beginning to grow.

## Causes of delayed puberty

- Constitutional delay (53%)
- Functional hypogonadotropic hypogonadism (HH) (19%)
- HH (12%)
- Hypergonadotropic hypogonadism (13%)
- Unclassified (3%).

## Arrested puberty

There may also be pubertal failure or arrest, when puberty begins but fails to progress adequately. This usually has a serious cause.

The causes of delayed puberty are classified as central or peripheral, i.e. depending on whether the problem is in the HP axis or in the gonads.

# Central causes of delayed puberty (hypogonadotropic hypogonadism)

HH may also be subdivided into functional (intact HP axis) or permanent (impaired HP axis).

## Intact HP axis—functional impairment

- Constitutional delay of growth and puberty (CDGP)
- Chronic disease: rheumatoid arthritis, diabetes mellitus, sickle cell disease, thalassaemia, eczema, asthma
- Poor nutrition: coeliac disease, cystic fibrosis, inflammatory bowel disease, anorexia nervosa, malnutrition
- Psychosocial deprivation
- Steroid therapy
- Hypothyroidism.

## Impaired HP axis (hypogonadotropic hypogonadism)—permanent impairment

- Tumours adjacent to HP axis:
  - craniopharyngioma
  - optic glioma
  - astrocytoma
- Developmental anomalies of HP axis:
  - septo-optic dysplasia (SOD)
  - hypopituitarism
- Irradiation and trauma/surgery
- Complete GnRH/LH/FSH deficiency:
  - idiopathic
  - Kallmann syndrome
  - Prader–Willi syndrome
  - Bardet–Biedl syndrome
  - CHARGE syndrome
- Partial or maturational GnRH/LH/FSH deficiency:
  - Idiopathic slow pubertal development (males > females); extreme of constitutional delay—see p. 72.
  - Hypothalamic gene variants (often familial).

# Peripheral causes of delayed puberty (hypergonadotropic hypogonadism)

## Males

- Bilateral testicular damage:
  - undescended testes
  - failed orchidopexy
  - torsion
  - chemotherapy
  - radiotherapy
- Syndromes associated with cryptorchidism:
  - Noonan syndrome
  - Prader–Willi syndrome
  - Bardet–Biedl syndrome
- Gonadal dysgenesis (➲ see Chapter 11).

## Females

- Disorders of sex development (DSD)
- Ovarian damage:
  - chemotherapy
  - radiotherapy
  - autoimmune ovarian failure
- Gonadal dysgenesis:
  - Turner syndrome
  - Noonan syndrome
- PCOS—usually delayed completion/menarche.

## Specific conditions

### Constitutional delay in growth and puberty

(➲ See also Chapter 1, p. 18.)

CDGP is by far the most common cause of delayed puberty in both sexes, but is more common in boys than girls (male-to-female ratio 7:1).

This is usually a diagnosis of exclusion. There is characteristically:

- a history of long-standing short stature during childhood
- poor growth, especially noticeable from about 9–11 years of age
- slow progression through puberty, and sexual development occurs later than expected
- family history of delayed growth and puberty in parents or siblings, but its presence or absence does not confirm or refute the diagnosis.

NB: it is not unusual to find early signs of puberty (e.g. testicular enlargement) which the boy himself or the initial examining doctor has not noticed.

### Central pubertal delay with intact HP axis

Any chronic disease can cause a delay in growth and puberty. Pubertal delay in undernutrition is likely to be a 2° adaptation to prevent reproduction in suboptimal circumstances.

- Impairment of linear growth and associated delay in pubertal development commonly complicate childhood Crohn's disease.

- Chronic renal insufficiency causes extensive neuroendocrine disturbance, including marked HP dysfunction.
- In some cases, therapy contributes to this, e.g. corticosteroids (inhaled or oral) can delay growth and epiphyseal and pubertal maturation in children with severe asthma.
- Hypothyroidism may be associated with not only delayed puberty but also precocious puberty.

### Central pubertal delay with impairment of the HP axis (hypogonadotropic hypogonadism)

Impairment of either hypothalamic GnRH or pituitary gonadotropins causes HH. This is dealt with in more detail in ➲ Chapter 3. The gonads themselves are normal but remain prepubertal because stimulation by gonadotropins is lacking.

Congenital or acquired lesions in or adjacent to the pituitary almost always result in deficiency of gonadotropins and other pituitary hormones. Isolated GnRH and gonadotropin deficiency is more common in boys than in girls.

### Peripheral pubertal delay (hypergonadotropic hypogonadism)

#### Turner syndrome
(➲ See also Chapter 1, p. 18.)

Turner syndrome occurs in 1 in 3500 live female births, and is the most common gonadal dysgenesis in females. Approximately 50% have a missing complete X chromosome (45,X).

- Although gonadal failure is common, a proportion of girls (~10–20%) show some spontaneous pubertal development, with both spontaneous menarche and unassisted pregnancy described.
- Streak ovaries are characteristically seen on pelvic USS.
- Oestrogen replacement is usually necessary to induce puberty.

#### Klinefelter syndrome (47,XXY)
(➲ See also Chapter 1, p. 38.)

Occurs in 1 in 600 males, and is due to an extra X chromosome (47,XXY). May cause delayed progress in puberty but NOT delayed onset.

Patients present with:
- antenatal diagnosis (usually unexpected)
- speech delay
- some degree of learning difficulty especially reading and writing
- behaviour problems, especially temper tantrums when frustrated
- tall stature
- eunuchoid proportions (increased arm span-to-height ratio)
- hypergonadotropic hypogonadism with characteristically small testes (2° to tubular hyalinization)
- persistent gynaecomastia (around 40%).

### Testosterone treatment

#### Biochemical hypogonadism
- Low testosterone: often not found before late puberty G4 around age 15 years. ► measure testosterone in morning 8–9am
- Prepubertal treatment subject to clinical trials.

### Clinical hypogonadism

- Slow virilization including small penis in childhood (➔ see p. 38)
- Low energy
- High BMI—'beer belly'
- Gynaecomastia
- Low bone density
- Poor muscle development/tone.

### Gynaecomastia

- Commence testosterone undecanoate or gel as soon as recognized.
- Administer *in the morning* to correct diurnal deficiency.
- Increase dose as per schedule (➔ see p. 76).
- Continue until late puberty >15 years.
- Re-evaluate treatment need then.

### Other reported benefits of testosterone

- Confidence boost
- Better moods
- Better concentration
- Better learning
- Better development.

Diagnostic evaluation of delayed puberty

### History

Detailed history including growth patterns, family details, evidence of chronic disease (especially gastrointestinal (GI)), psychosocial problems, and underlying conditions.

### Examination

- Weight, measured height of the child, parents, and siblings.
- BMI.
- Physical examination looking for chronic disease, evidence of underlying disease, dysmorphic features, and abnormal neurology.
- Pubertal staging.
- Micropenis and/or cryptorchidism may indicate congenital gonadotropin deficiency.
- Anosmia (lack of sense of smell) may indicate Kallmann or CHARGE syndrome.

### Investigations

- Bone age: characteristically delayed by at least 12 months.
- Baseline endocrine and other bloods including (where appropriate) FSH, LH, oestradiol, testosterone, growth factors (IGF-1), inhibin B, FBC, ESR, coeliac antibodies, and renal function.
- Thyroid function: late puberty may be the only symptom/clinical sign of acquired hypothyroidism.
- IGF-1 level may be low for age, but not for bone age/pubertal stage.
- Prolactin if indicated.
- Dynamic function testing: GnRH testing (both sexes) and hCG stimulation (males).
- If indicated, brain MRI to exclude intracranial lesions.

*Specific points for boys*
- Early-morning testosterone: the presence of a detectable level (usually >1 nmol/L) indicates nocturnal pituitary–gonadal activity; hence the imminent clinical signs of puberty.
- If negative, proceed to dynamic (GnRH) testing.
- hCG stimulation (both short and long tests); assess gonadal function.
- Karyotyping (microarrays) is indicated when there is evidence of gonadal dysfunction, or small testes and hypergonadotropic hypogonadism.

*Specific points for girls*
- Oestradiol (less useful than testosterone in boys).
- Karyotyping indicated as first-line investigation to exclude Turner syndrome/mosaic (45,X) or sex reversal (46,XY).
- Dynamic (GnRH) test.
- Pelvic USS: direct visualization of Müllerian structures (Fallopian tubes, uterus, cervix, upper vagina) and ovaries.

NB: if low gonadotropins/sex hormones or mismatch between growth and puberty, consider a central disorder. MRI scan is indicated.

## Constitutional delay treatment options

If the delay is a physiological variant, no treatment is required other than:
- reassurance and support
- understanding the difficulties from the patient's perspective
- counselling in lifestyle skills
- repeated assessment of progress for reassurance.

Short-term therapy (3–6 months until reviewed) may be required in some patients.

*Boys*
- Testosterone (e.g. 50–100 mg IM monthly, 40 mg orally, 10 mg transdermal) either on alternate days or daily if >13 years (➲ see p. 76).
- The response to therapy is often sustained in males with testicular volumes ≥8 mL.
- Oxandrolone 2.5 mg daily (1.25 mg if under 13)
- As oxandrolone is not aromatized, unlike testosterone it does not produce gynaecomastia.

*Girls*
- Oestradiol valerate 0.5 mg or ethinyloestradiol 2 mcg daily or oestradiol patch 25 mcg quartered, i.e. 6.25 mcg changed twice weekly.
- Therapy tends to be less effective for growth acceleration in females.

# Hormone therapies for induction of puberty and fertility

If spontaneous puberty is not expected (e.g. HP or gonadal dysfunction), plan to induce puberty within the physiological range, taking into account family timings and psychological maturity.

NB: dosage schedule and timings can be escalated in later presenting and larger individuals.

## Treatment schedule: males

Mainstay is testosterone by incremental dose; induction is more flexible with oral or transdermal preparations, but intramuscular is satisfactory and cheap despite poor pharmacokinetics.

### Long-acting testosterone esters (e.g. testosterone enantate) or ester mixtures (e.g. Sustanon®)

- Initially 50 IM monthly for 6 months.
- Increase every 6 months to 75–100–150–200 mg IM 4-weekly.
- Change to 250 mg IM 3-weekly after 2–3 years.
- Optional longer-term maintenance with Nebido® (testosterone undecanoate) 1000 mg IM every 12 weeks (repeat loading dose after first 6 weeks).

### Testosterone undecanoate (Restandol® Testocaps/Andriol®)

- Start at 40 mg initially alternate days for 6 months then increase to 40 mg once daily.
- Titrate up every 6 months to a maximum dose of 80 mg twice a day after 2–3 years.
- If ongoing treatment required, switch to full-dose gel or IM testosterone.

### Testosterone gel

- Tostran® 2% gel suggested starting dose 10 mg (1 metered pump) daily; can start lower, e.g. 1 pump alternate days if little previous exposure to testosterone or likelihood of behavioural issues.
- Increase by 10 mg (1 pump) every 6 months to 60–80 mg over 3 years.
- Testosterone level monitoring is helpful to prevent overdosing.
NB: apply to chest, abdomen, or thigh. If being applied by a parent (especially if mother), they need to wear latex gloves.
Testavan® 2% gel comes with a hands-free applicator:
- Dose 23–69 mg/day (1–3 pumps).
- This or Testogel (R) be more suitable for longer-term use as lower volume.

## Treatment schedule: females

- The mainstay of pubertal induction has been synthetic ethinyloestradiol, but smaller dose preparations are less available and now more expensive. Ethinyloestradiol cannot be measured by regular oestradiol assays so increments are made by clinical judgement.
- More experience has now been gained with 17-beta oestradiol preparations—transdermal or oral which are now the preferred options.

- Conjugated equine oestrogens are not recommended for adolescents as doses too high.

▶ NB: clinical examination of the speed of breast development is important to avoid areolar and glandular overgrowth due to too-rapid treatment (tubular breasts) which is disfiguring and irreversible.

### Oral oestradiol valerate

*1 mg and 2 mg tablet sizes*
- First 12 months: 0.5 mg alternate days
- Second 6 months: 0.5 mg daily
- Third 6 months: 0.75 mg daily
- Fourth 6 months: 1.0 mg daily
- Thereafter titrate against clinical assessment and serum oestradiol levels.

### Transdermal oestrogen patches 17-beta oestradiol (Evorel®)

25, 50, and 100 mcg/24-hour delivery patches. Start with 25 mcg patch:
- First 6 months: ¼ patch, 6.25 mcg 4 days/week
- Second 6 months: ½ patch for 3–4 days
- Third 6 months: ¼ patch for 3–4 days
- Fourth 6 months: 1 patch, 25 mcg twice/week
- Thereafter titrate against clinical assessment and serum oestradiol levels (adult range target 400–600 pmol/L).

### Ethinyloestradiol

Tablet sizes 2 and 10 mcg:
- Start at 2 mcg daily (0.1 mcg/kg/day).
- Increase dose by either doubling or increasing by 1–2 mcg at ~6–12-month intervals depending on pubertal, growth, and psychological response.
- The aim is to mimic the normal physical pattern of growth from the start of puberty—maturity in ~3 years.

## Treatment regime for growth and physical development in adolescents with constitutional delay of puberty

### Boys
- Continue as per induction of puberty.
- Approximately 6-monthly dose increases until evidence of testicular growth, which is evidence of endogenous gonadotropin secretion.
- May need several courses of testosterone with short breaks to assess spontaneous progress.

### Girls
- Continue as per induction of puberty.
- 6–12-monthly ovarian USS to look for follicular activity, which is evidence of endogenous gonadotropin secretion.
- Continuation usually only required if there is a defect in gonadotropin regulation or significant ovarian failure.

Induction of menstruation

When breast development is at stage B4 and height velocity is slowing, or if breakthrough vaginal bleeding occurs, increase oestradiol further towards adult dose ranges, target serum range 400–600 pmol/L.

Typical adult oestrogen doses:
- Evorel® 50–100 mcg twice weekly.
- Oestradiol valerate 4–8 mg daily.
- Equivalent dose of ethinyloestradiol is 20–30 mcg daily by clinical assessment.

Options:
- Add in oral cyclical progesterone (e.g. norethisterone 5 mg or medroxyprogesterone acetate 5 mg) day 14–21 of cycle.
- Switch to low-dose cyclical combined oral contraceptive pill, e.g. Loestrin® 20 (ethinyloestradiol 20 mcg–norethisterone acetate 1 mg) for 21 days of 28-day cycle
- Hormone replacement therapy (e.g. Cyclo-Progynova® (oestradiol valerate 2 mg–norgestrel 500 mcg)).
- Change to a combined HRT patch which included cyclical progesterone (e.g. Evorel® 50 Sequi).
- ▶ NB: women *without* a uterus do *not* need a progestogen added in.

Growth hormone

Not indicated in short normal/physiological delay patients.

Induction of gonadal development
in hypogonadotropic hypogonadism

- Mainly performed to initiate spermatogenesis in adolescent males as gametes in the ovary are more mature.
- May be required for cosmetic reasons to increase testicular volume.
- Recombinant human FSH (rhFSH) (Bemfola®, Follitropin Alfa®) and LH (equivalent is hCG (Pregnyl®, Gonasi®)) can be used to induce pubertal characteristics and spermatogenesis as follows:
- Start pubertal induction with testosterone (as per schedules given previously). When ready to comply with more involving schedule:
  - Start rhFSH 75 IU SC twice weekly.
  - Continue testosterone replacement.
  - After 3 months increase rhFSH to 150 IU twice weekly.
  - Stop testosterone.
  - Start hCG 1500–2000 IU SC twice weekly.
  - Measure FSH and testosterone after 3, 6, and 12 months. Titrate doses of rhFSH and hCG.
  - If evidence of testicular growth, consider semen analysis and repeat 3–6-monthly until positive.
  - If satisfactory semen sample eventually stored, stop rhFSH and hCG and return to previous full testosterone replacement.

# Other common pubertal problems

## Polycystic ovary syndrome

PCOS is diagnosed if two out of the following three criteria are present:
1. reduced or absent periods (oligomenorrhoea/amenorrhoea)
2. hyperandrogenism either clinical (hirsutism or male pattern alopecia), or biochemical (raised levels of testosterone)
3. polycystic ovaries on USS.

Excessive body hair occurs typically in a male pattern affecting the face, chest, and legs. Other features include:
- obesity
- acne
- oily skin
- infertility from chronic lack of ovulation.

PCOS is part of the metabolic syndrome and is associated with insulin resistance/type 2 diabetes, hypertension, raised lipids, and long-term cardiovascular disease (🔵 see also Chapter 6).

NB: reproductive function is not necessarily reduced in adolescents despite oligo/amenorrhoea.

### Investigation

Biochemistry reveals:
- raised LH and androgen levels, with raised LH:FSH ratio
- low sex hormone-binding globulin (SHBG)
- hyperinsulinism.

Pelvic USS may or may not show polycystic ovaries.

### Management

*Lifestyle intervention*
- Lifestyle intervention should be based on the combination of calorie-restricted diets, behavioural treatment, and exercise.
- Combined weight loss and physical exercise are the first-line therapy in overweight and obese girls. They decrease androgen levels, normalize menstrual cycles, and improve markers of cardio-metabolic health.
- Extremely obese adolescents respond poorly to lifestyle intervention.
- In normal-weight girls, increasing physical activity is effective in reducing the development of metabolic syndrome. However, the benefit of exclusive weight loss in these adolescents is not clear.

*Local therapies/cosmetic*
- Laser therapy is the first-line management of localized hirsutism in PCOS. Diode and alexandrite (superior) lasers are preferred.
- Topical eflornithine is recommended as an adjuvant to photoepilation in girls with laser-resistant facial hirsutism aged 16 years or older, or as monotherapy in those where laser therapy is not indicated.
- The use of topical finasteride is not recommended.

*Additive drugs*
- Metformin:
  - Metformin has beneficial effects in overweight or obese adolescents with PCOS, but only short-term data are available.

- In non-obese adolescents with PCOS and hyperinsulinaemia, metformin improves ovulation and testosterone levels.
- Antiandrogens:
  - Antiandrogens reduce androgen excess features more than metformin in monotherapy. Spironolactone is the most commonly used albeit data on efficacy compared to flutamide are limited.
  - Antiandrogens should only be used when contraceptive measures are guaranteed.
- Oral contraceptive pills:
  - No specific formulation can be recommended over another.
  - Those containing an antiandrogenic progestogen (e.g. Dianette®, Yasmin®) seem to confer efficacy in reducing androgen levels and producing regular cycles (and contraception).
- Combination treatments:
  - Triple low-dose combinations of insulin-sensitizing and antiandrogenic generics may normalize cardiovascular risk and body composition more than combinations of only metformin and an antiandrogen.

## Gynaecomastia in boys

- This occurs in up to 40% of early pubertal boys and is due to a temporary imbalance between androgens and oestrogen. In the vast majority it is self–limiting.
- Most settle within months or 1–2 years, but persistent or marked gynaecomastia, especially if associated with psychological problems, should be referred.
- Exclusion of any underlying disorder (such as Klinefelter syndrome or partial androgen insensitivity syndrome (PAIS)) should be considered if persistent.
- Medical treatment with antioestrogens or aromatase inhibitors is rarely effective
- Early- to mid-pubertal boys may benefit from a boost of testosterone: oral testosterone undecanoate 40 mg or testosterone gel 20 mg *given in the morning* for 6 months.
- Patients may be referred for either liposuction or subareolar mastectomy if persistent.

## Breast asymmetry in girls

This commonly occurs, especially early in puberty, and may well 'even up' as puberty progresses. Some degree of breast asymmetry is normal, and any therapy such as plastic surgery should only be considered once growth and puberty are complete, and usually not until late teens at least.

# Further reading

Carel JC, Eugster EA, Rogol A, et al. Consensus statement on the use of gonadotropin-releasing hormone analogs in children. *Pediatrics* 2009;123:e752–e762.

Dunkel L, Quinton R. Transition in endocrinology: induction of puberty. *Eur J Endocrinol* 2014;170:R229–R239.

Fuqua JS. Treatment and outcomes of precocious puberty: an update. *J Clin Endocrinol Metab* 2013;98:2198–2207.

Ibáñez L, Oberfield SE, Witchel S, et al. An international consortium update: pathophysiology, diagnosis, and treatment of polycystic ovarian syndrome in adolescence. *Horm Res Paediatr* 2017;88:371–395.

Lawaetz JG, Hagen CP, Mieritz MG, et al. Evaluation of 451 Danish boys with delayed puberty: diagnostic use of a new puberty nomogram and effects of oral testosterone therapy. *J Clin Endocrinol Metab* 2015;100:1376–1385.

Matthews D, Bath L, Högler W, et al. Hormone supplementation for pubertal induction in girls. *Arch Dis Child* 2017;102:975–980.

Rogol AD, Swerdloff RS, Reiter EO et al. A multicenter, open-label, observational study of testosterone gel (1%) in the treatment of adolescent boys with Klinefelter syndrome or anorchia. *J Adolesc Health* 2014;54:20–25.

Schoelwer M, Eugster EA. Treatment of peripheral precocious puberty. *Endocr Dev* 2016;29:230–239.

Wei C, Crowne EC. Recent advances in the understanding and management of delayed puberty. *Arch Dis Child* 2016;101:481–488.

# The pituitary and hypopituitarism

# Embryology

The pituitary gland (Fig. 3.1) consists of two main parts:
- the anterior pituitary, which arises from Rathke's pouch, an outpouch (pharyngeal stomodeum) of the oral ectoderm
- the posterior pituitary, which arises from the neural ectoderm (diencephalon).

In addition, there may be an intermediate lobe (pars intermedia) between the two lobes, although in humans this is often small.

The pituitary gland develops in response to a cascade of genes which regulate the differentiation of specific tissues and cell types. Much of the understanding of this process has been obtained from animal models and subsequent identification of their human homologues.

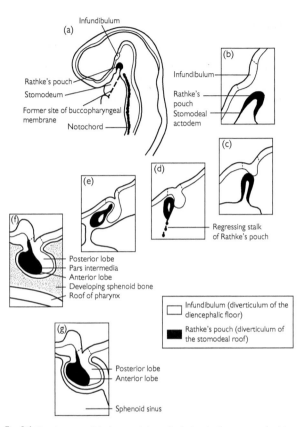

**Fig. 3.1** Development of the human pituitary gland, showing the compound origins of adeno- and neurohypophyses.

Reproduced from Wass JAH, Shalet SM (eds) (2002). *Oxford Textbook of Endocrinology and Diabetes*, Oxford University Press, Oxford. Copyright © 2002 OUP.

# Anatomy

The pituitary is connected to the hypothalamus by the pituitary stalk (hypophyseal–portal system) (Fig. 3.2).

The anterior pituitary secretes hormones itself under the influence of stimulatory and inhibitory peptides from the hypothalamus, whereas the posterior pituitary hormones are produced within the hypothalamus and transported down axons to be secreted from the gland.

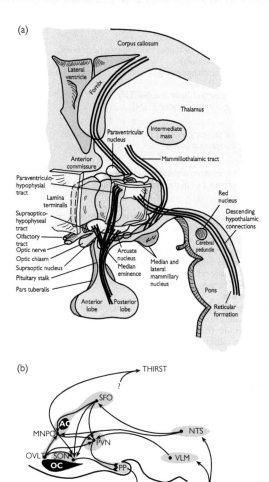

**Fig. 3.2** (a) The hypothalamic nuclei and hypothalamic–hypophyseal tracts in relation to the thalamus, ventricular system, and brainstem. (b) Schematic representation of the neurohypophysis and the major pathways regulating vasopressin release and thirst. Autonomic afferents project to the ventrolateral medulla (VLM) and the nucleus of the tractus solitarius (NTS). This sensory input is integrated with that from periventricular osmoreceptors in the subfornicular organ (SFO), the median pre-optic nucleus (MNPO), and the organum vasculosum of the lamina terminalis (OVLT). Further afferents project to the paraventricular (PVN) and supra-optic nuclei (SON), in addition to the higher centres responsible for processing thirst.

# Physiology

The anterior pituitary produces the following hormones:
- growth hormone (GH)
- the gonadotropins luteinizing hormone (LH) and follicle-stimulating hormone (FSH)
- adrenocorticotropic hormone (ACTH)
- thyroid-stimulating hormone (TSH)
- prolactin.

The posterior pituitary secretes the following hormones:
- arginine vasopressin (AVP)
- oxytocin.

Many of the hormones are under both stimulatory and inhibitory control by hormones secreted from the hypothalamus (Tables 3.1 and 3.2).

## Hypopituitarism

This refers to deficiency of one or more pituitary hormones (anterior and/or posterior). These deficiencies can be either isolated or multiple; the latter are often referred to as combined pituitary hormone deficiency (CPHD), multiple pituitary hormone deficiency (MPHD), or pan-hypopituitarism.

▶ There can be an evolving pattern of hormone deficiencies, so that what may initially present as an isolated hormone deficiency (often in GH) can develop further hormone deficiencies in time. Clinicians need to be mindful of this.

▶ Some hormones (e.g. GH) are more likely to present as isolated deficiencies, whereas others (e.g. TSH and ACTH) are more usually found in association with other hormone abnormalities.

The main causes of hypopituitarism are:
- genetic
- tumour (pituitary or para-pituitary)
- radiotherapy
- infiltration
- infection
- trauma, including surgery and traumatic brain injury
- idiopathic.

The symptoms of hypopituitarism are summarized in Table 3.3.

**Table 3.1** Anterior pituitary hormones

| Hormone | Cell | Stimulus | Inhibitory |
|---|---|---|---|
| GH (somatotropin) | Somatotroph | GHRH | Somatostatin |
| ACTH | Corticotroph | CRH (vasopressin) | |
| Prolactin | Lactotroph | TRH | Dopamine |
| LH/FSH | Gonadotroph | GnRH | |
| TSH | Thyrotroph | TRH | Somatostatin |

**Table 3.2** Posterior pituitary hormones

| Hormone | Site of production | Peptide size |
|---|---|---|
| Vasopressin | Supra-optic nucleus (hypothalamus) | Nonapeptide (9 peptides) |
| Oxytocin | Supra-optic nucleus (hypothalamus) Paraventricular area | Nonapeptide (9 peptides) |

**Table 3.3** Pituitary hormone deficiencies

| Hormone | Symptoms of deficiency |
|---|---|
| GH | Hypoglycaemia Growth failure, relative obesity |
| LH/FSH | Undescended testes and micropenis (boys) Pubertal failure, infertility |
| ACTH | Jaundice, hypoglycaemia Weakness, susceptibility to infection |
| TSH | Poor growth, intellectual disability |
| Prolactin | ? Lactation |
| ADH | Diabetes insipidus |
| Oxytocin | ? Parturition |

# Growth hormone deficiency (GHD)

GHD is the most common endocrine disorder presenting with short stature. It is estimated that ~25% of children with a height below −3 SDS have GHD (➔ see also Chapter 1). The frequency of GHD is estimated to be 1 in 3500–4000, although a milder phenotype may occur in up to 1 in 2000.

The most common causes of GHD are as follows.
- Congenital:
  - midline embryonic defect: septo-optic dysplasia (SOD), holoprosencephaly, pituitary aplasia/hypoplasia, Rathke's cyst
  - transcription factor mutations: *GH1, POU1F1, PROP1, HESX1.*
- Acquired:
  - pituitary/hypothalamic or midline tumour: craniopharyngioma, germinoma, pinealoma, optic nerve glioma
  - trauma: surgery, perinatal, traumatic brain injury
  - infiltration; Langerhans cell histiocytosis (LCH), lymphoma, leukaemia
  - infection: bacterial, viral, fungal
  - irradiation to intracranial, nasopharyngeal, and orbital tumours; cranial or craniospinal irradiation in acute leukaemia
  - temporary failure: peripubertal, emotional deprivation, hypothyroidism
  - idiopathic.

Most (50–70%) have an isolated GH deficiency (IGHD), but GHD can also occur as part of CPHD or MPHD.

The diagnosis of severe isolated GHD is relatively straightforward. The clinical phenotype, often present from birth or within the first years of life, includes:
- short stature (height more than −3 SDS below the mean, and more than −1.5 SDS below MPH)
- poor growth (a documented height velocity (HV) below the 25th centile for at least 1 year), and in severe GHD the HV may be <4 cm/year)
- delayed bone age (with associated delayed dentition and puberty)
- increased skinfolds
- mid-facial hypoplasia with frontal bossing ('doll-like facies')
- small hands and feet
- micropenis in males
- hypoglycaemia may occur (especially in the neonate).

Birthweight is characteristically low normal, confirming the limited role of GH in fetal growth. Association with breech delivery led to speculation that birth trauma has produced the GHD, although it is also postulated that the breech presentation may be a result of GHD and reduced fetal movement.

Milder forms of GHD may remain unrecognized until the child is older, and other clinical manifestations are much less obvious at this stage.

## Congenital GHD

### Isolated GHD

Between 3% and 30% of cases of isolated GHD are familial, with a number of genetic forms described.

- Type IA (autosomal recessive): absent GH levels and anti-GH antibodies when treated with GH; due to deletions and nonsense mutations in the *GH1* gene. Anterior pituitary hypoplasia (and ectopic posterior pituitary) is found.
- Type IB (autosomal recessive): low GH levels and no anti-GH antibodies when treated with GH; due to mutations in *GH1* (splice site, frameshift, and nonsense) and the GHRH receptor.
- Type II (autosomal dominant): low GH levels: due to mutations in the *GH1* gene intron 3 affecting splicing or GH secretion. May have significant variation in height deficit, with pituitary hypoplasia in up to 50%.
- Type III (X-linked recessive): low GH levels: associated with X-linked gammaglobulinaemia.

### MPHD including GHD

Mutations in various homeobox genes encoding pituitary transcription factors have been described with GHD in association with other variable pituitary hormone deficits. The genetic defects and endocrine clinical phenotypes are summarized in Table 3.4.

## Septo-optic dysplasia

SOD is a triad of:

- optic nerve hypoplasia

Table 3.4 Common genetic defects in hypopituitarism

| Gene | GH | LH/FSH | ACTH | TSH | Prolactin | Inheritance |
|------|-----|--------|------|-----|-----------|-------------|
| POU1F1 | − | + | + | ± | − | AD/AR |
| PROP1 | − | − | + | − | − | AR |
| HESX1 | − | ± | ± | ± | ± | (AR) |
| SOX2 | ± | − | + | + | + | AR |
| SOX3 | − | ± | + | ± | + | XL |
| OTX2 | − | ± | + | ± | ± | AD |
| LHX3 | − | − | + | − | − | AR |
| LHX4 | − | ± | + | ± | + | AD |
| PITX2 | − | ± | + | − | + | AD |

AD, autosomal dominant; AR, autosomal recessive; XL, X-linked.

+, hormone present, -, hormone always deleted, ±, hormone may be deleted

- absent septum pellucidum and other midline brain defects, including hypoplastic/absent corpus callosum
- hypopituitarism.

Although all may occur in isolation, at least two of the triad are required for the diagnosis of SOD. In one study, 62% of affected SOD individuals had hypopituitarism, with ~30% having all three parts of the triad. Although originally thought to be rare (~1 in 50,000), it is now recognized to be one of the more common identified causes of hypopituitarism, with a prevalence of ~1 in 12,000. It has been associated with reduced maternal age, primigravida birth, possible increased first-trimester bleeding, and adverse social circumstances (areas of high unemployment and high teenage pregnancy). A small minority have mutations in *HESX1* and other genes.

In addition to features of hypopituitarism, patients commonly present to ophthalmologists with visual defects (e.g. poor vision, nystagmus). Other neurological features may also be present, including developmental delay, autistic spectrum disorders, and epilepsy.

Other structural defects associated with GHD are cleft palate and single central incisor.

# Diagnosis of GHD

(➔ See also Chapter 14.)

Regulation of GH is shown in Fig. 3.3. As GH is secreted in a pulsatile fashion, random GH levels are of little diagnostic value outside of the neonatal period or if GH resistance is considered, and so a variety of different ways of assessing GH secretion have been utilized.

## Physiological

### Insulin-like growth factors

These GH-dependent peptides, produced in a paracrine or autocrine fashion, mediate much of the growth-promoting effects of GH. Low levels are seen in GHD, but also in malnutrition, hypothyroidism, liver disease,

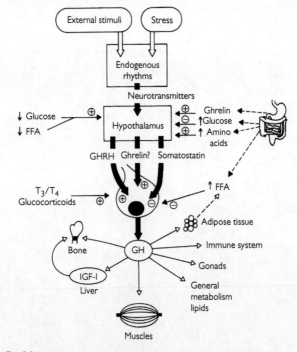

**Fig. 3.3** General scheme showing regulation of growth hormone secretion. FFA, free fatty acids.

Reproduced from Wass JAH, Shalet SM (eds) (2002). *Oxford Textbook of Endocrinology and Diabetes*, Oxford University Press, Oxford. Copyright © 2002 OUP.

and diabetes mellitus. Levels are affected by age and stage of puberty. There is a high specificity but poor sensitivity for GHD especially in younger children, i.e. a low IGF-1 level is predictive of GHD, while a normal level doesn't exclude it.

### Insulin-like growth factor-binding proteins

IGF-1 is carried in the circulation by at least six binding proteins, of which one (IGFBP3) is GH dependent. Although IGFBP3 levels are less dependent on nutrition than IGF-1, in practice its measurement offers little benefit over IGF-1. Levels are age dependent.

NB: both IGF-1 and IGFBP3 have relatively stable levels throughout the day, enabling random measurements to be used.

### Previously used tests

Exercise testing, urinary GH, and sleep studies are no longer routinely utilized.

Spontaneous GH secretion using profiling for 9–24 hours is still used routinely in some countries to diagnose GHD, but generally is only used in research settings or to diagnose neurosecretory dysfunction.

## GH stimulation testing

(⊙ See also 'Stimulation tests for growth hormone secretion', p. 388.)

A number of drugs which stimulate GH secretion, through either inhibition of somatostatin or stimulation of GHRH, are used. These tests may be performed on their own or in addition to other assessment of pituitary hormones (e.g. LHRH (GnRH) and thyrotropin-releasing hormone (TRH) testing).

It is important that patients should be carefully selected prior to doing these tests, and that those with a high likelihood of GHD clinically are identified and other causes of poor growth have been excluded. Tests should be performed in units with experience in performing them and expertise in interpreting the results.

The 'gold standard' is the insulin tolerance test (ITT) as:
- the hypothalamic–pituitary–adrenal (HPA) axis can be assessed at the same time, and the ITT has been validated against surgical stress, at least in adults
- insulin hypoglycaemia is a powerful stimulus to GH release, and consequently the range between normal and severe GHD is large
- even moderate hypoglycaemia is sufficient to elicit maximal GH responses.

However, this test conveys potentially significant morbidity and mortality, and therefore should only be performed in suitable (tertiary) units with very careful supervision and emergency back-up facilities. Previous convulsions are an absolute contraindication.

Other commonly used tests are:
- glucagon stimulation test: this is commonly used in younger children (i.e. <15 kg) and those in whom the ITT is contraindicated
- arginine stimulation
- clonidine
- (L-dopa)
- (GHRH).

Some of these tests have been used in combination and also consecutively. All tests have limited (<80%) sensitivity and specificity, with repeat testing showing concordance only 50–70% of the time.

Both spontaneous and stimulated GH secretion is a continuum between normality and abnormality, with (relatively) arbitrary cut-offs. Historically, peak GH levels <7 mU/L (<2.3 mcg/L) have been considered to represent severe GHD, and 7–15 mU/L (2.3–5 mcg/L) 'partial' GHD, although cut-offs are assay and laboratory specific.

As all children have a physiological reduction in GH secretion peripubertally, some, but not all, paediatric endocrinologists prime with sex steroids in prepubertal children above a certain chronological or bone age.

Some short slow-growing children also have an abnormal pattern of pulsatile GH release, but normal GH responses to stimulation tests. This is known as 'neurosecretory dysfunction'.

It is currently recommended by the National Institute for Health and Care Excellence (NICE) that diagnosis of GHD is confirmed by a peak plasma GH level <6.7 mcg/L (20 mU/L) (dependent on GH assay) to two provocative tests. Only one provocative test may be required for organic GH deficiency.

## Radiology

- Bone age is characteristically delayed, with the amount of delay related to both the duration and severity of GHD.
- MRI of the pituitary–hypothalamic region may show:
  - thinning or absence of pituitary stalk
  - aplastic or hypoplastic anterior pituitary
  - ectopically sited or absent posterior pituitary.

Broadly, the more severe the radiological abnormalities, the more likely it is that additional pituitary hormone deficiencies, other than GHD, are present.

Underlying pathology may also be noted (e.g. with associated tumour):
- a mass lesion (e.g. craniopharyngioma)
- thickening of the pituitary stalk (e.g. infiltration by LCH)
- bulky pituitary (e.g. pituitary germinoma, adenoma)
- or associated anomalies (e.g. SOD)
- abnormal midline structures (corpus callosum, septum pellucidum)
- hypoplastic optic nerves.

# Treatment of GHD

(➲ See also Chapter 1)

Historically, GHD patients have an untreated final height of 134–146 cm in males and 128–134 cm in females. With GH treatment, final height is improved by 8.7–10.7 cm in boys and 7.7–9.5 cm in girls.

## Recommended doses of GH

The recommended dose range for GHD is 23–39 mcg/kg/day (0.7–1.0 mg/m$^2$/day). Increasingly, IGF-1 titration is being used, with little supportive evidence, but may provide a guide to GH sensitivity and adherence issues.

NICE recommends that GH therapy should be re-evaluated, and potentially stopped if there is a poor response to treatment, judged as an increase in HV of <50% above baseline therapy. GH therapy should normally be stopped when adult height is achieved, i.e. HV <2 cm/year and fusion of the epiphyses.

International consensus guidelines for GH-treated patients have recently been produced.[1] These recommend that all patients should have their pituitary function re-evaluated at the completion of growth, with the only exceptions being those with severe congenital or acquired panhypopituitarism (i.e. four or five hormone deficiencies).

Re-evaluation after discontinuation of GH should be performed after at least 1 month, and GH reserve should be assessed by serum IGF-1 measurement and/or a GH stimulation test. The tests currently recommended for reassessment are the ITT, with the arginine or glucagon tests as alternatives; clonidine has been shown to be no better than placebo for GH stimulation during adulthood.

It has been proposed that the extent of GH–IGF-1 re-evaluation should depend on the likelihood of profound GHD on retesting, with two groups of patients.

- High likelihood:
  - severe GHD in childhood with/without two or three additional hormone deficits
  - due to a defined genetic cause
  - severe GHD due to structural HP abnormalities, CNS tumours, or patients having received high-dose cranial irradiation
- Low likelihood:
  - the remaining patients, including those with idiopathic GHD, either isolated or with one additional hormone deficit.

All patients previously treated with GH should be followed up long term, although in practice this often does not occur.

## Reference

1. Allen DB, Backeljauw P, Bidlingmaier M, et al. GH safety workshop position paper: a critical appraisal of recombinant human GH therapy in children and adults. *Eur J Endocrinol* 2016;174:P1–P9.

# Adult GHD

It is recognized that a proportion of patients who present with paediatric GHD will have persistence of this into adult life. This occurs more commonly in those patients with:

- MPHD
- genetic defects of GH production.

On retesting in adulthood, ~50–75% of patients previously diagnosed with isolated GHD in childhood are no longer GH deficient, using either the paediatric (<15–20 mU/L (<5–6.7 mcg/L) or adult cut-offs (<9 mU/L (<3 mcg/L)).

It is now well recognized that GH has other direct metabolic effects in addition to its effects upon growth, with the growth-promoting effects being mediated via IGF-1.

Patients with adult GHD show the following:

- Decreased:
  - lean body mass, in association with decreased exercise capacity
  - sweating
  - bone mineral density and increased fracture risk
  - psychological well-being
  - quality of life (QoL)
- Increased:
  - fat mass (especially central adiposity)
  - insulin resistance and glucose intolerance
  - cardiovascular mortality
- Adverse lipid profile
- Altered cardiac structure and function.

There is no specific symptom that is pathognomonic of adult GHD, especially in those with multiple pituitary deficiencies, and the profile in adults differs somewhat in those with childhood onset and adult onset.

NICE has stated that GH therapy should only be used in adults with severe GH deficiency which is severely affecting their QoL, namely[1]:

- 'have a peak growth hormone response of less than 3 mcg/L (9 mU/L) in the "insulin tolerance test" for growth hormone deficiency or a similar low result in another reliable test, and
- have an impaired quality of life because of their GH deficiency (judged using a specific questionnaire called the "Quality of Life Assessment of GH Deficiency in Adults" designed to assess the quality of life in people with growth hormone deficiency; a person should score at least 11 in this questionnaire), and
- already be receiving replacement hormone treatment for any other deficiencies of pituitary hormones if he or she has one or more other deficiencies.'

It is argued by some that a peak GH of <3 mcg/L (<9 mU/L) is too strict in the transition period, when GH levels are characteristically high, and that a level of <5 mcg/L (<15 mU/L) would be more appropriate. The current recommended cut-offs for adult GHD are:

- <3 mcg/L (NICE and USA)
- <5 mcg/L (European Society for Paediatric Endocrinology)
- <6 mcg/L (GH Research Society)

QoL should be checked after 9 months of therapy, which should be stopped if there has been insufficient improvement. GH should then be continued until at least 25 years of age, when peak bone mass is achieved.

## Treatment

Patients who satisfy the NICE guidelines for adult GH replacement[1] should be considered for therapy. As GH production rates are much lower in adults, the replacement doses required are much lower than seen in paediatric patients—characteristically a starting dose of 0.1–0.4 mg daily and maintenance doses of 0.2–0.6 mg daily. Women often require higher doses than men.

A low starting dose reduces the likelihood of side effects which, in addition to those seen in children, include:
- salt and water retention, producing oedema and carpal tunnel syndrome
- arthralgia
- myalgia.

Unlike paediatric practice, where dose is calculated on weight or body surface area, doses are usually titrated against serum IGF-1 levels, maintaining them within the top half of the normal range (IGF-1 SDS 0 to +2).

Yearly assessment of the following should be performed:
- height
- weight
- BMI
- waist and hip circumference
- blood pressure
- heart rate
- QoL.

The following should be assessed at baseline and every 2–5 years:
- bone densitometry
- lipids.

In view of the known effects of GH on carbohydrate metabolism, the following should be measured periodically:
- fasting plasma glucose
- insulin
- glycated haemoglobin (HbA1c).

Glucose tolerance testing (GTT) may be considered in obese patients and those with a family history of diabetes mellitus.

## Reference

1. National Institute for Health and Care Excellence (NICE). Human growth hormone (somatropin) in adults with growth hormone deficiency. TA64. NICE, 2003. ℛ https://www.nice.org.uk/guidance/ta64

# Adrenocorticotropic hormone deficiency

(➲ See also p. 35.)

ACTH deficiency usually occurs in association with other pituitary hormone deficiencies, and may occur in congenital forms of hypopituitarism (e.g. *HESX1* or *LHX4* mutations) or evolve with time (e.g. *PROP1* mutations).

Approximately 25% of patients with craniopharyngioma show ACTH deficiency at presentation, and this may be even higher in other tumours, such as germinoma and astrocytoma, and also following cranial tumour surgery and radiotherapy.

## Isolated ACTH deficiency

This congenital form is seen in mutations of *TPIT*, a T-box transcription factor. A hypoplastic pituitary gland may be found.

Mutations in *POMC* (pro-opiomelanocortin) are associated with rapid weight gain, hyperphagia, and red hair. In addition, adrenal insufficiency may be found along with central hypothyroidism, and gonadotropin and GH deficiency may also develop in adolescence.

Infants with extremely low birthweight may also demonstrate ACTH deficiency 2° to a sluggish HPA axis. In addition, there are extra-hypothalamic causes of acquired isolated ACTH deficiency:

- exogenous steroid administration
- steroid production from tumours
- sodium valproate administration.

as these suppress central corticotropin-releasing hormone (CRH) and ACTH secretion. As a result, recovery of the HPA axis from long-term steroid therapy may be prolonged.

## Features

ACTH deficiency results in deficient production of cortisol and androgens within the zona fasciculata and reticularis of the adrenal cortex. Unlike in 1° adrenal insufficiency:

- mineralocorticoid deficiency does not occur, as the renin–angiotensin–aldosterone axis (involving the zona glomerulosa) remains intact.
  Consequently, adrenal crisis with sodium loss leading to dehydration, hypotension, hyponatraemia, and hyperkalaemia is rarely seen.
  However, hyponatraemia alone may occur (see below)
- hyperpigmentation is not present because ACTH secretion is not increased
- hypoglycaemia, often severe, leading to convulsions and coma, may be the presenting symptom (➲ see 'Hypoglycaemia', Chapter 7).

In patients with ACTH deficiency there may be symptoms or signs of other pituitary hormone deficiencies, or clinical manifestations of a pituitary/hypothalamic lesion (e.g. signs of raised intracranial pressure, visual field defects).

Clinical features are often more non-specific in 2° adrenal insufficiency, but it must be remembered that patients may show hyponatraemia, which is dilutional, and may still develop hypotension and shock due to glucocorticoid deficiency, which can lead to death if untreated, especially during times of stress.

## Symptoms and signs
- Dry skin, decreased pubic/axillary hair, myalgia, arthralgia
- Hypotension and shock
- Anorexia, nausea, vomiting, abdominal pain, weight loss
- Headache, decreased consciousness
- Fatigue.

## Biochemical findings
- Hypoglycaemia
- Hyponatraemia (dilutional), but normal potassium levels
- Hypercalcaemia
- Low ACTH levels
- Low cortisol levels (basal and stimulated).

Special note: it is recognized that dynamic testing with pharmacological doses of Synacthen and also insulin hypoglycaemia may show normal responses. Physiological profiling of ACTH and cortisol are more rarely performed.

## Therapy
Physiological glucocorticoid replacement as with 1° adrenal insufficiency, i.e. hydrocortisone ~8–12mg/m$^2$/day given three times daily (early morning, lunch, evening), often with a larger dose in the morning to mimic physiological levels. This can be monitored and adjusted by means of a modified day curve of serum or salivary cortisol.

Patients need to take the same precautions as those with 1° adrenal insufficiency:
- increased doses during infection and stress; systemic steroids if unwell and vomiting
- steroid cards and either a steroid medallion or a bracelet (e.g. SOS Talisman).

Mineralocorticoid replacement is not required.

Although patients may show evidence of androgen deficiency at puberty (e.g. reduced pubic and axillary hair), androgen replacement is not routinely given to children and adolescents with ACTH deficiency.

# Gonadotropin deficiency

(⊃ See also Chapter 2, pp. 76–8.)

Physiology

- The gonadotropins (LH and FSH) are produced under the influence of GnRH, which is secreted from the arcuate nucleus and pre-optic area of the hypothalamus.
- The gonads (ovary and testis) are the site of action of the gonadotropins.
- LH stimulates the Leydig cells of the testis and the theca cells of the ovary to produce hormones (testosterone and oestradiol).
- FSH stimulates maturation of germ cells in both sexes. In males, it facilitates sperm production from the testis, and in females, growth of Graafian follicles in the granulosa cells of the ovaries.
- In turn, in the male, gonadal androgens produced from the Leydig cells under the influence of LH are involved in the last phase of testicular descent from the inguinal canal into the scrotum. In addition, testosterone is converted into its more active metabolite dihydro-testosterone (DHT) by the enzyme 5α-reductase, and this is responsible for development of the external genitalia, seminal vesicles, and prostate gland in the male.

Deficiency

This frequently occurs in association with other pituitary hormone deficiencies, as gonadotropin secretion is often lost early in destructive lesions and following radiotherapy, although precocious puberty may also initially be seen in the latter.

As a result, patients with mass lesions of the pituitary or hypothalamus may present with gonadotropin deficiency but preservation of ACTH and TSH. Gonadotropin deficiency may also occur as part of MPHD due to transcription factor defects (most commonly *PROP1* mutations).

Causes of gonadotropin deficiency may be further subdivided into impaired and intact HP axis.

## Impaired HP axis

### Idiopathic hypogonadotropic hypogonadism (IHH)

IHH has an incidence of ~1 in 10,000 in males and 1 in 50,000 in females. Most cases (~80%) are sporadic, indicating either that they are not due to a genetic disorder or that spontaneous mutations are common.

Fertile eunuch syndrome is a form of incomplete GnRH deficiency in which normal testicular growth and spermatogenesis may occur during puberty, although it is insufficient to produce full virilization. Homozygous mutations in the GnRH receptor gene (*GnRHR*) have been described.

### Congenital adrenal hypoplasia

(⊃ See also Chapter 8, p. 279.)

This is an X-linked condition in which HH occurs in association with adrenal insufficiency. The phenotype is heterogeneous, with some patients having IHH but normal adrenal function, while others show the syndrome of adrenal insufficiency in childhood and have subsequent hypogonadism at puberty. This condition is due to mutations in the *DAX-1* gene.

*Kallmann syndrome (KS)*

The association of HH with anosmia (absent sense of smell) was first described by Kallmann in 1944. In this condition, GnRH neurons fail to migrate *in utero* from the olfactory placode. Other associated features are cleft lip and palate, sensorineural deafness, cerebellar ataxia, and in X-linked forms renal agenesis, undescended testes, and synkinesia (mirror movements).

  Genetics:
- May have autosomal dominant (AD), autosomal recessive (AR), and X-linked recessive inheritance.
- The *KAL1* gene is implicated in the X-linked recessive form of KS, which may also occur as part of a contiguous gene syndrome including ichthyosis, intellectual disability, glycerol kinase deficiency, chondrodysplasia punctata (skeletal dysplasia), and short stature.
- Autosomal genes include *FGFR1* (*KAL2*: AD inheritance), which causes up to 10% of cases of KS, with *PROKR2* (AR), *PROK2* (AR), and *FGF8* (AD) also implicated.

Radiology:
- MRI scanning usually reveals normal pituitary and hypothalamic morphology, but absent olfactory bulbs.

*CHARGE syndrome*
- First described in 1979, this condition occurs in ~1 in 25,000.
- Over 90% with characteristic features have mutations in the chromodomain gene *CHD7*.
- This name is an acronym describing clinical features: Coloboma (eye defect), Heart problems, Atresia choanae (blockage/narrowing of nasal passages), Retarded growth and development, Genital abnormalities, Ear abnormalities.
- Initially four of six features of the acronym were required to make the diagnosis; now there are new diagnostic criteria, major and minor.
- Major criteria (with frequencies) are:
  - coloboma (80–90%)
  - choanal atresia (50–60%)
  - cranial nerve dysfunction: I (frequent), VII (40%), VIII (70–85%), IX/X (70–90%)
  - characteristic CHARGE ear (90%):
    —external: cupped, snipped off helix, triangular helix
    —middle: abnormal stapes, cochlear abnormalities.
- Minor clinical features include characteristic face and hand, congenital heart disease, facial clefting, hypotonia, tracheo-oesophageal fistula, genital anomalies, and short stature.
- Micropenis and/or cryptorchidism occur in 70–85% of males; labial hypoplasia in girls is also very common.
- Short stature is common, with ~50% of adults having heights <2nd centile. Growth failure is probably multifactorial, due to:
  - infantile: SGA and poor feeding/gastro-oesophageal reflux, frequent hospitalizations

- childhood: increased incidence of hypopituitarism (including GHD)
- puberty: absent/delayed/arrested puberty (in nearly all boys and ~2/3 of girls).
- HH is common, especially in males, who often present with absent pubertal development; while females may have delayed or arrested puberty. HH is often associated with anosmia, as with KS.

*Other conditions*

Isolated congenital HH with *normal* sense of smell (normosmia) may result from mutations in GNRH1, TAC3, TACR3, and KISS1R.

Mutations in the GnRH receptor (GNRHR) and in both LH-β and FSH-β subunits have also been reported in HH, and are also described in PWS and Bardet–Biedl syndrome.

*Intact HP axis*

Functional HH with an intact HP axis may occur in the following:
- constitutional delay of growth and puberty (CDGP)
- exercise
- weight loss/anorexia
- stress (both physical and psychological)
- psychosocial deprivation
- systemic disorders
- critical illness.

## Presentation

The clinical presentation of HH is heterogeneous, and depends on:
- age of onset (e.g. congenital vs acquired)
- duration (e.g. functional vs permanent)
- severity (e.g. partial vs complete).

*Neonatal period*

- Males: micropenis (stretched penile length <2.5 cm) and cryptorchidism (described in up to 50% of males with KS and IHH)
- Females: hypoplastic labia.

*Puberty*

- Delayed/arrested puberty in both sexes.
- Typically males with gonadotropin deficiency do not spontaneously achieve testicular volumes >4 mL.
- Gynaecomastia characteristically does not occur in the untreated patient.

As most growth during puberty is in the spine, adult patients with untreated hypogonadism have eunuchoid proportions (upper-to-lower body ratio <1 with an arm span 6 cm greater than standing height). In addition, delayed fusion of the epiphyses will occur, with long-term osteoporosis.

## Investigation

(⮕ See also Chapter 14.)

The postnatal surge of gonadotropins is a 'mini-puberty' which provides a window of opportunity to investigate this group of patients in the first 6 months of life, with the ideal time at 6–8 weeks. Bloods for baseline gonadotropins, plus testosterone (and inhibin B) in boys, can be taken.

There is considerable overlap of hormone levels between prepubertal and hypogonadotropic children, which means that there are no baseline levels or stimulation tests which will distinguish between the two. In these patients it may be necessary to treat through puberty, and then stop therapy and reassess at the end.

### Suggested tests

- Baseline testosterone (male) and oestradiol (female)
- Inhibin B
- LHRH (GnRH) test
- hCG stimulation test: short (several days) and long (several weeks), ↪ see Chapter 14.

Although spontaneous pulsatile secretion of gonadotropins is reduced in HH, long-term profiling is rarely performed outside research studies.

### Radiology

- US scanning:
  - pelvic/ovarian in females (visualizing ovaries and uterus)
  - inguinal/intra-abdominal in males (looking for testes)
- MRI scanning: looking for testes in males (this is probably better than US scanning)
- Bone age: characteristically delayed by several years in older patients
- Bone density (e.g. dual-energy X-ray absorptiometry (DXA)): reduced in older patients.

### Therapy

#### Micropenis

Although hCG can be used, both diagnostically and therapeutically, this involves regular (i.e. twice- or thrice-weekly) injections. In practice, either topical testosterone gel or monthly testosterone injection (e.g. 12.5–25 mg IM for 3 months) is commonly used.

hCG therapy may also be used to assist with descent of testes prior to surgery. Again, prolonged courses are often given (e.g. 500–2000 IU twice weekly for 3 weeks).

No treatment is usually given for hypoplastic labia in girls.

#### Pubertal induction

(↪ See also Chapter 2.)

- Treatment with hypothalamic GnRH or pituitary hormones (e.g. recombinant human FSH with the addition of hCG; LH equivalent) is the most physiological.
- The earlier induction of the reproductive process starts Sertoli cell maturation and differentiation of the germ cells into mature spermatozoa which can be preserved for future use as a back-up. Earlier initiation of this process, despite a hiatus on return to simple testosterone replacement in late adolescence/early adulthood, permits an easier and more rapid re-awakening of spermatogenesis when conception is to be attempted.

- However, these require parenteral therapy involving pump therapy (GnRH) or regular (e.g. twice-weekly) injection (gonadotropins). In patients with HH there is no evidence of the benefit of pulsatile GnRH over gonadotropin therapy, and both will induce testicular growth and fertility in a third to half of patients.
- In practice, for ease in males, when pubertal induction is required, the same regimens as in 1° hypogonadism are used (i.e. increasing doses of testosterone given by monthly IM injection (depot) or transdermally/ orally), initially, and testicular development can be initiated from mid-puberty onwards (➡ see Chapter 2, p. 76).
- In females, oestrogen therapy is commonly given first, and recombinant gonadotropin therapy or pulsatile GnRH is reserved for the time of fertility induction as oocytes are already at a later stage of maturation than spermatic germ cells.

# Thyroid-stimulating hormone deficiency (central hypothyroidism)

- TSH deficiency most commonly occurs in association with other pituitary hormone deficiencies (especially GH and gonadotropins), and acquired causes include:
  - tumours (especially craniopharyngioma)
  - granulomatous disease
  - infection (including meningitis)
  - surgery
  - cranial irradiation
  - trauma.
- Congenital TSH deficiency has an incidence of 1 in 16,000 births, and also occurs in combination with other pituitary hormone deficiencies, usually due to developmental abnormalities of the pituitary gland or hypothalamus.
- These abnormalities may be due to mutations in one of a number of transcription factors (e.g. *POU1F1, PROP1, HESX1, LHX3, LHX4, SOX3m, OTX2*), although idiopathic cases also occur.
- Isolated TSH deficiency is rare, with an incidence quoted at ~1 in 65,000.
- Genetic causes of isolated TSH deficiency are due to mutations in the:
  1. TSH beta subunit (*TSHB*) gene
  2. TRH receptor (*TRHR*) gene
  3. immunoglobulin superfamily member 1 (*IGSF1*) gene.
- Isolated TSH deficiency has been described in patients with empty sella syndrome, pituitary tumour, and diabetes, although in most cases no cause has been found.

## Diagnosis

- TSH deficiency will not be picked up on routine neonatal thyroid screening as (in most countries including the UK) this is dependent on a significantly raised TSH level.
- Demonstrating an inappropriately low serum TSH concentration in the presence of subnormal serum levels of free $T_4$ and free $T_3$ concentrations is characteristic of central hypothyroidism. However, TSH may be raised in some patients, although usually only mildly so, and inappropriate for the thyroid hormone concentrations.
- The TRH test is of little benefit in making the diagnosis, or for distinguishing between hypothalamic TRH deficiency and pituitary TSH deficiency, although some have argued that both the TRH test and nocturnal surge of TSH should be used in oncology survivors to identify subclinical cases.
- In contrast with congenital 1° hypothyroidism, the thyroid hormone levels are often just below the lower end of the normal range (characteristically, free $T_4$ levels are 8–10 pmol/L).
- Consequently, the clinical features seen in 1° hypothyroidism are usually less severe. Goitre is never present. The outcome in terms of intellectual development is usually good.

### TSHB mutations

- Inherited in an AR fashion.
- Associated with severe central hypothyroidism; as patients present late, neurodevelopmental issues are common and correlates with the length of delay in diagnosis.
- Additional biochemical features include:
  - elevated pituitary glycoprotein $\alpha$ subunit,
  - impaired TSH response to TRH, but normal rise in serum prolactin.

### TRHR mutations

- The least common form of isolated central hypothyroidism.
- Has only been described in four cases from three families.
- Likely AR inheritance.
- Low $T_4$ levels (~75% of normal) are associated with detectable TSH, normal prolactin. and normal pituitary MRI.

### IGSF1 mutations

- Also known as central hypothyroidism/testicular enlargement syndrome (CHTE).
- Estimated to affect 1 in 100,000 people. X-linked inheritance with incomplete penetrance. More common in males than females.
- Hypothyroidism is variable, but most males require treatment with thyroxine.
- Hypoprolactinaemia occurs in up to 75%.
- Also have delayed puberty and macro-orchidism from ~11 years of age.
- No evidence long term of fertility problems.

### Therapy

- As with 1° hypothyroidism, treatment is with L-thyroxine.
- Unlike 1° hypothyroidism, monitoring of TSH levels in TSH deficiency are of no use in assessing the response to thyroxine replacement.

▶ NB: *if there is a likelihood of ACTH deficiency, this should also be investigated.* If confirmed, hydrocortisone therapy should be started first as otherwise the increased metabolic rate produced by L-thyroxine may precipitate an adrenal crisis.

## Prolactin deficiency

The lactotroph axis is shown in Fig. 3.4.

- Elevations in prolactin are commonly seen in hypothalamic damage, and are thought to be due to damage to inhibitory dopaminergic neurons.
- Prolactin deficiency itself nearly always occurs in association with other anterior pituitary hormone deficiencies (either congenital or acquired).
- The clinical manifestation of prolactin deficiency is probably limited to lack of post-puerperal lactation, although menstrual disorders, delayed puberty, infertility, and problems with subfertility are also associated with hypoprolactinaemia through poorly understood mechanisms.

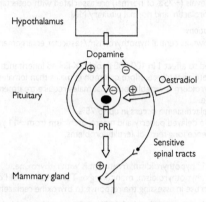

**Fig. 3.4** General scheme showing regulation of the lactotroph axis.

Reproduced from Wass JAH, Shalet SM (eds) (2002). *Oxford Textbook of Endocrinology and Diabetes*, Oxford University Press, Oxford. Copyright © 2002 OUP.

# Prolactin excess (prolactinomas)

Prolactinomas are rare tumours in childhood and adolescence (0.1 per 1,000,000) and rare before age 10 years.

Most likely pituitary tumour. Usually sporadic. May be part of MEN1 sequence (< 25%) or mutations in the aryl hydrocarbon receptor-interacting protein (AIP).

## Diagnosis

Prolactin significantly raised. Macroprolactin (inactive polymer of prolactin bound to IGG, needs to be excluded by laboratory).

### Definition of prolactinoma
- <1 cm: microprolactinoma (more common in girls)
- >1 cm: macroprolactinoma (more common in boys).

### Presenting symptoms
- Headache
- Fatigue
- Hypogonadism
- Pubertal delay ± short stature
- Pubertal arrest
- Gynaecomastia
- Galactorrhoea.

### With macroprolactinoma: pressure effects
- Visual loss
- Raised intracranial pressure
- Other anterior pituitary hormone deficiencies.

## Treatment
- Cabergoline (dopamine agonist):
  - starting dose 0.5 mg orally twice weekly
  - titrate against prolactin levels
- Microproactinoma: review after 2 years of normal prolactin
- Macroprolactinoma: maintenance prolactin in normal range long term
- Surgery: only required for urgent decompression, e.g. acute visual loss or failure to respond to cabergoline (unusual).

# Posterior pituitary

(→ See also Chapter 14, p. 396.)

Vasopressin physiology

- AVP, also known as antidiuretic hormone (ADH), is a nonapeptide produced within the supra-optic and paraventricular nuclei of the hypothalamus.
- It is then transported in neurosecretory granules down axons of the hypothalamic neuron to the posterior pituitary lobe for storage.
- Release of AVP occurs in response to changes in osmolality, detected in osmoreceptors within the hypothalamus. The hypothalamus also regulates thirst by sensing increases in serum osmolarity within the ventromedial nucleus.
- In addition to changes in osmolality, AVP is also secreted in response to reductions of ~5–10% in intravascular volume. Nausea, vomiting, stress, and exercise also release vasopressin, which may be of importance in postoperative fluid balance. Other non-osmotic releasers of AVP are acute hypoxia and hypercapnia, hypoglycaemia, and various drugs (this may be mediated via emetic and haemodynamic routes).
- AVP is also inhibited in response to alcohol and caffeine.
- AVP acts on the renal collecting ducts, specifically the aquaporin channels, to produce absorption of water. It is the major determinant of water excretion via the kidney, and hence fluid balance. It also has some effect as a pressor and as an ACTH secretagogue.

Secretion of vasopressin in response to osmolality is shown in Fig. 3.5.

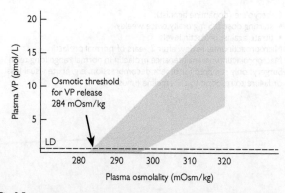

**Fig. 3.5** Relationship between plasma osmolality and plasma vasopressin (VP) concentration during progressive hypertonicity induced by infusion of 855 mmol/L saline in a group of healthy adults.

Reproduced from Wass JAH, Shalet SM (eds) (2002). *Oxford Textbook of Endocrinology and Diabetes*, Oxford University Press, Oxford. Copyright © 2002 OUP.

### Deficiency

Abnormal vasopressin secretion or action results in diabetes insipidus (DI), a condition characterized by the passage of large volumes of dilute urine. DI is often subdivided as follows:

- Cranial diabetes insipidus (CDI). This arises due to deficiency of AVP.
- Nephrogenic diabetes insipidus (NDI), in which AVP is produced but the kidney is unable to respond to it.
- 1° polydipsia, occurring 2° to consumption of large volumes of liquid. This can arise from a deficiency of AVP production 2° to excess water intake. Only one form (dipsogenic DI) is due to a 1° defect in the thirst mechanism.

Causes of DI/polyuric syndromes are shown in Table 3.5.

### Arginine vasopressin deficiency (cranial diabetes insipidus)

Various definitions of polyuria exist, including >4 mL/kg/hour, >120 mL/m²/hour, and 2 L/m²/day. The normal urine output often considerably exceeds normal urine output, which ranges with age from 2–3 mL/kg/hour in infants to 1–2 mL/kg/hour in children and adults.

Often several litres a day of urine are passed in older patients.

Other features include:

- dehydration
- failure to thrive
- weight loss
- constipation
- fever.

Following lesions to the HP area there may also be a triphasic response:

1. An initial diuretic phase lasting from hours to days.
2. A period of antidiuresis and hyponatraemia due to vasopressin release from injured axons (syndrome of inappropriate ADH secretion (SIADH)). In addition, hyponatraemia may be due to coexisting cerebral salt wasting.
3. Final CDI; dependent on extent of lesion, but may take several weeks to develop.

The aetiology of CDI is similar to other causes of hypopituitarism, with the following differences:

- LCH and pituitary germinoma may characteristically present with CDI.
- The posterior pituitary is particularly radioresistant, and therefore CDI usually does not occur after cranial irradiation.

Up to 50% of cases are considered to be idiopathic.

### Investigation

- On MRI scanning, the posterior pituitary usually has a hyperintense appearance on sagittal $T_1$-weighted scans.
- Although the frequency of hyperintensity decreases with age, ~80% of children with CDI show an absent posterior pituitary signal.
- A thickened infundibulum or pituitary stalk, or both, may indicate an infiltrative disease. If this is associated with a bulky pituitary (in association with precocious puberty) then this may indicate a germinoma.

**Table 3.5** Causes of diabetes insipidus

| Pituitary | | |
|---|---|---|
| Genetic | Autosomal dominant (occasionally recessive) neurophysin gene | |
| | Autosomal recessive: DIDMOAD (*WFS1* gene) | |
| | X-linked recessive | |
| Congenital | Septo-optic dysplasia | |
| | Holoprosencephaly | |
| | Other cranial midline defects | |
| Acquired | Tumour: craniopharingioma, germinoma | |
| | Infiltration: LCH, leukaemia, lymphoma, sarcoidosis | |
| | Infection: meningitis, encephalitis | |
| | Vascular: hypoxia, haemorrhage | |
| | Trauma | |
| | Drugs: narcotic agonists | |
| | Idiopathic | |
| **Nephrogenic** | | |
| Genetic | Autosomal recessive (occasionally dominant) aquaporin 2 gene | |
| | X-linked recessive (vasopressin receptor-2 gene) | |
| Acquired | Drugs: lithium, tetracyclines, rifampicin, cisplatin | |
| | Renal: urinary tract obstruction, chronic renal disease | |
| | Metabolic: hypokalaemia, hypercalcaemia | |
| | Vascular: sickle cell disease/trait | |
| **Primary polydipsia** | | |
| | Psychogenic | |
| | Iatrogenic | |
| **Dipsogenic (abnormal thirst)** | | |
| | Granuloma (sarcoid) | |
| | Infection: tuberculosis meningitis | |
| | Trauma | |
| | Multiple sclerosis | |
| | Drugs: lithium | |
| | Idiopathic | |

## Diagnosis

- Fluid intake and urine output should be ascertained to confirm that excessive volumes are being consumed/passed. If intake is normal, further investigation of DI is not required unless there is evidence that features may be masked by other disease (e.g. adrenal insufficiency or hypo/adipsia), in which case the underlying defect should be corrected first.
- In order to exclude DI from other forms of polyuria, baseline measurement of blood glucose, bicarbonate, and calcium should also be performed.
- Under normal circumstances, AVP is not stimulated at physiological osmolality (i.e. <284 mOsmol/kg), so random plasma and urine are often not useful.
- Early-morning split osmolalities (urine and plasma): if the plasma osmolality is raised (>295 mOsmol/kg) with a urine osmolality <300 mOsmol/kg, there is no need to continue investigation.

## Dynamic function

### Water deprivation test

(See also 'Water deprivation test', p. 396.)

If fluids are withheld for a number of hours, under normal circumstances plasma osmolality will rise, leading to production of AVP, with concentration of the urine. Strict fluid balance and regular measurement of plasma and urine osmolality are required throughout the test, which must only be performed in specialist centres.

- The test should be concluded if there is weight loss of >5%, thirst can no longer be tolerated, or at the end of a fixed period (usually 8–12 hours).
- If fluid restriction fails to result in concentration of urine to >300 mOsmol/kg before plasma osmolality reaches 300 mOsmol/kg, DI is likely, and 1° polydipsia and partial defects of AVP secretion and action are unlikely. Subsequent administration of DDAVP (1-deamino-8-D-arginine vasopressin) (e.g. 1–2 mcg SC) resulting in >50% increase in urine osmolality confirms CDI; <50% is indicative of NDI.

▶ Partial concentration of urine in response to fluid restriction is unable to distinguish between partial defects in AVP secretion and action and 1° polydipsia. Ideally, measurement of AVP during increased plasma osmolality is required, although its very short half-life means that increasingly copeptin, the C-terminal moiety of provasopressin, is measured as it is stable for several days.

### Hypertonic saline infusion

As high levels of hypertonic dehydration may be difficult to achieve with fluid restriction alone, an alternative test is hypertonic saline infusion. In this, hypertonic (3%) saline is infused for up to 60–90 minutes. This produces a controlled increase in plasma osmolality, allowing concomitant measurement of AVP/copeptin and assessment of defects of osmoreceptor function.

Plasma osmolality tends to rise higher with hypertonic saline infusion, with no rise in AVP/copeptin in patients with CDI. This may distinguish mild forms of CDI.

## Therapy

### CDI

Desmopressin (DDAVP) has a preferential effect on the $V_2$ receptors of the kidney, and therefore has a reduced pressor effect and longer duration of action than the natural hormone. Treatment of CDI is with DDAVP either intranasally via a rhinal tube, metered spray, or orally (Desmotabs® or Desmomelts®). The oral route is probably preferred as it tends to produce less hyponatraemia than the intranasal route. Characteristically, at least 10× the dose of DDAVP is required via the oral rather than the intranasal route. Given its short half-life DDAVP usually needs to be given twice or thrice daily. For those unable to tolerate oral or intranasal DDAVP, it can also be administered parenterally (IV or IM).

The assessment of the response to DDAVP treatment involves:
- clinical: resolution of symptoms, with normal fluid intake and urine output
- biochemical: U&E, urine and plasma osmolality.

▶ In patients with 'isolated DI', where no underlying cause has been found, periodic (i.e. initially yearly, and subsequently every few years) rechecking of baseline endocrinology and MRI scanning are warranted, as evolution of infiltrative lesions such as LCH can often take many years.

Patients with destructive lesions involving the hypothalamus may also have an abnormal sense of thirst (hypodipsia or adipsia). In these patients, a fixed fluid regimen may be required in addition to DDAVP therapy to avoid wide fluctuations in plasma sodium and osmolality, as this can produce the rare but potentially fatal complication of acute pontine myelinolysis.

### NDI

- Treat the underlying cause (e.g. metabolic or drug-related)
- Desmopressin, even in high dose, is rarely effective
- Reduce intravascular volume with thiazide diuretics
- Prostaglandin synthase inhibitors such as indometacin.

### Primary polydipsia

Treatment can be challenging. Only offering water if the child demands drinks, and also gradually reducing the volume of fluids offered, can be beneficial.

DDAVP has little or no effect on psychogenic polydipsia, and only partly inhibits thirst and polydipsia in dipsogenic DI. Administration often leads to water intoxication.

## Other posterior pituitary hormones

### Oxytocin

- In males, oxytocin has no known effect.
- In females, oxytocin produces contraction of both the uterus and smooth muscle during breastfeeding. The only symptom of oxytocin deficiency is usually failure of lactation postpartum, and there appears to be no effect on labour and delivery.

# Further reading

Alatzoglou KS, Webb EA, Le Tissier P, et al. Isolated growth hormone deficiency (GHD) in childhood and adolescence: recent advances. *Endocr Rev* 2014;35:376–432.

Breil T, Lorz C, Choukair D, et al. Clinical features and response to treatment of prolactinomas in children and adolescents: a retrospective single-centre analysis and review of the literature. *Horm Res Paediatr* 2018;89:157–165.

National Institute for Clinical Excellence (NICE). Human growth hormone (somatropin) in adults with growth hormone deficiency. TA64. NICE, 2003. ℜ https://www.nice.org.uk/guidance/ta64

National Institute for Health and Care Excellence (NICE). Human growth hormone (somatropin) for the treatment of growth failure in children. TA188. NICE, 2010. ℜ https://www.nice.org.uk/guidance/ta188

Romero CJ, Nesi-Franca S, Radovick S. The molecular basis of hypopituitarism trends. *Endocrinol Metab* 2009;20:506–516.

Schoenmakers N, Alatzoglou KS, Chatterjee VK, et al. Recent advances in central congenital hypothyroidism. *J Endocrinol* 2015;227:R51–R71.

# Chapter 4

# Endocrine effects of other diseases and treatments

# Statistics

There are now a substantial number of children with endocrine dysfunction arising from malignant disease and its treatment during childhood.

- 1 in 500–600 children develop cancer by 15 years: 120–140 cases/million children/year. In the UK this represents 1600 children/year.
- Survival rates for children's cancer have more than doubled over the last 50 years, and 82% of all children are now cured. This varies from cancer to cancer: the survival rate for acute lymphoblastic leukaemia is >80%, while that for non-Hodgkin's lymphoma is >90%.
- Second only to accidents as the leading cause of death in this age range.
- 1 in 715 young adults are childhood cancer survivors: currently >33,000 in the UK.

Improved survival is due to a variety of factors:

- radiotherapy
- chemotherapy
- multimodal therapy
- supportive care
- centralization of services in large specialist centres.

The improved survival does, however, carry both an increased risk of premature death and also physical and psychosocial problems compared to the general population.

## Radiotherapy

Radiotherapy can be used:

- on its own
- along with chemotherapy and/or surgery, often after non-curative surgery.

It is used to:

- shrink the 1° tumour
- reduce tumour regrowth
- treat hormone hypersecretion.

The potential for damage with radiotherapy is related to:

- the dose of radiotherapy used
- the protocol used (i.e. single dose or fractionated)
- the site of the 1° lesion.

Radiation-induced hormonal defects are both progressive and irreversible. Commonly used radiotherapy doses are:

- >30 Gy: cranial irradiation for brain and head and neck tumours
- 20–30 Gy: abdominal irradiation for intra-abdominal tumours
- 18–24 Gy: craniospinal irradiation (CSI) for CNS leukaemia prophylaxis and therapy (now less used in the former in favour of intrathecal drugs)
- 750–1600 cGy: total body irradiation (TBI).

NB: newer forms of irradiation such as proton beam therapy may reduce unnecessary irradiation to normal tissues by >50%. While this may reduce some of the sequelae of irradiation, the higher dose to the tumour itself may increase the risks and rapidity of development of endocrine dysfunction in tumours involving the pituitary and hypothalamus.

Chemotherapy
- Does not usually cause as extensive endocrine damage as radiotherapy.
- The main endocrine late effects observed following chemotherapy are gonadal dysfunction, osteopenia/osteoporosis, and dyslipidaemia, although direct effects on the growth plate have also been implicated in poor growth.
- Damage depends on both the type and dose of chemotherapy used, and may be reversible in some cases.
- Some evidence that cytotoxic drugs may potentiate irradiation effects to the pituitary and hypothalamus.
- In addition to conventional chemotherapy, increasingly the newer agents such as immune-modulating therapies and tyrosine kinase inhibitors are also being implicated in endocrine late effects.

# Late effects

A late effect is defined as any physical, psychological, or social consequence of either the disease itself or its treatment.

- Almost any organ system can be affected.
- Aetiology, onset, and severity are highly variable.
- Around 2/3 of paediatric cancer survivors will develop at least one late effect (medical issue or disability) by 30 years from diagnosis, and most of this is due to previous cancer therapy, and ~20% have three or more.

Endocrine dysfunction as a late effect occurs in between 20% and 50% of patients, depending on the treatment received. This is related to:
- the underlying malignancy
- surgery
- radiotherapy
- chemotherapy.

These factors are further modified by:
- the age at which treatment was initiated
- the length of time since treatment
- gender.

Those patients exposed to radiotherapy and alkylating chemotherapy are at highest risk.
- Multiple endocrine late effects occur in over 1/5 of patients in some studies.

Almost all the endocrine organs can be affected either directly or indirectly by cancer treatment. The endocrine effects of radiotherapy are shown in Table 4.1 and those of chemotherapy in Table 4.2.

**Table 4.1** Endocrine effects of radiotherapy

|  | Radiotherapy: irradiation | | | |
|---|---|---|---|---|
|  | Cranial | Craniospinal | Total body | Target organ |
| **Growth hormone** | | | | |
| GH deficiency | + | + | + | + |
| **Thyroid** | | | | |
| 1° hypothyroidism | | + | + | + |
| 2°/3° hypothyroidism | + | | | |
| Hyperthyroidism | + | + | | |
| Thyroid nodule or carcinoma | | + | + | + |
| **Adrenal** | | | | |
| 1° hypoadrenalism | | | | |
| 2°/3° hypoadrenalism | + | | | |
| **Gonads** | | | | |
| 1° hypogonadism | | + | + | + |
| 2°/3° hypogonadism | + | | | |
| Precocious puberty | + | + | | |
| Infertility | + | + | + | + |
| **Hyperprolactinaemia** | + | + | | |
| **Obesity/metabolic syndrome** | + | + | + | |

**Table 4.2** Endocrine effects of chemotherapy

|  | 1° hypogonadism | Infertility | Osteopenia | Dyslipidaemia |
|---|---|---|---|---|
| Alkylating agents | + | + | | |
| Heavy metals | + | + | | + |
| Antimetabolites | | | + | |
| Corticosteroids | | | + | |

# Specific endocrine problems

## Growth

Poor growth in childhood cancer survivors is multifactorial. Causes include the following:

- *Non-hormonal*:
  - poor nutrition
  - corticosteroids
  - chemotherapy and radiotherapy causing bone and soft tissue damage.
- *Hormonal*:
  - GHD
  - pubertal defects: delayed and premature
  - hypothyroidism.

Characteristically, patients may lose up to 1 SD in height prior to diagnosis of GHD and institution of GH therapy.

The loss of spinal height with radiotherapy depends on both the age at irradiation and the type of irradiation (Table 4.3).

Boys tend to have a greater reduction in height than girls.

## Hypopituitarism

### Irradiation to the hypothalamus

- Produces disruption of feedback mechanisms.
- Damage occurs as the hypothalamus is more radiosensitive than the pituitary gland.
- Total dose of irradiation determines both speed and incidence of hormone deficits.
- Generally the pattern of hormone loss is GH then LH/FSH then ACTH then TSH.
- Pre-existing hypopituitarism may also contribute.
▶ Posterior pituitary dysfunction is very rare.
▶ May have 2° temporary mild hyperprolactinaemia, which usually gradually returns to normal.

## Growth hormone deficiency

GHD is the most common central endocrine defect following cranial irradiation. It depends on both total dosage and fractionation:

- high dose (>30 Gy): usually by 2 years
- lower doses: incidence variable up to 50%. In patients treated with 18 Gy, ~1/3 are GHD 5 years post irradiation.

**Table 4.3** Loss of spinal height with radiotherapy

| Loss of height (cm) | | |
|---|---|---|
| Age at irradiation (years) | Abdominal irradiation | Craniospinal irradiation |
| 1 | 10 | 9 |
| 5 | 7 | 7 |

More subtle forms of GHD may also be found:
- normal stimulated GH levels on provocative testing, but abnormal physiological GH secretion—'growth hormone neurosecretory dysfunction (GHNSD)'. May present at puberty with increasing GH secretory needs. More likely to be seen after lower dose irradiation, e.g. cranial prophylaxis for leukaemia or TBI.
- screening IGF-1 levels may be normal, even in the face of impaired provocative testing.

### GH and malignancy
- *In vitro* and animal experiments:
  - increased risk of hyperplasia and malignancy
  - increased chromosome fragility.
- *In vivo*:
  - increased IGF-1 levels associated with malignancy: prostate, premenopausal breast, and colon cancer (and also, in some studies, with low IGFBP3)
  - acromegaly (GH excess due to pituitary-secreting tumour) is associated with increased colon cancer risk.

### GH therapy and malignancy
- Possible increase in some specific cancers in GH-treated patients in some studies. Numbers are too few to be predictive. Although GH increases IGF-1 levels, it also increases the levels of IGFBP3, which may be protective.
- No overall increase in 1° tumour recurrence in GH-treated patients, especially if low-normal replacement doses of GH are used.
- No requirement to delay GH therapy until the patient has been tumour free for a year.
- Survivors have an increased risk of developing a 2° malignancy (cumulative risk 4.3% within 25 years).
- Most common CNS second tumour is meningioma, but this is related to previous cranial radiotherapy and not GH treatment.

### Thyroid
#### Radiation-induced primary hypothyroidism
There is an increased risk of 1° hypothyroidism from CSI because of radiation scatter. This may also result from:
- TBI prior to bone marrow transplantation (BMT); occurs in 20–30%
- neck/mantle irradiation for Hodgkin's lymphoma (30–50%). NB: this may also produce hyperthyroidism (relative risk = 8).
This may coexist with central hypothyroidism due to 2° pituitary TSH deficiency and/or 3° hypothalamic TRH deficiency.

#### TSH deficiency
- Occurs less commonly than GHD and CPP following hypothalamic–pituitary irradiation.
- Reported in 6–36% following irradiation doses >30–40Gy.
- Not seen with lower-dose irradiation, e.g. cranial prophylaxis or TBI.
- Implementation of GH therapy may unmask central hypothyroidism.

- TSH can be high, low, or normal depending on the relative contribution of the above-listed factors.
- Some dispute as to whether the TRH test is beneficial in distinguishing between forms of central hypothyroidism with inappropriately low TSH levels in both, but which fail to increase after TRH administration (2° TSH deficiency) or show a normal or late/exaggerated response (3° TRH deficiency) (→ see also 'TRH test', p. 128).
- Free thyroxine ($T_4$) may also be in the normal range (but often in the lower third). There is some argument as to whether all patients with free $T_4$ levels in this range need L-thyroxine replacement.
- Evidence that patients with increased TSH levels post irradiation have increased risk of thyroid carcinoma in the long term. Treatment with suppressive doses of thyroxine is recommended in this group, and should reduce this risk.

*Thyroid malignancy*

- Thyroid neoplasia (both benign and malignant) may arise following either direct or scatted irradiation to the thyroid gland.
- Palpable nodules are found in 20–30% of patients who receive neck irradiation.
- Relative risk overall of thyroid malignancy is 15; more common in:
  - children treated <10 years of age and/or
  - irradiation doses of 20–29 Gy.
- Most thyroid cancers are differentiated (papillary and follicular).

## Adrenal

*Primary adrenal insufficiency*

- The adrenal gland itself is resistant to both radiotherapy and chemotherapy.

*ACTH deficiency*

- May occur transiently due to prolonged used of pharmacological doses of glucocorticoids.
- Long term is uncommon, arising as disruption of the hypothalamic–pituitary axis due to:
  - tumour
  - surgery
  - high-dose (>30 Gy) irradiation (in ~19%). Rarely seen with doses <24 Gy.
- Features of central hypoadrenalism are often relatively non-specific (e.g. tiredness, lethargy, feeling unwell).

*Testing*

(→ See p. 388.)

- The insulin tolerance test (ITT) is probably the 'gold standard' as it tests the full integrity of the hypothalamic–pituitary–adrenal axis (and has also been validated against surgical stress). It also appears to be more sensitive to irradiation effects than other tests such as arginine and GHRH.
- The Synacthen (ACTH) test assesses the readily releasable pool of cortisol within the adrenal.

- Discrepancies between ITT and Synacthen:
  - failed ITT, but passed Synacthen test
  - ? partial defect; give hydrocortisone only at times of stress.

## Puberty

Pubertal disorders may involve:
- CPP due to cranial irradiation
- hypogonadism:
  - 1° due to organ irradiation or chemotherapy
  - 2° to central gonadotropin deficiency due to cranial irradiation.

### Precocious puberty

Both low- and high-dose cranial irradiation are associated with CPP, probably because of disinhibition of cortical influences.
- More likely if radiotherapy at young age.
- Girls are affected more than boys with irradiation doses <30 Gy.
- At higher doses CPP occurs equally in both sexes, with a correlation between the age of irradiation and the age of pubertal onset.

Often coexists with GH deficiency, producing a relatively 'normal' growth rate (although inappropriate for stage of puberty) resulting in:
- premature epiphyseal fusion
- attenuated pubertal growth spurt leading to unanticipated adult short stature.

### Gonadotropin deficiency

- Caused by high-dose cranial irradiation (>30 Gy). This produces CPP followed by gonadotropin deficiency in 25–50%, resulting in failure of pubertal progression after cessation of GnRH therapy.

### Primary hypogonadism: male

*Sex hormone production*
- Leydig cell dysfunction and androgen deficiency are uncommon, and are due to damage from high-dose chemotherapy or radiotherapy (>20 Gy).

Radiotherapy damage is greatest at higher doses and at younger age at irradiation. Characterized by:
- raised levels of LH plus
- low levels of testosterone

but these may not become apparent until mid-adolescence, and there may be progressive decline.

*Spermatogenesis*

Sertoli and germ cells are more susceptible than Leydig cells to many chemotherapy agents and low-dose radiotherapy (>2 Gy). This is both dose and age related, as there is evidence that the pubertal and adult germinal epithelium is more susceptible to damage than the prepubertal testis. Despite this, young age at exposure is not protective. In post-pubertal males, testicular volume <10 mL is associated with impaired spermatogenesis, and testicular damage with raised FSH and reduced inhibin-B levels.

*Primary hypogonadism: female*

As there is both structural and functional interdependence of the sex hormone cells and oocytes within the ovarian follicle, damage to germ cells results in:

- endocrine dysfunction
- hypogonadism and subsequent infertility.

The prepubertal ovary is more resistant to chemotherapy-induced damage, with frequent post-treatment recovery of function.

Ovarian failure with both inability to produce sex steroids and anovulation is seen following:

- high-dose myeloablative chemotherapy (e.g. BMT)
- irradiation to the abdomen, pelvis, or spine.

In both irradiation- and chemotherapy-induced ovarian damage, the susceptibility of the ovary to damage, onset of amenorrhoea, and recovery potential are dependent on age and cumulative dosage.

*Fertility*

In survivors of childhood cancer:

- 40–60% of adult males have impaired fertility, with a high probability of oligo- or azoospermia. As a result, semen cryopreservation should be offered to at-risk teenage boys. Risk is dependent on the chemotherapeutic agent used, and the cumulative dose.
- ~6% of adult females develop persistent ovarian failure.

*Pregnancy*

- Early menopause reduces fertility.
- Pregnancy outcome is otherwise good.

However, abdominal irradiation (20–30 Gy) impairs uterine growth, reduces uterine blood flow, with failure of the endometrium to respond to oestrogen and progesterone and produces an increase in:

- abortion rate
- low birthweight babies
- premature delivery
- positional deformity
- perinatal mortality.

## Prolactin

### Hyperprolactinaemia

- Described in both sexes and at all ages, but is more commonly found in young women, usually following high-dose cranial irradiation.
- It is usually subclinical.

## Other endocrine late effects

### Metabolic syndrome and hypothalamic obesity

Obesity in children with brain tumours is multifactorial. It includes hypothalamic dysfunction with:

- insulin hypersecretion and resistance
- hypopituitarism
- hyperphagia with poor satiety
- reduced activity due to obesity and visual problems.

Obesity is found in up to 75% of children treated for craniopharyngioma, with predictive features being:
- postoperative hypothalamic damage on MRI scans
- higher BMI at presentation.

These patients often show features of the metabolic syndrome with:
- decreased insulin sensitivity
- abnormal lipid profiles.

The prevalence of metabolic syndrome is also
- ~10% in acute lymphoblastic leukaemia (ALL)
- ~20% in BMT survivors.

### Bone health

Patients undergoing cancer treatments and also long-term survivors are at risk of:
- low bone mass
- increased fractures
- avascular necrosis (usually affecting the knees and hips).

The aetiology is usually multifactorial due to a combination of:
- poor nutrition (including low vitamin D levels)
- reduced weight-bearing
- catabolism
- glucocorticoids (reduced bone formation and increased bone resorption)
- endocrine dysfunction (including iatrogenic hormone inhibition with GnRH)
- radiotherapy (probably via indirect effects including GH resistance at the epiphysis)
- chemotherapy (direct effects via reduction of stromal progenitor cells, decrease in osteogenesis, and promotion of osteoclast formation).

### Second malignancy

Development of subsequent malignant neoplasms:
- is 10× the background rate
- exceeds 20% at 30 years after the 1° malignancy.

# Management of late effects

Hold joint clinics with an endocrinologist and an oncologist (regular follow-up every 3–6 months). At each visit:

- measure height, sitting height, and weight (BMI)
- calculate height velocity
- pubertal staging is mandatory.

## Baseline testing (yearly)

- IGF-1, TFTs, cortisol (ideally 9 am), and prolactin (LH, FSH, testosterone, oestradiol)
- Bone age.

### Provocative anterior pituitary function tests

These tests are performed in children with:

- suboptimal growth for age and pubertal stage
- precocious puberty
- low random cortisol levels and/or symptoms of adrenal insufficiency.

Educational materials available to patients and families are summarized in Table 4.4.

**Table 4.4** Problems associated with cancer treatments

| Endocrine problem | Associated cancer treatment |
| --- | --- |
| Obesity and reduction of physical activity | All treatments |
| GH deficiency | Cranial irradiation; TBI |
| Hypopituitarism | Cranial irradiation; TBI |
| 2° adrenal insufficiency | High-dose cranial irradiation |
| Hyperprolactinaemia | Cranial irradiation and surgery |
| Hypothyroidism | Cranial and spinal irradiation; TBI |
| Male and female reproduction | Cranial irradiation; TBI; gonadal/pelvic/bladder irradiation; chemotherapy especially alkylating agents and heavy metals |
| Precocious puberty | Cranial irradiation |
| Bone health | TBI; bone marrow transplant; corticosteroids; antimetabolites |

# Further reading

Allen DB, Backeljauw P, Bidlingmaier M, et al. GH safety workshop position paper: a critical appraisal of recombinant human GH therapy in children and adults. *Eur J Endocrinol* 2016;174:P1–9.

Chow EJ, Stratton KL, Leisenring WM, et al. Pregnancy after chemotherapy in male and female survivors of childhood cancer treated between 1970 and 1999: a report from the Childhood Cancer Survivor Study cohort. *Lancet Oncol* 2016;17:567–576.

King AA, Seidel K, Di C, et al. Long-term neurologic health and psychosocial function of adult survivors of childhood medulloblastoma/PNET: a report from the Childhood Cancer Survivor Study. *Neuro Oncol* 2017;19:689–698.

Rose SR, Horne VE, Howell J, et al. Late endocrine effects of childhood cancer. *Nat Rev Endocrinol* 2016;12:319–336.

Scottish Intercollegiate Guidelines Network (SIGN). SIGN 132: Long term follow up of survivors of childhood cancer. 2013. ℰ http://www.sign.ac.uk/assets/sign132.pdf

Swerdlow AJ, Cooke R, Beckers D, et al. Cancer risks in patients treated with growth hormone in childhood: the SAGhE European cohort study. *J Clin Endocrinol Metab* 2017;102:1661–1672.

Wei C, Hunt L, Cox R, et al. Identifying cardiovascular risk in survivors of childhood leukaemia treated with haematopoietic stem cell transplantation and total body irradiation. *Horm Res Paediatr* 2017;87:116–122.

Wells EM, Ullrich NJ, Seidel K, et al. Longitudinal assessment of late-onset neurologic conditions in survivors of childhood central nervous system tumors: a Childhood Cancer Survivor Study report. *Neuro Oncol* 2018;20:132–142.

# Diabetes mellitus

# Introduction

## Definition

Diabetes mellitus is a group of metabolic disorders characterized by chronic hyperglycaemia. This hyperglycaemia arises from defects in:

- insulin secretion
- insulin action
- both of these.

## Aetiological classification of disorders of glycaemia

(As classified by WHO (2014).[1])

### Type 1

β-cell destruction, usually leading to absolute insulin deficiency:

- autoimmune
- idiopathic.

### Type 2

May range from predominantly insulin resistance with relative insulin deficiency to a predominantly secretory defect with/without insulin resistance.

### Other specific types

- Genetic defects of β-cell function: e.g. maturity-onset diabetes of the young (MODY)), neonatal diabetes, mitochondrial diabetes
- Genetic defects in insulin action: e.g. Donohue syndrome (leprechaunism) and Rabson–Mendenhall syndrome
- Diseases of the exocrine pancreas: e.g. pancreatitis, trauma, pancreatectomy, infection
- Endocrinopathies: e.g. Cushing syndrome, phaeochromocytoma, growth hormone excess
- Drug or chemical induced: e.g. glucocorticoids, thyroxine, thiazides, diazoxide
- Infections: e.g. congenital rubella, Coxsackie B, mumps, adenovirus, cytomegalovirus
- Uncommon forms of immune-mediated diabetes: e.g. anti-insulin receptor antibodies
- Other genetic syndromes sometimes associated with diabetes: e.g. Down, Klinefelter, Turner, Wolfram syndromes
- Gestational diabetes.

## Diagnosis

Diagnosis is based on both on symptoms and biochemical confirmation. The American Diabetes Association (ADA)[2] recommends the following criteria:

- symptoms of diabetes plus casual (i.e. any time of day without regard to time since last meal) blood glucose ≥11.1 mmol/L

or

- fasting (i.e. no caloric intake for at least 8 hours) plasma glucose ≥7.0 mmol/L

or

- 2-hour plasma glucose ≥11.1 mmol/L during an oral glucose tolerance test (OGTT).

The 2-hour plasma glucose test should be performed as described by WHO[1] using a glucose load containing the equivalent of 75 g anhydrous glucose dissolved in water.

Plasma glucose thresholds are defined as follows[1,2]:
- diabetes mellitus:
  - fasting plasma glucose ≥7.0 mmol/L
  - 2-hour plasma glucose ≥11.1 mmol/L.

Other abnormalities of glucose homeostasis:
- impaired glucose tolerance (IGT):
  - fasting plasma glucose <7.0 mmol/L
  - 2-hour plasma glucose ≥7.8 mmol/L and <11.1 mmol/L
- impaired fasting glycaemia (IFG):
  - fasting plasma glucose 6.1–6.9 mmol/L
  - 2-hour plasma glucose (if measured) <7.8 mmol/L.

Both the ADA[3] and the International Society for Pediatric and Adolescent Diabetes (ISPAD)[4] have now recommended decreasing the threshold for IFG from 6.1 to 5.6 mmol/L. It is unclear whether lowering the threshold will aid predicting progression to frank diabetes or a reduction in adverse outcomes.

IFG and IGT are referred to as pre-diabetes, indicating an increased risk of developing diabetes, and each represent different abnormalities in glucose homeostasis:
- IFG represents abnormal glucose metabolism in the basal state
- IGT represents abnormal glucose dynamics.

A raised glycated haemoglobin level (HbA1c ≥6.5% (48 mmol/mol)) (➲ see 'Glycated haemoglobin', p. 163) is now accepted in the diagnosis of diabetes in adults, although its diagnostic value in children and adults is unclear.

## References

1. World Health Organization. *Definition and Diagnosis of Diabetes Mellitus and Intermediate Hyperglycaemia: Report of a WHO/IDF Consultation.* Geneva: WHO, 2006.
2. American Diabetes Association. 2. Classification and diagnosis of diabetes: standards of medical care in diabetes—2018. *Diabetes Care* 2018;41(Suppl. 1):S13–S27.
3. American Diabetes Association. Impaired fasting glucose and impaired glucose tolerance: implications for care. *Diabetes Care* 2007;30:753–759.
4. International Society for Pediatric and Adolescent Diabetes (ISPAD). Clinical Practice Consensus Guidelines 2018: Chapter 1: Definition, epidemiology, and classification of diabetes in children and adolescents *Pediatr Diabetes* 2018;19 (Suppl. 27):7–19. ➶ https://www.ispad.org/page/ISPADGuidelines2018/page/ISPADGuidelines2018

# Type 1 diabetes

- Type 1 diabetes mellitus (T1DM) is the third most common chronic disorder in childhood (after asthma and epilepsy). Occurs in ~1 in 400 children.
- Currently 25.1 new cases per 100,000 children aged 0–15 years in England and Wales.[1]
- Increasing in prevalence, especially in children 5–9 years old.
- Associated with a mean reduction in lifespan of 23 years.
- Overall standardized mortality rate is 2.3, and is highest in the 1–4-year age group at 9.2.
- Currently only 28.6% of children and young people in the UK achieve appropriate diabetic control (HbA1c <58 mmol/mol or <7.5%).

## Epidemiology

### Age

Most (50–60%) patients with T1DM are diagnosed in childhood (<15 years of age), and currently T1DM accounts for >95% of children with diabetes in the UK, although in other countries the incidence of non-T1DM (especially type 2 diabetes mellitus (T2DM)) is higher.

The incidence of T1DM has two major peaks:
- at 4–6 years of age
- at 10–14 years of age (puberty)—the highest prevalence is at this age.

### Sex

- Slightly more prevalent in males than females (especially older adolescents and young adults) in contrast to most other autoimmune disorders.

### Seasonal variation

- In presentation of diabetes, with a peak in the winter months (especially January) (in the UK) and lower rates in the summer months. Postulated that this might reflect the time of increased exposure to potential pathogens such as viruses.
- At birth, with some studies showing increased risk of T1DM in babies born in the spring and summer. Postulated that these babies have a shorter period of breastfeeding than babies born at other times.

### Geographical distribution

- Geographical variation in the incidence of T1DM is well recognized (Fig. 5.1).
- While no population worldwide is completely exempt from T1DM, there is a >350-fold difference in incidence rates (20-fold in European Caucasians).
- Generally, the further from the equator, the higher the incidence of T1DM, although there are notable exceptions to this (e.g. Sardinia).
- Evidence indicates that migration from one country to another broadly confers the diabetes risk of the new country within a generation.

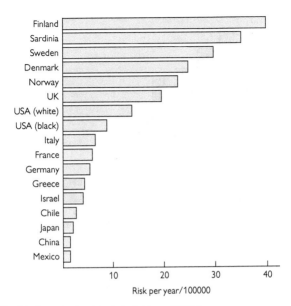

**Fig. 5.1** Geographical variation in the incidence of T1DM.

Reproduced from Wass JAH, Shalet SM (eds) (2002). *Oxford Textbook of Endocrinology and Diabetes*, Oxford University Press, Oxford. Copyright 2002 © OUP.

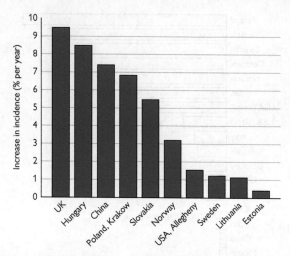

**Fig. 5.2** Incidence of T1DM.

Reproduced with permission from Devendra D, Liu E, Eisenbarth GS (2004). Type 1 diabetes: recent developments. *BMJ* 328: 750. Copyright © 2004 BMJ Publishing Group Ltd.

### Incidence of T1DM

- Rising over the last decades, with a mean increase/year of 3.4% (Fig. 5.2) although there is wide variation between countries, and some evidence of plateauing in high-incidence areas, including the UK.
- Downward shift in age of incidence, with increasing numbers <5 years, although presentation <1 year remains uncommon.

**Reference**

1. National Paediatric Diabetes Audit (NPDA). Annual report 2017–18. NPDA, 2019. ↗ https://www.rcpch.ac.uk/resources/npda-annual-reports#downloadBox

# Pathophysiology of type 1 diabetes

T1DM is:
- due to lack of insulin
- a complex process whereby environmental factors operate in a genetically susceptible individual to produce autoimmune destruction of the islets of Langerhans in the pancreas.

Although the environmental triggers are poorly understood, it is recognized that this process may occur months or even years before the onset of clinical symptoms. This is because there is considerable reserve within the pancreas, so that most (>70–90%) of the endocrine pancreatic function needs to be lost before blood sugar levels rise.

- Histologically, autoimmune destruction is shown by mononuclear infiltration of the insulin-producing islets of Langerhans within the pancreas; so-called insulitis, leading ultimately to destruction of the β-cells. Much of the understanding of this process has come from animal (murine) models.

A scheme of the development of endocrine pancreatic failure over time is shown in Fig. 5.3.

## Serological markers

A variety of serological markers are found in patients with T1DM, with antibodies to:
- islet cell (ICA)
- insulin (IAA)
- tyrosine phosphatase-like molecule (IA$_2$)
- glutamic acid decarboxylase (GAD)
- zinc transporter-8
- tetraspanin-7

being detected in 85–90% of patients with T1DM at diagnosis. Each autoantibody is found in 50–75% of individual patients.

Development of diabetes over the next 10 years is seen in:
- 15% of patients with single islet autoantibodies
- 70% of patients with multiple islet autoantibodies.

A number of stages of T1DM are therefore recognized:

Stage 1: islet autoantibodies, normal blood glucose, pre/asymptomatic
Stage 2: islet autoantibodies, raised blood glucose, pre/asymptomatic
Stage 3: islet autoantibodies, raised blood glucose, symptomatic
Stage 4: longstanding T1DM.

When the clinical presentation is typical of T1DM, but autoantibodies are not present, this is classified as type 1b diabetes mellitus. This represents ~5% of T1DM in white populations, but is more common in other parts of the world, such as Japan.

## Potential pathogens implicated in T1DM

### Infections

Viral infections (both RNA and DNA) are diabetogenic in both humans and animals. These probably initiate the autoimmune process rather than precipitate diabetes in subjects with autoimmunity. Two or more infections with similar viruses may be needed.

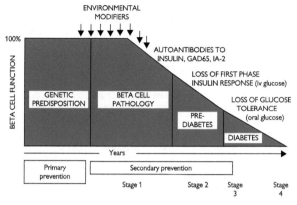

**Fig. 5.3** Stages of T1DM.

Reproduced with permission from Harrison, LC. Vaccination against self to prevent autoimmune disease: the type 1 diabetes model. *Immunology and Cell Biology*, 2(86). Copyright © 2008 John Wiley and Sons.

- Mumps: association both from case reports and epidemiological studies.
- Rubella: up to 25% of affected children with congenital rubella syndrome subsequently develop diabetes, often insulin dependent, and at an older age. ICA may be found in this group.
- Enterovirus links include:
  • viral RNA and enterovirus detection via immunohistochemistry in pancreas of children with T1DM
  • virus isolated from the pancreas of childhood diabetics produces diabetes in animals
  • diabetes described following enterovirus infection, and patients may demonstrate ICA
  • increased enterovirus infection and antibodies in children developing T1DM compared with non-diabetics.

*Cow's milk protein, wheat, and breastfeeding*
- Cow's milk introduced at weaning triggers insulitis and diabetes in animal models.
- Early exposure in humans to cow's milk at <3–4 months of age is also associated with an increased risk of developing T1DM, with casein, bovine insulin, and bovine serum albumin all potentially implicated.
- In humans, breastfeeding for >2 weeks may have a protective effect, and also if continued at the time of weaning in susceptible infants.
- At weaning, ingestion of root vegetables, wheat storage globulin, gluten/gliadin, and casein have also been implicated in development of T1DM.

*Vitamin D*
- Deficiency in mothers during pregnancy increases T1DM incidence in offspring, whereas high-dose vitamin D supplementation to the mother and in early childhood may be protective.
- In addition, low levels of vitamin D are found in newly diagnosed patients with T1DM compared to controls.

*Immunizations*
None of the routine childhood immunizations have been shown to increase the risk of diabetes or pre-diabetic autoimmunity.

*Chemicals*
Streptozotocin and dietary nitrates induce β-cell autoimmunity in animal models. In humans, there is a connection between T1DM and consumption of foods and water containing nitrates, nitrites, and nitrosamines.

*Others*
- Blood group incompatibility; ABO more so than Rhesus.
- Pre-eclampsia, neonatal respiratory distress and infections, Caesarean section.

## Other hypotheses

In addition to postulated environmental triggers, there are also several hypotheses to account for the increase in T1DM. These include:

*Molecular mimicry*
Various islet cell proteins share structural homology with postulated antigens, e.g. Coxsackie B virus and bovine serum albumin, so autoimmune destruction of islet cells may be due to a misguided immune response.

*Hygiene hypothesis*
A reduced number of infections in early life leads to increased risk of developing T1DM in later life. It is postulated that too clean an environment may not allow the immune system to develop appropriately, putting individuals at risk of immune-regulated illnesses. Conversely, infections which elicit Th2 (allergic)-like immunity such as pinworm are associated with decreased risk.

*Accelerator and overload hypotheses*
Increased levels of environmental stress (e.g. moderate excess growth in childhood, even if not associated with obesity), especially in early life, may overload the β-cells, accounting for both the rise in diabetes and its earlier onset.

*Fertile field hypothesis*
A microbial infection induces a temporary tolerance state allowing other antigens to act to generate autoreactive T cells.

### 'Old friends' hypothesis

This implicates dietary exposure and normal gut microbes as a possible direct regulator of the immune system and of self-tolerance.

### Threshold hypothesis

A mathematical model which calculates the risk of T1DM based on the contributions of environment and genetics.

# Risks of developing type 1 diabetes

- In general public: 0.2–0.25%
- Father affected: 3.6–8.5%
- Mother affected: 1.3–3.6% (lower if child is born at maternal age >25 years)
- Sibling affected: ~4% by aged 20 years, and 9.6% by 60 years
- Both parents affected: ~30%.

NB: ~10–15% of newly diagnosed T1DM cases have an affected first-degree relative.

## Identical twins and T1DM

- Identical twin affected: ~36% of cases (range 17–70%).
- Risk of developing T1DM in a second monozygotic twin is >50% if the index case develops the disease before 5 years of age, but only 10% if after 25 years.
- The fact that concordance is not 100% indicates that factors other than genes are involved in the aetiology of T1DM.

## Susceptibility genes

More than 60 genetic variants have now been identified through genome-wide linkage studies. Details of these can be found at ℘ http://www.immunobase.org/.

The first two susceptibility loci were located in the human leucocyte antigen (HLA) region (*IDDM1*) and the insulin gene (*INS*) locus (*IDDM2*). These two loci contribute most familial clustering in T1DM (~50% for *IDDM1* and ~10% for *INS*):

- *IDDM1*. The HLA genes (*IDDM1*) are associated with both predisposing and protective genes.
  - More than 90% of patients developing T1DM have either DR3, DQ2 or DR4, DQ8 haplotypes, compared with <40% of normal controls. Odds ratios for developing diabetes range from 0.02 to >11 for specific DR–DQ haplotypes.
  - DR3 and DR4 heterozygosity is found in 2.4% of the general population, but in 50% of children who develop T1DM before 5 years of age, and 20–30% of adults presenting with T1DM. Heterozygotes have a 30-fold increase in the risk of developing ICA and diabetes.
- *IDDM2*. This is a polymorphic region with variable numbers of tandem nucleotide repeats (VNTR) of the insulin gene. Allele frequencies cluster at 30–60 repeats (class I alleles) or 120–170 repeats (class III alleles). Homozygosity for short class VNTR I alleles is found in ~75–85% of patients with T1DM compared with 50–60% in the general population, suggesting that this predisposes to T1DM, whereas the class III VNTR allele may confer a protective effect. In large population studies the VNTR confers an odds ratio of 2.38.

- Other susceptibility loci have also been identified, including:
  - *PTPN22* (protein tyrosine phosphatase non-receptor type 22), encoding a lymphocyte-specific phosphatase involved in T-cell function
  - *IL2RA/CD25*, encoding the interleukin (IL)-2 receptor
  - *IDDM12*, encoding a cytotoxic T-lymphocyte antigen 4 (CTLA4) which plays a role in response to antigens through T-cell activation
  - *IF1H1/MDA5*, interferon-induced helicase 1 gene region.

Only *PTPN22* and *IL2RA* have odds ratios for developing T1DM >1.5; the remaining genes range from 1.1 to 1.3.

# Clinical features and development of type 1 diabetes

This is divided into several different phases:
- preclinical phase
- presentation with clinical features of diabetes
- partial remission phase ('honeymoon period')
- chronic phase of insulin dependence.

## Preclinical diabetes

See also Fig. 5.3.
- This refers to the period before clinical presentation of diabetes when genetic predisposition and autoimmune phenomena can be identified.
- Although frank biochemical changes are not apparent at this stage, initial insulin release during an IV GTT may have prognostic significance long term; impaired IV GTT confers a 60% chance of developing T1DM over the next 5 years.
- In high-risk individuals, prospective follow-up can identify patients prior to them developing overt T1DM, reducing the risk of diabetic ketoacidosis (DKA). In these children insulin should be considered if the HBA1c level is >6.5%.

## Presentation with clinical features of diabetes

Many children present with the classical features of diabetes mellitus over the preceding weeks:
- polyuria
- polydipsia
- weight loss
- lethargy.

Diagnosis is usually easy in these cases, and once biochemical confirmation of diagnosis has been made urgent (i.e. same-day) referral to a centre with expertise is mandatory.

### Points
- Some high-risk patients (especially younger ones) can present with a rapid onset of symptoms and DKA, while others may have a much slower onset, with symptoms over a number of months.
- A small number may also have symptoms of hypoglycaemia.

Other presenting features (and misdiagnoses) include:
- 2° enuresis (urinary tract infection)
- vomiting (gastroenteritis)
- abdominal pain ('acute abdomen')
- hyperventilation (Kussmaul breathing) (asthma or pneumonia)
- chronic weight loss (anorexia)
- vaginal candidiasis ('thrush') in prepubertal girls.

## Partial remission phase ('honeymoon period')

- In ~80% of children with T1DM, insulin requirements fall following institution of insulin therapy.
- Although different definitions of partial remission are used, an insulin requirement of <0.5 U/kg/day with HbA1c level <7.0% is often used.
- This phase usually commences shortly after insulin is started, and may last for weeks or months.
- The presence of DKA at presentation and younger age make this phase less likely.
- Insulin requirements may occasionally reduce to the point where insulin can be temporarily stopped, although it must be made clear that this does not represent a 'cure'.
- β-cell destruction is complete within 3 years of diagnosis in most young children, especially those with the HLA DR3/4 phenotype.
- It may be slower and partial in older patients, with 15% still showing β-cell function (positive C-peptide) 10 years after diagnosis.

Total and partial remissions have been reported in, respectively, 2–12% and 18–62% of young T1DM patients. The following are associated with deeper and longer remission:

- older age
- less severe initial presentation of diabetes, i.e. without DKA
- absent or low levels of autoantibodies ICA or IA-2.

It has been postulated that preservation of β-cell function is associated with better glycaemic control (lower HbA1c).

The prevalence of ICA (but not GAD) antibodies decreases from 87% at the time of diagnosis of T1DM to 38–62% 2–3 years later, and is more rapid in:

- young boys
- patients lacking HLA DR3 and HLA DR4
- those diagnosed between July and December.

Natural remission is always temporary, ending with a gradual or abrupt increase in insulin requirements.

## Prevention/modulation of T1DM

Treatment has been attempted at several stages of diabetes.

- At a preclinical stage to prevent or modulate autoimmune phenomenon. This can be done before (1° prevention) and after development of islet autoantibodies (2° prevention) to delay the onset.
- *1° prevention* (to delay onset of islet autoantibodies):
  - reduction of antigen exposure (delayed gluten, modified formulae, omission of cow's milk within first year)
  - modulation of the immune response, e.g. nicotinamide, metformin, nasal/oral insulin.
- *2° prevention* to delay onset of clinical diabetes (stages 1–2):
  - anti-CD3 monoclonal antibodies, CTLA4 immunoglobulin (Ig), oral/intranasal/low-dose SC insulin, metformin.

At present, no interventions have been clearly shown to either prevent or postpone the onset of T1DM.

To prolong remission phase (stage 3):

* *Immune-modulation*: fusion protein abatacept, rituximab (anti-CD20 monoclonal antibody), antithymocyte globulin, granulocyte colony stimulating factor (GCSF), stem cell transplantation
* *Antigen-based therapies*: DiaPep277, GAD aluminium hydroxide treatment
* *Cell therapies*: autologous regulatory T cells, infusion of umbilical cord blood infusion
* *Anti-inflammatory agents and GLP-1 agonists*.

NB: as 70–90% of islet cell function has already been lost by the time clinical features appear, any effect of immunomodulation is lost when treatment ceases.

# Therapy of type 1 diabetes

Insulin

### Principles of therapy

As T1DM is due to insulin deficiency, therapy must be with insulin. Several different insulin regimens have been established, all of which mimic physiological insulin secretion to some degree or other (Fig. 5.4).

### Insulin therapy

Although no one regimen is ideal, the aim is to:
1. mimic physiological insulin secretion as much as possible
2. obtain optimal glycaemic control.

Three main types of insulin regimen exist:
1. Multiple daily injection (MDI) basal–bolus insulin regimens: injections of short- or rapid-acting insulin/insulin analogue before meals, plus 1 or more injections of intermediate/long-acting insulin/insulin analogue a day.
2. Continuous subcutaneous insulin infusion (CSII); insulin pump: a programmable pump of rapid-acting insulin analogue or short-acting insulin giving SC baseline insulin infusion along with boluses for meals and snacks.
3. One, two, or three insulin injections per day: these are usually injections of short-acting insulin or rapid-acting insulin analogue mixed with intermediate-acting insulin.

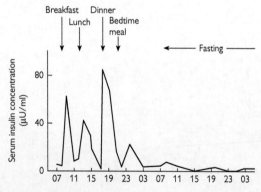

**Fig. 5.4** Physiological secretion of insulin.

Reproduced from Lee WL, Zinman F (1998). From insulin to insulin analogies: progress in the treatment of type 1 diabetes mellitus. *Diabetes Rev* 6: 73–88. Copyright American Diabetes Association.

The insulin regimen should, however, be individualized for each patient, based on:
- personal and family circumstances
- personal preferences

Over the last few years there has been a move towards more intensive insulin regimens. Generally it is recommended to offer newly diagnosed patients MDI from diagnosis; if this is not appropriate then to consider CSII (insulin pump) therapy.

# Insulins

Virtually all children within the UK are now treated with authentic sequence human insulin. Insulins are available from several manufacturers, with differences in the onset and duration of action. These include natural insulins, as well as insulin analogues (both short and long acting).

## Short-acting insulins

These have been superseded in most developed countries by the rapid analogues (see following section).

These start working within 30–60 minutes, have a peak action at 2–4 hours, and last for 5–8 hours. Examples are Actrapid® (Novo Nordisk) and Velosulin® (Lilly).

As these short-acting insulins (e.g. Actrapid®) require dissociation in SC tissue before onset of action, they should be administered at least 20 minutes before a meal, and often snacks are required several hours later (e.g. mid-morning and before bed) to avoid postprandial hypoglycaemia.

## Rapid-acting analogues

These start working within 15 minutes, have a peak action at 1–3 hours, and last for up to 5 hours. Examples are insulin aspart (Novo Nordisk), insulin lispro (Lilly), and insulin glulisine (Sanofi-Aventis). All have a more rapid onset and shorter duration of action than soluble insulin.

These insulins are an essential component of most insulin regimens:
- in combination with an intermediate-acting insulin (either free or premixed) in a twice-daily regimen
- as pre-meal boluses within a basal bolus regimen
- in CSII (insulin pump).

Rapid analogues and soluble insulin can both be used in situations where IV insulin is administered, e.g. DKA or surgery.

Advantages of rapid analogues over soluble insulin are:
- rapid action, so that:
  - they can be given with, or even immediately after meals
  - there is less postprandial hyperglycaemia
- shorter duration of action, so that:
  - postprandial and nocturnal hypoglycaemia are reduced
  - mid-morning and bedtime snacks may not be required.

Ultra-rapid analogues are also being developed including Fiasp (Novo Nordisk): fast-acting insulin aspart, containing niacinamide and L-arginine which speed monomer formation.

## Intermediate-acting insulin

Isophane insulin starts working after 2–4 hours, has a peak of action at 4–12 hours, and lasts for 12–24 hours. Examples are Humulin® I (Lilly) and Insulatard® (Novo Nordisk).

Isophane insulin can be used in children, either within twice-daily premixed insulin regimens or as a basal bolus (although in the latter it has been superseded by the long-acting analogues). Unlike lente preparations, isophane insulin will not react with short-acting insulin, blunting its short-acting properties.

### Long-acting analogues

These have an onset of action after 2–4 hours, do not have a peak action (especially with glargine), and last for up to 24 hours.

There are now two long-acting insulin analogues; both are licensed for use from 2 years of age within Europe (glargine from 6 years in the USA).

- Insulin glargine: formation of micro-precipitates produces an almost constant background of insulin over 24 hours.
- Insulin detemir: insulin is acylated and bound to albumin, producing a mean duration of action of 12–16 hours.

*Points*
- Glargine is usually given once daily, but detemir may need to be administered once or twice daily.
- The low pH of glargine produces local stinging, and it needs to be given at a separate site from the short-acting insulin to avoid inactivation.
- Detemir may be associated with less weight gain.

### Very long-acting insulins/analogues

- Ultralente insulin was devised to have an action of >24 hours, although its action is variable, with the potential for dose accumulation.
- Degludec is an ultra-long-acting analogue. Slow dissociation of soluble multihexamers into stable monomers after SC injection produces an action up to 40 hours. Other very long-acting analogues are also in development including glargine U300 (Table 5.1).

### Premixed insulins

- *Biphasic insulins*: mixtures of short- and intermediate-acting insulins in different proportions, such as 30:70. Examples are Humulin® M3 (Lilly), Insuman® comb 25 (Sanofi-Aventis).
- *Biphasic insulins with analogues*: there are also mixtures of rapid-acting analogues and intermediate-acting insulins. Examples are NovoMix® 30 (Novo Nordisk) and Humalog® Mix 25 (Lilly).

Fixed-ratio mixtures of short-acting or rapid analogue plus isophane are still popular in some countries, especially in prepubertal children. While they

**Table 5.1** Types of insulin

| Insulin type | Onset of action (hours) | Peak action (hours) | Duration of action (hours) |
|---|---|---|---|
| Rapid acting | 0.15–0.35 | 1–3 | 3–5 |
| Regular acting | 0.5–1 | 2–4 | 5–8 |
| Intermediate (isophane) | 2–4 | 4–12 | 12–24 |
| Long-acting analogue: *glargine* | 2–4 | 8–12 | ~24 |
| Long-acting analogue: *detemir* | 1–2 | 4–7 | 20–24 |
| Ultra-long analogue: *degludec* | 0.5–1.5 | – | Up to 42 |

reduce errors in drawing up insulin they also reduce flexibility. Premixed insulins are generally no longer recommended for routine paediatric use, but may be beneficial where adherence is a problem.

## Free mixing

Free mixing of short- and long-acting ('*clear*' and '*cloudy*') insulins in a syringe is now much less commonly used, with increased use of premixed insulins, MDI and CSII. Usually the clear insulin is drawn up first. The cloudy insulin needs to be gently but thoroughly mixed before adding to the clear.

## Insulin doses (rough guides)

- ~0.5 U/kg/day initially during honeymoon period
- ~0.7–1.0 U/kg/day after honeymoon period (prepubertal)
- Usually >1.2 and up to 2.0 U/kg/day after honeymoon period (pubertal)

If there is poor glycaemic control with an insulin requirement >1.5 units/kg/day, consider non-adherence with therapy.

## Commonly used regimens

### Multiple daily injections

- Long-acting insulin once (occasionally twice) daily (usually at bedtime); usually analogue (glargine or detemir).
- Short-acting insulin (analogue) before meals and snacks (anything containing 10 g of carbohydrate).
- Of total daily doses of insulin:
  - ~30–50% as intermediate insulin or long-acting analogue
  - ~50–70% as short-acting insulin or rapid-acting analogue, given in three or four divided boluses before meals (often higher percentage of total if a rapid-acting analogue is used).

Doses need to be individualized; previously broad recommendations were:
- 1 U of short-acting insulin for ~10 g of carbohydrate.
- 1 U of short-acting insulin to lower blood sugar by ~2.5 mmol/L (correct to 7.5 mmol/L).
- Both pre- and postprandial blood glucose testing are required to assess an individual's sensitivity.
- Advantage: more flexibility in lifestyle (e.g. meals, lie-ins on holidays/at weekends).
- Disadvantage: at least four injections a day, including at school/college.

While on MDI:
- insulin dose adjustment can be performed if appropriate after each blood glucose measurement.
- injecting rapid-acting insulin analogues before rather than after food reduces postprandial blood glucose levels and optimizes blood glucose control.

## Continuous subcutaneous insulin infusion

SC cannula *in situ* for ~3 days to give:
- background basal SC infusion of insulin
- boluses of insulin given via insulin pump to cover meals and snacks.

*Points*

- Can be removed for up to an hour (e.g. sport, bathing). Some pumps are waterproof.
- Offer setting temporary basal rates and different patterns of bolus insulin administration.
- Its use has increased in England and Wales from ~1–2% of patients a decade ago to >35% in 2017–2018: equivalent to numbers in Europe and the USA.
- Low rates of hypoglycaemia make CSII attractive, especially for young children. It is now the preferred method of insulin administration for children <7 years with T1DM.

Despite increasing use of CSII, there are few randomized studies, with some studies clearly showing improvement in HbA1c in CSII compared with analogue-based MDI. Meta-analyses have however shown reductions in HBA1c, total insulin daily dose, and severe hypoglycaemia (Box 5.1).

The most recent NICE guidelines[1] also clarified that CSII should be considered in children or young people of all ages with T1DM if MDI is not appropriate.[2]

## Less intensive regimens

*Twice-daily insulin*

- Free-mixing or premixed insulins: contain short-acting insulin or short-acting analogue, e.g.:
  - ~30% short-acting:70% intermediate-acting (e.g. Humulin® M3 (short-acting insulin), NovoMix® 30, Humalog® Mix 25 (short-acting analogue).
- Characteristically about two-thirds of the daily dose is given in the morning, and about one-third in the evening:
  - advantage: only twice-daily injection
  - disadvantage: rigid regimen regrading timings of injections, meals, and snacks.

In addition, combination of waning overnight insulin, early morning rises in counter-regulatory hormones (GH, cortisol, and catecholamines), and increased resistance to insulin action and hepatic glucose production often produces a rise in the blood sugar evident on waking (the 'dawn phenomenon'). Increasing the previous evening dose of insulin or giving thrice-daily insulin to try and overcome this may still produce nocturnal hypoglycaemia.

Where appropriate, patients on a twice-daily insulin regimen should be encouraged to adjust the insulin does according to blood glucose levels (including occasional night-time levels).

*Thrice-daily insulin (occasionally used in adolescents)*

- Insulin mixture in morning
- Short-acting insulin with afternoon snack or evening meal
- Intermediate-acting insulin at bedtime.

**Box 5.1 The NICE guidelines (2008) for CSII (updated in 2015) recommended**

'Continuous subcutaneous insulin infusion or "insulin pump" therapy is recommended as a possible treatment for adults and children 12 years and over with type 1 diabetes mellitus if:

- attempts to reach target haemoglobin A1c (HbA1c) levels with multiple daily injections result in the person having "disabling hypoglycaemia,"

or

- HbA1c levels have remained high (8.5% or above) with multiple daily injections (including using long-acting insulin analogues if appropriate) despite the person and/or their carer carefully trying to manage their diabetes.

Insulin pump therapy is recommended as a possible treatment for children under 12 years with type 1 diabetes mellitus if treatment with multiple daily injections is not practical or is not considered appropriate. Children who use insulin pump therapy should have a trial of multiple daily injections when they are between the age of 12 and 18 years.

"Disabling hypoglycaemia" is when hypoglycaemic episodes occur frequently or without warning so that the person is constantly anxious about another episode occurring, which has a negative impact on their quality of life.

Insulin pump therapy should only be started by a trained specialist team. This team should include a doctor who specialises in insulin pump therapy, a diabetes nurse and a dietitian (someone who can give specialist advice on diet). This team should provide structured education programmes and advice on diet, lifestyle and exercise that is suitable for people using insulin pumps.

Insulin pump therapy should only be continued in adults and children 12 years and over if there has been a sustained improvement in the control of their blood glucose levels. This should be shown by a decrease in the person's HbA1c levels or by the person having fewer hypoglycaemic episodes. Such goals should be set by the doctor through discussion with the person or their carer.'

ℛ http://www.nice.org.uk

## Which insulin regimen?

There is still debate about the optimal regimen, and few randomized studies have been performed. Insulin treatment which more closely mimics normal physiological secretion has, however, become the 'gold standard'.

Current regimen use in England and Wales[3] is:

- One to three injections a day (5.2%)
- MDI (57.9%)
- CSII (35.7%)
- Other (including missing data) (1.2%).

### Alternatives

*Islet cell transplantation*: usually via infusion of donor islet cells into the liver, remains experimental. Islet cell supplies are limited, and immunosuppressants need to be given, but most patients remain insulin free after 1 year, although this falls to 1/4 after 5 years. Currently the main indication for islet-cell transplantation is in adults to treat hypoglycaemic unawareness unresponsive to other measures.

*Pancreatic transplant*: as it requires immunosuppression this is usually reserved for those diabetic patients who also require renal transplantation for end-stage renal failure.

*Closed-loop systems* (either hybrid or full) using a glucose sensor and insulin pump along with an algorithm determining insulin delivery have been trialled. The FDA (2016) has now approved the first system (Minimed® 670 G hybrid pump with the Guardian Sensor® 3 continuous glucose monitoring (CGM)) in children >14 years, although paediatric trials are ongoing on this and other closed-loop systems.

### Injection sites

- Arms (lateral aspect)
- Stomach
- Legs (front/lateral part of thigh)
- Buttocks (upper outer quadrant).

*Points*

- Absorption is more rapid from arms and stomach, and slower from legs and buttocks.
- Arms and stomach are often used for morning injections, when more rapid absorption is required.

NB:

- Use of the abdomen may be less affected by muscle activity or exercise.
- The thigh is the preferred injection site for longer-acting insulins.
- Stomach and arms are often used for MDI as they are easily accessible.
- Younger children often have injections in legs and buttocks, as these have more SC tissue. Injection into other sites might result in IM injection, with rapid absorption and bruising.
- At a particular time of day patients should inject consistently the same site, but not into the same spot to avoid lipohypertrophy (see following section).
- Cleaning or disinfection of sites is not required.

*Common injection problems*

- *Lipohypertrophy* (lumpy sites) due to accumulation of fat and fibrous tissue at site of repeated injection. Often more easily palpated than seen. Occurs in up to 48% of children with T1DM, and is seen most often in those with:
  • higher HbA1c
  • longer duration of diabetes
  • larger number of injections.

As failure to rotate injection sites, using only small areas for injections, and reusing needles are also independent risk factors these should be avoided.

If lumpy sites are used repeatedly, absorption is erratic and variable (e.g. reduction in absorption by up to 25%), and diabetic control often worsens. Omitting the site until the lump disappears (usually for at least 2–3 months) usually results in spontaneous resolution.

- *Painful injections*: usually due to IM rather than SC injection. It is important to check both needle length and angle of injection.
- *Bruising and bleeding*: more common after IM injection.
- *Air bubbles*: if large, these should be removed as they may affect the dose of insulin administered.
- *Lipoatrophy* is now uncommon (1–2% of diabetic patients) with highly purified authentic sequence human insulins, although it is described with both newer rapid-acting analogues lispro and aspart (including via CSII), and also the long-acting analogues glargine and detemir. It is also described in association with the autoimmune disorders coeliac disease and also Hashimoto's thyroiditis.
- *Local hypersensitivity reactions* may occur with insulin or preservative. Changing the insulin preparation may be all that is required.
- *Skin infection and abscess formation* may occur with CSII if poor sterile technique is used for cannula insertion.
- *Skin irritation* may occur with CGM.

There is considerable variation in the age at which children will self-inject.

- Broadly, most children over the age of 10 years can either administer or assist with their own injections.
- Self-injection is often precipitated by an external event (e.g. sleepover, school trip, diabetes camp). In addition, MDI injections will need to be given at school.

Some devices (e.g. Novo Nordisk PenMate®) assist with needle insertion, although needle-free devices have not proved particularly popular in diabetes.

References

1. National Institute for Health and Care Excellence (NICE). Diabetes (type 1 and type 2) in children and young people: diagnosis and management. NG18. NICE, 2015. ℘ https://www.nice.org.uk/guidance/ng18
2. National Institute for Health and Care Excellence (NICE). Continuous subcutaneous insulin infusion for the treatment of diabetes mellitus. TA151. ℘ NICE, 2008. https://www.nice.org.uk/guidance/ta151
3. National Paediatric Diabetes Audit (NPDA). Annual report 2017–18. NPDA, 2019. ℘ https://www.rcpch.ac.uk/resources/npda-annual-reports#downloadBox

# Diabetes monitoring

## Control (self-monitoring of blood glucose (SMBG))

Assessed using SMBG to:
- help monitor short- and longer-term levels of control
- maintain euglycaemia (e.g. blood sugars in range 4–7 mmol/L)
- detect hypoglycaemia
- allow safe and appropriate management of hyperglycaemia
- assess the individual's blood glucose response to insulin, food, and exercise
- allow optimal growth and development.

## Timing

- Regular blood glucose monitoring is usually performed preprandially.
- Some postprandial bloods may be necessary in MDI and CSII to determine individual insulin sensitivity. Also commonly performed in cystic fibrosis-related diabetes (CFRD).
- The current NICE recommendations for all patients with T1D is a minimum of 5 blood sugars a day,[1] but others recommend 6–10 times in intensive management.
- Although optimal target ranges for plasma glucose vary from unit to unit, they are of the order of:
  - fasting level of 4–7 mmol/L on waking
  - 4–7 mmol/L before meals at other times of the day
  - 5–9 mmol/L after meals
  - at least 5 mmol/L when driving.

Achieving and maintaining levels towards the lower end of the optimal range will achieve the lowest attainable HbA1c level, although it is also important to avoid problematic hypoglycaemia or emotional distress.

- Increased frequency of SMBG correlates with both improved diabetes control, and concordance with treatment. In one study, the HbA1c level fell by 0.3% for each additional SMBG each day.
- Although many patients state that they can 'feel' what their blood sugar is at any time, this has not been supported by studies.

More frequent blood glucose testing is required during:
- hypoglycaemia (and also following)
- intercurrent illness, along with assessment of ketones (either in the urine or blood)
- vigorous sport or exercise.

## Sites

- The usual site for SMBG is the fingertips, although other sites can also be used (e.g. palm or forearm).
- In the fasting state, glucose readings from forearm and fingertips are equivalent, but as rapidly falling blood sugars may not be reflected in alternative sites, it is still recommended that fingertips are used if symptoms of hypoglycaemia are present.
- If the fingertips are used, it is important that the hands are washed properly, as glucose residue can produce false high results.

Regular review of blood glucose is recommended, recording the blood sugars (ideally daily) by downloading from the meter using software or manually writing in a blood glucose diary allows much clearer visualization of any trends in blood glucose.

Other advantages are:

- enabling any variations in normal routine (exercise, illness, unusual food intake (e.g. parties)) to be documented
- documentation and description of the severity of any hypoglycaemic episodes, plus any precipitants or changes in routine.

## Other ways of assessing glycaemic control

### Glycated haemoglobin

As glucose attaches itself to the red blood cell (RBC) or erythrocyte during the lifespan of the cell, the HbA1c concentration is a reflection of overall glycaemic control during the preceding 4–12 weeks, although it is weighted towards the preceding 4 weeks.

- HbA1c monitoring is the most useful measure for evaluating metabolic control (especially long term). The previous normal range for HbA1c is ~3.9–6.2% (depending on assay). The assay units have now been changed to mmol/mol. The association between HbA1c (%), HbA1c (mmol/mol), and average blood sugar (in mg/dL (divide by 18 for mmol/L)) can be found at ℛ http://www.ngsp.org/convert1.asp.
- HbA1c is measured using international (Diabetes Control and Complications Trial (DCCT)) standards either via venesection (lab based) or at the bedside (e.g. Bayer DCA® meter).
- Each child should have at least four HbA1c measurements per year, although in England and Wales only just over half of patients do (54.6%).[2]
- Ideally, HbA1c results should be available at the clinic visit, so that they can be used to inform adjustments of care.
- HbA1c is the only measure for which good data for its association with later microvascular and macrovascular complications are available.

### Points

- HbA1c is a measure of 'average' blood sugar, and not variation within blood sugars. Therefore, a patient with repeated hypoglycaemia and rebound hyperglycaemia ( see 'Rebound phenomenon', p. 170) may have a relatively normal HbA1c LEVEL, even if few of the blood sugars fall within the acceptable range.
- Evidence from studies such as the DCCT[3,4] indicate that the better the control, the lower the risk of complications and the progression of existing complications. The current recommendation for good control (HbA1c <7.5% or <58 mmol/mol) is only achieved by ~28.6% of paediatric patients in England and Wales (2017–2018); this is, however, improved since 2011–2012 (15.8%) but is still much lower than other countries, e.g. 60% of children <13 years in Sweden. As HbA1c rises to >58 mmol/mol (7.5%), the risk of developing later microvascular complications increases steeply ( see Fig. 5.5, p. 164). Currently, 16.5% of patients in England and Wales have an HbA1c concentration

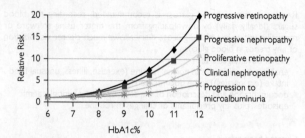

**Fig. 5.5** Risks of diabetic complications with differing levels of control.

Adapted from Skyler JS (1996). Diabetic complications: glucose control is important. *Endocrinol Metab Clin N Am* 25: 243–54 (based on data from DCCT Research Group (1993)). The effect of intensive treatment of diabetes on the development and progression of long-term complications of insulin-dependent diabetes mellitus. *N Engl J Med* 329: 977–86, 1993.

>80 mmol/mol (>9.5%), although this has also improved from 28.7% in 2011–2012.

- With newer regimens compared to those previously available in the DCCT, tighter control of diabetes is possible. As a result, an HbA1c target level of ≤48 mmol/mol (≤6.5%) should be aimed for[1]; this is currently achieved in 7.2% of patients in England and Wales.[2]
- Any reduction in HbA1c is, however, to be encouraged. Patients should attempt to achieve the lowest attainable HbA1c level without inducing severe hypoglycaemia, and this may need to be based on the individual's personal circumstances.

### Fructosamine

- This measures serum protein glycation, reflecting glycaemic control over the previous 3–4 weeks.
- Although proposed as an assessment of long-term control, in practice most units still use HbA1c.
- Its main use is in assessing long-term control in diabetic patients with haemoglobinopathies (e.g. β-thalassaemia major and sickle cell disease).

### Continuous glucose monitoring system (CGMS)

Now standard of care in many countries
Can be:
- blinded/retrospective
- real time
- intermittently scanned or viewed.

### Indications

- Assessing the impact of any adjustment in therapy
- Achieving tighter blood glucose control without producing hypoglycaemia
- Diagnosing and/or prevention of hypoglycaemia during sleep or hypoglycaemic unawareness

- Quantifying the response in clinical trials.

CGMS and SMBG produce similar profiles in terms of blood sugars and correlation with HbA1c.

*Advantages*
- Increased density of data
- Better detection of postprandial blood glucose peaks
- Real-time or retrospective data can be produced.

*Disadvantages*
- Lag time of 15 minutes between interstitial glucose (measured in CGMS) and blood glucose, and even longer if blood glucose levels are changing rapidly.
- May overestimate the frequency of low blood glucose levels, especially overnight.
- CGMS is increasingly being used with CSII to provide sensor-augmented pump therapy (SAPT), with pumps showing real-time blood glucose data from a separate sensor.

The has been English (NICE) guidance[5] in 2016 regarding the use of SAPT (specifically the integrated Minimed Paradigm Veo® insulin pump and CGMS), under the care of an appropriately experienced and trained multi-disciplinary team. The patient should use the sensors for at least 70% of the time, and also have a structured education programme on diet and lifestyle, and counselling.

CGMS in both patients using CSII and MDI has been shown to improve HbA1c without increasing the number of severe hypoglycaemic episodes.

Real-time CGMS with alarms should be offered to children with:
- frequent and severe hypoglycaemia
- impaired awareness of hypoglycaemia
- inability to recognize or communicate regarding hypoglycaemic symptoms.

Real-time CGMS should also be considered in:
- neonates, infants, and preschool children
- those having high levels of physical activity
- those with comorbidities (e.g. anorexia nervosa) or on treatment which may affect blood glucose control.

Intermittent (real-time or retrospective) CGMS may help improve blood glucose control in those struggling with hyperglycaemia despite additional support and insulin adjustment.[1]

### Flash glucose scanning

A sensor is worn on the upper arm for up to 14 days, and although continuous readings or alarms are not provided, the previous 8 hours of glucose levels can be shown by scanning. There is currently one system available, the Freestyle Libre®. Unlike other sensors for blinded or real-time CGMS this does not require recalibration against fingertip glucose monitoring.

An implantable sensor (Eversense XL®) which gives readings for up to 180 days is now licensed in patients >18 years of age.

*Non-invasive glucose monitoring*

This remains one of the 'holy grails' of diabetes.

A number of technologies including iontophoresis and other ways of drawing glucose through the skin, near infrared, and other spectroscopies have been attempted but are not currently accurate or commercially viable.

*Ketone testing*

Ketones are produced from free fatty acids when there is a lack of glucose due to inadequate intake or utilization inability due to insulin deficiency.

While starvation ketones are produced when the blood glucose is low, high levels of ketones (e.g. 4 to >8 mmol/L in blood (moderate to high in urine)) indicate insulin deficiency and the risk of metabolic decompensation.

- It is recommended that patients should be offered ketone testing strips along with a meter, and be advised to test for ketonaemia if they are ill and/or are hyperglycaemic.[1]
- Some blood glucose meters (e.g. Optium Xceed® (Abbott)) measure both blood glucose and blood ketones.
- In most developed countries, blood ketone testing has superseded urine testing. Moreover, blood ketone testing has been shown to be more cost-effective than urine ketone testing for preventing hospital admission during intercurrent illness.

Ketone testing should be performed:

- during hyperglycaemia for whatever reason, including intercurrent illness
- with symptoms of impending DKA: polyuria, drowsiness, rapid breathing, and abdominal pain
- for avoidance and early treatment of DKA.

Some units also recommend routine ketone testing at breakfast to identify overnight insulin deficiency ('dawn phenomenon').

*Equivalent levels of ketones (rough guide only)*

| Blood (3-β hydroxybutyrate) | Urine (acetoacetate) |
| --- | --- |
| 0.1–0.9 mmol/L | Small |
| 0.2–1.8 mmol/L | Moderate |
| 1.4–4.2 mmol/L | Large |

**References**

1. National Institute for Health and Care Excellence (NICE). Diabetes (type 1 and type 2) in children and young people: diagnosis and management. NG18. NICE, 2015. https://www.nice.org.uk/guidance/ng18
2. National Paediatric Diabetes Audit (NPDA). Annual report 2017–18. NPDA, 2019. https://www.rcpch.ac.uk/resources/npda-annual-reports#downloadBox
3. DCCT Research Group. The effect of intensive treatment of diabetes on the development and progression of long-term complications of insulin-dependent diabetes mellitus. *N Engl J Med* 1993;329:977–986.
4. DCCT/EDIC Research Group. Beneficial effects of intensive therapy of diabetes during adolescence; outcomes after the conclusion of the Diabetes Control and Complications Trial. *J Pediatr* 2001;139:804–812.
5. National Institute for Health and Care Excellence (NICE). Integrated sensor-augmented pump therapy systems for managing blood glucose levels in type 1 diabetes (the MiniMed Paradigm Veo system and the Vibe and G4 PLATINUM CGM system). DG21. NICE, 2016. https://www.nice.org.uk/guidance/dg21

# Hypoglycaemia

⮕ See also Chapter 7.
- This is the commonest acute complication in T1DM.
- The most commonly used definition of hypoglycaemia in children with diabetes is a blood glucose concentration <4.0 mmol/L. This '4 is the floor' in diabetes provides a safety margin, and should not be confused with the lower level of 2.5–2.8 mmol/L used for patients without diabetes. Many would treat a diabetic child if blood sugar is <4 mmol/L if symptomatic, or <3.5 mmol/L if asymptomatic.
- Rapid falls of blood sugar, even if the absolute level is not low, may also produce symptoms, especially in patients with poor control (i.e. high HbA1c).

Hypoglycaemia is commonly subdivided depending on whether the child can self-treat and whether parenteral therapy is required.

## Severity of hypoglycaemia
- *Mild (grade 1):* the patient is aware and can treat themselves.
- *Moderate (grade 2):* the child requires assistance from another person, but oral therapy is sufficient.
- *Severe (grade 3):* the child is either semiconscious or unconscious, and assistance from others is required with parenteral therapy (e.g. IV glucose or IM glucagon). Hypoglycaemic convulsions may also occur.

NB: children <5–6 years old cannot usually self-treat, whatever the circumstances. For this reason mild and moderate hypoglycaemia are often considered together.

## Causes
Mismatch between insulin, food, and exercise may be due to:
- taking too much insulin
- missing or delaying a meal
- vigorous exercise (may occur immediately afterwards, or be delayed by several hours)
- alcohol (especially in excess).

Incidence of hypoglycaemia is higher in younger children, as there is:
- lack of/reduced awareness of hypoglycaemia
- unpredictable food intake
- unpredictable physical activity.

## Symptoms
Symptoms are 2° to autonomic overacting or neuroglycopenia, and also result in behavioural changes, see Table 5.2.[1]

As every child is different, it is important that both children and carers recognize their specific early warning signs, so that hypoglycaemic episodes can be treated early before the blood sugar falls too low.

Although occasional hypoglycaemia is probably inevitable to maintain good blood glucose control (especially in twice-daily and MDI regimens), historically the tighter the glycaemic control, the greater the likelihood of severe hypoglycaemia. In the DCCT, adolescents in the intensively treated group (MDI or CSII) had a ~85% chance each year of a severe

**Table 5.2** Symptoms of hypoglycaemia

| Autonomic | Neuroglycopenic | Behavioural |
| --- | --- | --- |
| Pallor | Headache | Irritability |
| Sweating/clamminess | Confusion | Mood change |
| Hunger | Weakness | Erratic behaviour |
| Tremor | Glazed expression | Nausea |
| Restlessness | Lethargy | Combative behaviour |
| Palpitations | Visual/speech disturbance | |
| | Seizures | |
| | Loss of consciousness | |

hypoglycaemic episode. With newer regimens, even though tighter overall blood glucose control is achievable, there is some evidence that the incidence of severe hypoglycaemia is decreasing.

Hypoglycaemia has three potential adverse effects:
1. the episodes themselves
2. patient and family fear of recurrence of severe hypoglycaemic episodes
3. long-term complications resulting from poor diabetic control in order to avoid hypoglycaemia.

### Nocturnal hypoglycaemia

- ~50% of episodes of severe hypoglycaemia are nocturnal and may be asymptomatic, with children sleeping through the episode. Although daytime exercise is a risk factor, they may also occur after non-exercise days.
- Counter-regulatory homeostatic responses to hypoglycaemia are attenuated during sleep and diabetic patients are less likely to be woken than non-diabetics.
- Overnight profiles show a high frequency of hypoglycaemia, especially if less physiological replacement regimens are used (e.g. twice-daily premixed insulins). This should be considered in patients with low blood sugars pre-breakfast, although rebound hyperglycaemia (the Somogyi phenomenon) may also be seen.
- In addition, nightmares, sweating, and somnambulism may occur in the night, or lethargy, confusion, and headaches on waking.
- Regular nocturnal blood sugar testing or a CGMS may be required to demonstrate hypoglycaemia. It may also be reduced by SAPT with low-glucose suspension, or closed-loop systems.

As the major metabolic fuel of the brain is glucose, hypoglycaemia is potentially damaging, especially to the younger developing brain. Reductions in reading skills and IQ (by 10–20 points) are described in diabetic children, with poor cognitive performance related to:
- age of onset of diabetes (more if diagnosed at <5 years)
- extent of severe hypoglycaemic episodes
- number of hypoglycaemic seizures
- nocturnal hypoglycaemic episodes.

Both hypo- and hyperglycaemia have been shown to produce white and grey matter changes on brain imaging.

Overall in younger children (<5 years) it is felt that optimal glycaemic control involves maintaining the lowest HbA1c level without disabling or severe hypoglycaemia, chronic hyperglycaemia, or DKA.

## Rebound phenomenon

- Also known as the Somogyi phenomenon, after the doctor who first described it.
- Unlike the physiological rise in glucose overnight due to hormonal changes ('the dawn phenomenon'), in this situation overnight hypoglycaemia (which may be asymptomatic) leads to glycaemic rebound with apparent hyperglycaemia on waking.
- Increasing the evening insulin will, if anything, worsen the situation.

The HbA1c may give some indication, with a (relatively) low HbA1c in the face of high blood sugars. Either checking blood sugars during the night or CGMS may be required to distinguish between dawn and rebound phenomena. This is less common now with more physiological insulin replacement, but changes in the timing, dose, and/or type of insulin may be required.

## Hypoglycaemia unawareness

Loss of the usual warning symptoms of hypoglycaemia can occur, leading to sudden loss of consciousness, often with little or no warning, producing considerable anxiety and distress.

- A sudden drop in blood sugar can also bypass the usual warning symptoms.
- Severe hypoglycaemia is 3–6× more common in people with hypoglycaemic unawareness.
- Those with tight control and frequent hypoglycaemic episodes are more susceptible.
- The cause is unclear, but may be related to the frequency of previous hypoglycaemic episodes, with resetting of the threshold for activation of the autonomic nervous system. As a result, autonomic symptoms are lost before neuroglycopenic ones.
- Can be reversed by avoidance of hypoglycaemia for 2–3 weeks.

### Treatment
Initially oral glucose 10–20 g. 10 g of glucose approximates:
- 2 teaspoons of sugar
- 3 sugar lumps
- non-diet versions of Lucozade® 112 mL, Coca-Cola® 90 mL, Ribena® Blackcurrant drink 100 mL or Original 13.5 mL (to be diluted).
  NB: sugar content of some drinks has fallen in the UK following introduction of a 'sugar tax' in 2018
- GlucoGel® (formerly known as Hypostop Gel®); dextrose 40% (10 g/25 g oral ampoule) may also be used.

NB: due to their high fat content, chocolate and milk are not good treatments for hypoglycaemia.

- Recheck blood sugar after 10–15 minutes, and if necessary, hypoglycaemia treatment may be repeated.
- NB: British Society for Paediatric Endocrinology and Diabetes (BSPED)/ Association of Children's Diabetes Clinicians (ACDC) guidance recommends a blood glucose level post-treatment of >4 mmol/L, while ISPAD recommends 5.6 mmol/L.[1,2]
- After initial hypoglycaemia treatment, unless the child is about to eat anyway or on CSII, a snack containing 10–15 g carbohydrate should be given (e.g. milk and biscuits, sandwich, cereal bar) as soon as the child can eat or they may become hypoglycaemic again.

If the child is unconscious or unable to take anything orally, glucagon can be given IM or by deep SC injection in acute insulin-induced hypoglycaemia but is not appropriate for chronic hypoglycaemia. Recommended doses are:

- 0.5 mg <8 years or bodyweight <25 kg
- 1 mg ≥8 years or bodyweight ≥25 kg
- or 10–30 mcg/kg bodyweight.

Alternatively, 200–500 mg/kg glucose, e.g. 5 mL/kg of 10% glucose, may be given IV as a slow bolus. Higher concentrations of glucose are no longer recommended. Because this concentration is irritant, especially if extravasation occurs.

Appropriate treatment of hypoglycaemia should increase the blood sugar by 3–4 mmol/L. The blood sugar should be rechecked repeatedly to check whether additional glucose is required, especially in those who have a reduced conscious level after a severe hypoglycaemic episode.

Close observation is also required during recovery from severe hypoglycaemia, as glucagon (especially) causes rebound hyperglycaemia and nausea and vomiting. Further glucose, either orally or IV (e.g. 10% glucose 1–3 mL/kg/hour) is usually required.

Patients and carers (including at school) should always have immediate access to a source of fast-acting glucose and also blood glucose monitoring equipment. They should also be trained in the identification and appropriate management of hypoglycaemia (including administering IM glucagon).

## References

1. Association of Children's Diabetes Clinicians (ACDC). Management of hypoglycaemia in children and young people with type 1 diabetes. ACDC, 2016. ℛ http://www.a-c-d-c.org/wp-content/uploads/2012/08/Management-of-Hypoglycaemia-in-Children-and-Young-People-with-Type1-Diabetes2.pdf
2. International Society for Pediatric and Adolescent Diabetes (ISPAD). Clinical Practice Consensus Guidelines 2018. Chapter 12: Assessment and management of hypoglycemia in children and adolescents with diabetes. *Pediatr Diabetes* 2018;19(Suppl. 27):178–192. ℛ https://www.ispad.org/page/ISPADGuidelines2018.uk

# Diabetic ketoacidosis

(➲ See also p. 360.)

Pathophysiology

Arises due to:
- absolute or relative deficiency of insulin
- combined effects of the counter-regulatory hormones: GH, glucagon, catecholamines, and cortisol.

Absolute insulin deficiency occurs in:
- patients with previously undiagnosed T1DM
- existing diabetic patients who are non-compliant with insulin therapy
- CSII patients whose pump becomes disconnected (NB: this can occur rapidly).

Relative insulin deficiency occurs in situations of:
- increased counter-regulatory hormones
- stress such as intercurrent illness.

The frequency of DKA at the onset of T1DM varies widely worldwide, with rates of 15–70% inversely correlated with incidence of the disease. In England and Wales it is currently 18.2%.[1]

DKA is more common at presentation in children who are:
- younger (<2 years of age)
- from families with poor access to medical care as a result of socioeconomic status
- from ethnic minorities
- without a first-degree relative with T1DM.

NB: delayed or misdiagnosis is associated with increased DKA risk.

5–25% of patients with T2DM within certain ethnic groups also have DKA at presentation.
- DKA in existing diabetic patients:
  • accounts for ~60% of cases
  • in England/Wales, Austria/Germany, and USA occurs in 5–7% of patients/year; more common in females, ethnic minorities, and those with a raised HbA1c
  • 5% of patients account for >25% of admissions with DKA.
- Infection is the most likely precipitant in the prepubertal child.
- Missed injections, alcohol, or emotional upset are most common causes in the older teenager, usually female.

In existing patients the risk of DKA is increased in children:
- with poor metabolic control or previous episodes of DKA
- who omit insulin
- with gastroenteritis and persistent vomiting who are adolescent and peripubertal (especially girls)
- with psychiatric problems, including eating disorders
- with difficult/unstable family circumstances
- with limited access to medical resources (for whatever reason)
- with interruption of insulin pump therapy (for whatever reason).

## DKA: osmotic diuresis

- When glucose exceeds the fixed maximum for tubular reabsorption (usually 10 mmol/L), this leads to glucose loss in the urine, in turn producing an osmotic diuresis with accompanying water loss.
- Although glucose and water losses are initially compensated for by compensatory fluid intake (polydipsia) this ultimately fails, leading to dehydration and acidosis.

## DKA: acidosis

- Initial insulin deficiency leads to lipolysis.
- Excess free fatty acids overwhelm muscle and liver gluconeogenesis, condensing to form ketone bodies.
- Hydrogen ions are also produced, leading to metabolic acidosis.
- Hyperventilating; so-called Kussmaul breathing may maintain the pH, but lowers the plasma bicarbonate.
- As dehydration progresses, it is accompanied by peripheral circulatory failure and 2° tissue anoxia, leading to anaerobic metabolism and further acidosis.

## DKA: metabolic decompensation

- Vomiting may result from:
  - central effects of ketosis on vomiting centres
  - overdistension of the atonic stomach
  - an underlying illness.
- Vomiting prevents further oral replacement of fluids, leading to a further decrease in circulating blood volume. If untreated, it results in progressive tissue perfusion failure, electrolyte imbalance, coma, and ultimately death.

## Diagnosis

### Biochemical features of DKA

- Hyperglycaemia (blood glucose >11 mmol/L).
  - Some children who have had little carbohydrate intake, or who have been vomiting, may have only a modest increase in blood glucose ('euglycaemic ketoacidosis').
- Ketosis: raised blood ketones (β-hydroxybutyrate) >3 mmol/L.
- Acidosis (venous pH <7.30 and/or bicarbonate <15 mmol/L): based on these, DKA may also be further subdivided by severity:
  - UK guidelines (2015)[2] indicate pH:
    - —≥7.1: mild/moderate DKA
    - —<7.1: severe DKA
  - ISPAD guidance (2018)[3]:
    - —Mild: pH <7.3, bicarbonate <15.0 mmol/L
    - —Moderate: pH <7.2, bicarbonate <10.0 mmol/L
    - —Severe: pH <7.1, bicarbonate <5.0 mmol/L.

The pathophysiology of DKA is shown in Fig. 5.6.

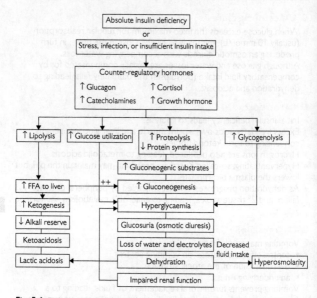

**Fig. 5.6** Pathophysiology of DKA.

Copyright 2006. American Diabetes Association. From *Diabetes Care*, vol 29, 2009; 1150–1159. Reprinted with permission from the American Diabetes Association. Reproduced with permission.

## Symptoms and signs of DKA

- *Hyperglycaemia*: polyuria/polydipsia, 2° enuresis, weight loss
- *Acidosis and dehydration*: abdominal pain, rapid (Kussmaul) breathing, confusion, and coma
- *Others*: nausea and/or vomiting, signs of underlying infection, drowsiness, weakness, and non-specific malaise.

NB: even if euglycaemic, DKA should be suspected if known diabetic patient and any of the following:

- nausea and/or vomiting
- abdominal pain
- hyperventilation
- dehydration
- reduced conscious level.

## Management of DKA

(⊖ See also 'Diabetic ketoacidosis', p. 360 and BSPED DKA guidelines.[2])

### Clinical

- Evaluation to confirm diagnosis and ascertain the cause

- Weigh the patient
- Assess level of consciousness (using the Glasgow Coma Scale (GCS)) and evidence of cerebral oedema
- Evidence of ileus
- Assess severity of dehydration.

*Points*
- 3% is probably the minimum dehydration detectable
- 5% dehydration for mild and moderate DKA
- 10% dehydration for severe DKA.

Most useful clinical indicators of dehydration are:
- prolonged capillary refill time (>1.5–2 seconds)
- abnormal skin turgor
- other useful signs are dry mucous membranes, sunken eyes, and cool peripheries.
- More severe dehydration (~10%) is characterized by:
  - weak or absent peripheral pulses
  - hypotension
  - oliguria.

Initial assessment of ABC: Airway, Breathing, and Circulation.

Children with severe DKA should be considered for treatment in a paediatric intensive care unit. Will also need to seek paediatric critical care/anaesthetic review if the child:
- has a reduced level of consciousness and is unable to protect their airway
- is in hypotensive shock, and may require inotropes.

Successful treatment of DKA requires careful monitoring of the clinical and biochemical response to therapy. The following should be performed:
- hourly (or more frequently if required):
  - vital signs: heart rate, blood pressure, respiratory rate
  - neurological observations
  - fluid input and output
  - capillary blood glucose
  - amount of administered insulin
- 2–4-hourly:
  - electrolytes, glucose, calcium, blood gases
  - blood ketones.

*Fluids*

Patients with DKA are often 5–10% dehydrated (moderate to severe), although it is recognized that subjective assessment of dehydration is often inaccurate. Objectives of fluid and electrolyte replacement are:
- restoration of circulating volume
- replacement of sodium
- replacement of extracellular and intracellular deficit of water
- improved glomerular filtration, enhancing clearance of glucose and ketones from the blood
- reduction of risk of cerebral oedema.

*Principles of fluid replacement*
- It should be commenced before insulin therapy.

- Unlike previous recommendations IV fluid boluses should not be given routinely to children with mild/moderate or even severe DKA.
- If shocked, a bolus of 10 mL/kg 0.9% NaCl should be given. Further boluses should not be given without discussion with a senior paediatrician.
- Subsequent rehydration should be performed evenly over 48 hours, at a rate that does not exceed 1.5–2× the usual daily maintenance.
- Volume expansion should be performed with normal saline, and deficit replacement should be initially with normal saline (N/saline) (Ringer's solution also recommended internationally).
- Unlike previous guidance, N/saline can be given throughout, rather than changing to ½ N/saline. Use 0.9% NaCl with 40 mmol KCl/L until blood glucose levels <14 mmol/L, then add glucose and added potassium. NB: international guidelines[3] still also recommend 0.45% saline.
- If hypernatraemia occurs this should not be problematic, and may protect against cerebral oedema.

NB:
1. IV fluids may not be required in children who are alert, not clinically dehydrated, not nauseated or vomiting, even if they have ketonaemia. These children usually tolerate oral rehydration and SC insulin but require regular monitoring to ensure that they are clinically and biochemically improving.
2. If the child is hyperosmolar with a blood glucose level >30 mmol/L, with little or no acidosis or ketones, this represents hyperosmolar hyperglycaemia. This requires different treatment, and can be very difficult to manage.

*Insulin therapy*
- Although rehydration may cause a fall in blood glucose, insulin therapy is needed both to normalize blood glucose and to suppress lipolysis and ketogenesis.
- As there is some evidence that cerebral oedema is more likely if insulin is started early, IV insulin infusion should be started 1–2 hours after beginning IV fluids.
- Soluble insulin should be infused at a starting dose between 0.05 and 0.1 U/kg/hour until resolution of DKA has occurred. There is no evidence that one of these doses is superior to the other.
- The plasma glucose should fall at 2–5 mmol/L/hour.
- More rapid falls should be prevented by either decreasing the rate of insulin infusion (e.g. to 0.05 U/kg/hour) or increasing the strength of the glucose solution (e.g. to 10%).

NB:
- Bolus doses of IV insulin should not be given.
- If on CSII (insulin pump), the pump should be stopped when starting IV insulin.
- If on long-acting insulin (especially glargine (Lantus®)), this may be continued in addition to the IV insulin infusion, to shorten the length of stay on recovery from DKA.

*Potassium replacement*

- Children with DKA usually have a potassium deficit of 3–6 mmol/kg.
- Despite total body depletion, movement of potassium from the intracellular to the extracellular space may produce hyperkalaemia, while other mechanisms such as vomiting or $2°$ hyperaldosteronism may produce hypokalaemia.
- Administration of insulin and correction of acidosis promotes movement of potassium into cells, and serum potassium levels may fall precipitously, producing cardiac arrhythmia.
- All fluids (except any initial boluses) should contain 40 mmol/L KCl, unless there is evidence of renal failure.
- If hypokalaemia ($K^+$ <3 mmol/L) develops, consider:
  - temporarily suspending the insulin infusion
  - insertion of a central venous catheter, which is required for higher concentrations of KCl.
- If the patient is hyperkalaemic, potassium replacement can be delayed until the patient has passed urine. Most would use a potassium concentration of 40 mmol/L in the rehydration fluids.

NB: international guidance[3] recommends replacement therapy whatever the potassium level is, unless there is renal failure.

*Phosphate*

- As with potassium, there is phosphate depletion in patients with DKA.
- In addition, phosphate levels fall after onset of therapy, stimulated by insulin which promotes passage of phosphate into the cell.
- Despite this, studies have shown no benefit of phosphate replacement in DKA. Rather, there is evidence that it may induce hypocalcaemia.

*Acidosis*

- The severe acidosis of DKA can usually be readily reversed by appropriate administration of fluid and also by insulin replacement.
- Bicarbonate administration shows no benefit and may cause paradoxical CNS acidosis.

NB:

- The 2015 UK guidelines[2] state that bicarbonate should *not* be given IV in DKA.
- International guidelines (2018)[3] indicate that very occasionally bicarbonate may be appropriate in patients with life-threatening hyperkalaemia or severe acidosis (pH <6.9) compromising cardiac contractility. If bicarbonate is considered absolutely necessary, cautious administration of 1–2 mmol/kg over 60 minutes should be considered.

## Complications of DKA

- Cerebral oedema
- Hypoglycaemia
- Hypokalaemia
- Inadequate rehydration
- Hyperchloraemic acidosis.

The mortality rate for DKA is 0.13–0.3%:

- Cerebral oedema accounts for 60–90% of all DKA deaths.

*Cerebral oedema*

Although rare (0.68% of cases of DKA), cerebral oedema has a high mortality rate (21–24%), with significant morbidity in 10–25%. Increased risk of cerebral oedema occurs with:

- younger age
- new onset of diabetes
- longer duration of symptoms.

Other predictors of cerebral oedema:

- *At presentation*:
  - more severe acidosis
  - hypocapnia, even after adjustment of acidosis
  - raised urea.
- *During therapy*:
  - attenuated rise in serum sodium
  - bicarbonate therapy for acidosis
  - increased volumes of fluid given in the first 4 hours
  - administration of insulin in the first hour of fluid treatment.

NB: cerebral oedema often occurs during recovery from DKA.

*Symptoms*

- Headache, lethargy, and failure to regain consciousness.

*Warning signs*

- Headache
- Bradycardia
- Hypertension
- Neurological: restless, irritability, drowsiness, incontinence
- Reduction in oxygen saturation.

*Late signs*

- Papilloedema
- Convulsions
- Respiratory arrest.

All carry very poor prognosis.

If cerebral oedema is suspected, treat immediately with the most readily available of:

- mannitol (20% 0.5–1 g/kg over 10–15 minutes) or
- hypertonic saline (2.7% or 3% 2.5–5 mL/kg over 10–15 minutes).

Fluids should be restricted to half maintenance rates.

Inform senior staff immediately and seek specialist advice.

- Intubation and ventilation should not be carried out until an experienced doctor is available.
- Once the child is stable, exclude alternative diagnoses by CT scan, as other intracerebral events may occur and present similarly.
- A further dose of mannitol may be given after 2 hours if no response.

*Other complications*

*Hypoglycaemia and hypokalaemia*

- Regular monitoring and adjustment of infusion.

*Aspiration pneumonia*
- A nasogastric tube may be required in a child who is vomiting, especially if consciousness is impaired.
▶ Antibiotics are not routinely given.

## Hyperosmolar hyperglycaemic state (HHS)

Previously known as hyperosmolar non-ketotic coma (HONK).

May be found in T1DM, T2DM, and 6q24-related neonatal diabetes. Consists of a triad of:

1. marked hyperglycaemia (blood sugar >33.3 mmol/L or more)
2. severe dehydration but no significant acidosis or hyperketonaemia (pH >7.25, bicarbonate >15 mmol/L)
3. hyperosmolar state (plasma osmolality usually >320 mOsmol/kg or more).

NB: altered consciousness and seizures.

### Treatment

*Fluids*
- Fluid replacement should be more rapid than in DKA, aiming for a decrease in serum sodium of 0.5 mmol/L/hour.
- Assume fluid deficit of ~12–15%.
- Initial fluid bolus should be ≥20 mL/kg of N/saline (further boluses may be required) and then fluid replacement of the deficit over 24–48 hours with 0.45–0.75% NaCl plus added potassium.[4]

*Insulin therapy*
- Early insulin administration is unnecessary as fluids alone cause a fall in blood glucose.
- If the glucose falls rapidly (>5 mmol/L/hour) then glucose (2.5–5%) may need to be added to the replacement fluids.
- Insulin should be instituted when the blood sugar is no longer falling at >3 mmol/L. Low-dose insulin infusion (0.025–0.05 U/kg/hour) can be used initially.[4]

### References

1. National Paediatric Diabetes Audit (NPDA). Annual report 2017–18. NPDA, 2019. ℘ https://www.rcpch.ac.uk/resources/npda-annual-reports#downloadBox
2. British Society for Paediatric Endocrinology and Diabetes (BSPED). BSPED recommended guideline for the management of children and young people under the age of 18 years with diabetic ketoacidosis 2015. BSPED, 2015. ℘ https://www.bsped.org.uk/media/1629/bsped-dka-aug15_.pdf
3. International Society for Pediatric and Adolescent Diabetes (ISPAD). Clinical Practice Consensus Guidelines 2018. Chapter 11: Diabetic ketoacidosis and hyperglycemic hyperosmolar state. *Pediatr Diabetes* 2018;19(Suppl. 27):155–177. ℘ https://www.ispad.org/page/ISPADGuidelines2018
4. Ng SM, Edge JA. Hyperglycaemic hyperosmolar state (HHS) in children: a practical guide to management. *Paediatrics and Child Health* 2017;17:S1751–7222.

# Diabetic management

## Diabetes teams

Current guidelines are that children with diabetes mellitus should be managed in 2°/3° care by specialist multidisciplinary teams.

- The management team involves:
  - the child
  - their family
  - paediatric diabetologist or paediatrician 'with an interest' in diabetes
  - paediatric diabetes specialist nurse (PDSN) or paediatric diabetes nurse (PDN) educator
  - dietician
  - psychological support
  - social worker.

Current international recommendations[1] are that in order to obtain sufficient experience the clinic should contain at least 150 patients.

Suggested recommendations for staffing per 100 diabetic patients are:

- 0.75–1.0 paediatric diabetologist
- 1.0–1.25 PDSN/PDN educator
- 0.5 dietitian
- 0.3 social worker/psychologist.

Structured educational programmes need to be tailored and individualized, bearing in mind factors such as:

- Personal preferences
- Emotional well-being
- Age and maturity
- Cultural considerations
- Existing knowledge
- Current/future social circumstances
- Life goals.[2]

## Home or hospital management?

The principles of initial diabetes management are teaching:

- the child and family how to inject insulin
- the child and family how to perform blood glucose monitoring
- dietary modification to adhere to a diet containing healthy food choices.

Since most children with T1DM do not need hospital admission at diagnosis for medical reasons, if suitable facilities are available then home care from diagnosis can be offered, based on:

- availability of well-trained staff
- time of presentation
- individual family circumstances
- parental choice.

There are also intermediate options for these patients, such as ambulatory care whereby the patient only attends the hospital for injections.

Hospital management at diagnosis should be offered:

- to children <2 years of age
- if there are factors (including social or emotional) which would make home-based management inappropriate, or
- if children live far from the hospital.

A UK survey in 2010, however, indicated that only 28% of units offered home management from diagnosis.

### Follow-up

- Routine visits need to be at least 3-monthly, with evidence that more frequent follow-up by the multidisciplinary team are associated with better metabolic control (using HbA1c) than fewer visits (e.g. once or twice per year).
- Annual visits need to include:
  - expanded physical assessment
  - additional self-management assessments
  - comorbidity and long-term risk factors screening.
- Emergency 24-hour support (at least by telephone) needs to be provided to all patients.

## Infection and 'sick day' management

- There is no evidence that children with well-controlled diabetes have more infections and illness than children without diabetes.
- Poorly controlled diabetes may result in increased susceptibility to infection because of reduced neutrophil phagocytosis 2° to hyperglycaemia.

The effect of intercurrent illness on blood sugars may be:

- an increase, e.g. viral or bacterial infections, through secretion of counter-regulatory hormones, and also gluconeogenesis
- a decrease, e.g. vomiting and/or diarrhoeal infections, with poor food intake
- no effect, e.g. trivial intercurrent illness.

## Management

Children and their families need to be provided with clear advice about managing T1DM during intercurrent illness or episodes of hyperglycaemia ('sick-day rules'), including:

- regular monitoring of blood glucose
- monitoring and interpreting blood ketones
- adjusting insulin regimen and food and fluid intake
- when and where to seek further advice or help.

### General principles

- Treatment of underlying illness
- Providing adequate nutrition and hydration
- Avoidance of hypoglycaemia and DKA.

### Specific principles

1. *Close contact with the diabetes team.*
2. *Monitoring of glucose and ketones.*
   - Frequent assessment of blood glucose and ketones (urine and/or blood). Even if the child does not feel like eating, insulin should *never* be stopped. Insulin doses often need adjustment (both up and down) dependent on blood glucose and ketone levels.

   NB:

- Check blood ketone levels whenever a child is ill, regardless of blood glucose level, as these may be elevated even if the blood glucose is normal, e.g. in gastroenteritis.
- If ketones are present when blood glucose is low, these represent starvation ketones and respond to drinking extra sugar containing fluids. Extra insulin may be required when the blood glucose starts rising.

3. *Insulin (BSPED/ACDC guidance (2018)[3]).*
   - Give additional fast-acting insulin every 2 hours if blood glucose is above target.
     - If ketones <0.6 mmol/L, then give the usual correction insulin dose.
     - If ketones are 0.6–1.5 mmol/L, then advise giving 10% of total daily dose of insulin (TDD), or 0.1 U/kg, as additional fast-acting insulin.
     - If ketones are >1.5 mmol/L, then advise giving 20% of TDD, or 0.2 U/kg as additional fast-acting insulin.
   - The same principles apply to patients on insulin pumps. Even when unwell, if blood glucose levels remain high, standard checks should be made for pump occlusions, disconnection, battery failures, etc.

4. *Fluids.*
   - Keep well hydrated by drinking plenty of fluids.
   - Water, or sugar-free fluids appropriate in most cases when the blood glucose levels are normal or high.
   - If blood glucose levels are low, glucose-containing drinks or oral carbohydrate are required. Carbonated drinks should be avoided.
   - Hospital referral should be considered if:
     - there is any change in child's response/conscious level or respiration
     - the child is becoming dehydrated
     - parents are not happy to continue home management (e.g. inability to maintain blood sugar)
     - fluids are not tolerated.

UK national[3] and international guidelines[4] are available.

### References

1. International Society for Pediatric and Adolescent Diabetes (ISPAD). Clinical Practice Consensus Guidelines 2018. Chapter 7: The delivery of ambulatory diabetes care to children and adolescents with diabetes. *Pediatr Diabetes* 2018;19(Suppl. 27):84–104. ℘ https://www.ispad.org/page/ISPADGuidelines2018

2. National Institute for Health and Care Excellence (NICE). Diabetes (type 1 and type 2) in children and young people: diagnosis and management. NG18. NICE, 2015. ℘ https://www.nice.org.uk/guidance/ng18

3. British Society for Paediatric Endocrinology and Diabetes (BSPED). Management of type 1 diabetes mellitus during illness in children and young people under 18 years (sick day rules). BSPED/ACDC, 2018. ℘

4. International Society for Pediatric and Adolescent Diabetes (ISPAD). Clinical Practice Consensus Guidelines 2018. Chapter 13: Sick day management in children and adolescents with diabetes. *Pediatr Diabetes* 2018;19(Suppl. 27):193–204. ℘ https://www.ispad.org/page/ISPADGuidelines2018

# Other problems

Exercise

- Diabetic patients probably do similar amounts of exercise compared with non-diabetic counterparts.
- Although exercise is encouraged, there is little published information on its metabolic effects in diabetes. Due to its effect on long-term cardiovascular disease, all diabetic patients should, however, be encouraged to exercise regularly. They should be able to take part in all forms of exercise as long as appropriate attention is paid to insulin and dietary management.

The glucose response to exercise is based on both duration and intensity:

- anaerobic exercise may last seconds but may increase blood sugar for 30–60 minutes due to glucagon and epinephrine release
- aerobic exercises lowers blood sugar both during and afterwards.

Strategies need to be put in place to avoid hypo- and/or hyperglycaemia both during and after physical activity. Nearly all exercise >30 minutes will require adjustment to food and/or reduction in insulin.

- Mild/moderate exercise may produce hypoglycaemic unawareness through blunting of counter-regulatory hormones.
- Exercise should however be avoided if pre-exercise blood sugars are >14 mmol/L with ketones >0.5 mmol/L.

*Practicalities*

- A mixed meal containing fats, protein, and carbohydrate should be consumed 3–4 hours prior to exercise or competition to allow digestion and maximize energy stores.
- Carbohydrate-based foods should be available both during and after exercise. In addition, carbohydrate is also required before exercise if glucose levels are <7 mmol/L.

Regular blood glucose testing both before and during exercise can enable:

- appropriate changes to be made in insulin and food intake
- identification of glycaemic response to different amounts and periods of exercise, as hypoglycaemia may occur several hours after prolonged exercise.

NB: a there is a time lag between blood and interstitial levels, CGM may misrepresent true dynamic changes in blood glucose concentrations.

- Short-term exercise is best managed by ingestion of additional carbohydrate, while for exercise >30 minutes there should also be reduction in rapid insulin (e.g. ~25–75%).
- Consensus guidelines recommend 1–1.5 g carbohydrate/kg/hour during peak insulin action; often given in beverage form if pre-exercise insulin is not reduced. If blood sugar is <7 mmol/L, additional treatment may be required.
- Late hypoglycaemia (including nocturnal) may occur many hours post exercise and reflect depleted glycogen stores.

## Travelling

This can be challenging, especially when involving:

- changing time zones (especially if on twice-daily insulin)
- increased physical activity and exercise
- different climate (both hot and also cold weather)
- travel to areas with limited access to health resources.

Prior to any trip a travel plan needs to be organized with the diabetes team. A covering letter is also required to explain the medical condition and to allow supplies through Customs.

NB: medical supplies need to be carried as hand luggage in an insulated container, and it is also recommended that duplicate supplies are carried in the event of any accident.

NB: more frequent blood glucose measurement is required, especially during travel and 24 hours after arrival.

## Immunization

It is recommended that diabetic patients are routinely immunized and that they should also receive:

- influenza vaccine yearly above the age of 6 months
- pneumococcal vaccine.

## Fasting and feasting

- In religions such as Judaism and Islam, periods of fasting are held, often with subsequent feasting.
- In the Jewish faith, where characteristically fasting occurs for 24 hours, children and those who are unwell are exempt, but adolescents are not.
- In the Muslim faith, Ramadan lasts for 30 days, with periods of strict fasting (no food or drink) for 11–19 hours. As with the Jewish faith, children and those who are unwell are exempt.
- It is usually recommended that diabetic patients who wish to fast should be on MDI. Reduction in basal bolus insulin may be required, with increases in rapid-acting insulin to cover feasting.

## Surgery

Optimal management includes:

- adequate hydration
- maintenance of normoglycaemia, with minimization of hypo- and hyperglycaemia.

### Recommendations

*Preoperatively*

- Whenever possible, surgery on children and adolescents with diabetes should be performed in centres with appropriate facilities and personnel to care for children with diabetes.
- To ensure the highest levels of safety, careful liaison is required between surgical, anaesthetic, and children's diabetes care teams before admission to hospital for elective surgery, and as soon as possible after emergency surgery.

- Elective surgery should be scheduled as the first case on a surgical list, preferably in the morning. It should be postponed if glycaemic control is poor, and if necessary admission to hospital for stabilization may be required.

NB: for T2DM, metformin should be discontinued:
- 24 hours before major surgery
- on the day for minor surgery

and other hypoglycaemic agents on the day of surgery.

*Perioperatively*
- IV access, infusion of glucose, and frequent blood glucose monitoring is essential in all situations when general anaesthesia is given, to maintain the blood sugar between 5 and ~10 mmol/L. 5% glucose is usually sufficient, although 10% may be necessary where there is risk of hypoglycaemia.
- Elevated blood ketone (beta-hydroxybutyrate ($\beta$-OHB)) and blood glucose concentrations require extra insulin and possibly IV fluids for correction, with consideration of delaying and rescheduling an elective surgical procedure.

*Postoperatively*
- Once the child is able to tolerate normal nutrition then the usual diabetes regimen should be recommenced.
- Centres performing surgical procedures on children with diabetes should have available written protocols for operative management on the wards where children are admitted. UK national[1] and international guidelines[2] are available.

## Nutrition and diabetes
- Patients and their carers/families should be supported to develop a good understanding of nutrition and its effect on their diabetes.
- Children with T1DM have similar nutritional requirements as other children, and require sufficient calories and nutrients for growth and development.
- Healthy eating (including low glycaemic index (GI) foods, fruit and vegetables, and appropriate types and amounts of fats) is recommended, also for their effect on reducing cardiovascular disease risk, and in the case of low GI foods, hyperglycaemia.
- Patients should be encouraged to eat a minimum of five portions of fruit and vegetables daily.
- The UK national 2016 guidance (NICE)[3] is that level 3 carbohydrate counting from diagnosis (including of snacks) with adjustment of insulin dosage according to agreed insulin:carbohydrate ratios should be used in those on MDI and CSII, with regular updates, and dietary advice should also be provided in those changing their insulin regimen.

Principle:
- Total energy intake needs to be adequate to promote optimal growth, development, and health, but not so excessive as to produce obesity.

Encourage:
- sensible and healthy eating, with a low-fat, high complex-carbohydrate diet

- patients to achieve and maintain an ideal body weight
- patients to maintain optimal blood glucose control:
  - to prevent and also treat acute complications of diabetes, both hypoglycaemia and also hyperglycaemia
  - long term to prevent micro- and macrovascular complications of diabetes.

Total energy requirement should be distributed roughly as follows:
- carbohydrate 45–50%
- fat <35%:
- protein 15–20%.

*Carbohydrate*
- Given as complex and unrefined high-fibre, low-GI carbohydrate, with reduced refined sugar intake.
- Non-starch polysaccharides may be soluble or insoluble.
- Complex carbohydrate with soluble fibre (e.g. vegetables, fruits, and oats) has a low GI, reducing the speed of carbohydrate absorption and rapid rise in blood sugar. This may improve both glycaemic control and lipid metabolism.
- No more than 10% of total calories should be taken as refined carbohydrate (sucrose).
- While calorie-free artificial sweeteners can be used, especially for diet fizzy drinks, there are worries that they produce a 'sweet tooth'. In addition, many bulk sweeteners, such as sorbitol, have a laxative effect when consumed in large amounts.
- In order to match carbohydrate intake to insulin requirement, various assessments of carbohydrate are used; grams, portions/servings, or exchanges. This is needed when intensive insulin regimens are used (e.g. MDI and CSII), where quantification of carbohydrate is required to tailor the short-acting insulin dose (e.g. 1–2 units of short-acting/rapid analogue insulin per 10 g carbohydrate).
- For patients on twice-daily insulin (especially with a short-acting component rather than a rapid-acting analogue), frequent and regular carbohydrate intake, including snacks, is required to reduce the risk of hypoglycaemia postprandially.
- In addition, extra carbohydrate (both short acting and complex) is required to cover exercise and sport.

*Fat*
- Should contain <10% saturated fat.
- Reductions from infantile proportions of fat (~50% of total) occur variably from 2–5 years of age depending on recommendations.
- Unsaturated fatty acids containing omega-3 may be beneficial in T1DM: recommendations are to consume oily fish twice a week (80–120 g).

*Protein*
- Since animal protein is often associated with increased fat (especially unsaturated fat), consumption of large amounts is not recommended.

- If microalbuminuria or nephropathy occurs, further reductions may be required.

NB: some centres internationally not only count carbohydrate but also protein and fat in assessing insulin requirements when using CSII. One fat–protein unit (FPU) = 100 kcal of fat or 115–134 kcal of protein, and is equivalent in terms of insulin to 10 g of carbohydrates.

*Other nutritional intake*

- Although the benefits of various trace elements have been promoted in diabetes (e.g. chromium, vanadium), there is no evidence that additional supplementation with vitamins, minerals, or trace elements is required unless there is significant nutritional deficiency.
- As vegetables and fruits are a natural source of antioxidants, their use in diabetes is encouraged. As with other children, at least five portions of fruit and vegetables are recommended in diabetics as these may provide some protection against long-term cardiovascular disease.

## References

1. Association of Children's Diabetes Clinicians (ACDC). Care of children under 18 years with diabetes mellitus undergoing surgery. ℔ http://www.a-c-d-c.org
2. International Society for Pediatric and Adolescent Diabetes (ISPAD). Clinical Practice Consensus Guidelines 2018. Chapter 15: Management of children & adolescents with diabetes requiring surgery. *Pediatr Diabetes* 2018;19(Suppl. 27):227–236. ℔ https://www.ispad.org/page/ISPADGuidelines2018
3. National Institute for Health and Care Excellence (NICE). Diabetes in children and young people. QS125. NICE, 2016. ℔ https://www.nice.org.uk/guidance/qs125/chapter/Quality-statement-3-Intensive-insulin-therapy-and-level-3-carbohydratecounting-education-for-type-1-diabetes

# Autoimmune disorders and diabetes

- Other organ-specific autoantibodies (thyroid, adrenal, antigliadin, gastric parietal cell) are found more commonly in children with T1DM than in the general population (Table 5.3).
- ~ 25% of all patients (children and adults) with T1DM are diagnosed with another autoimmune condition.
- Increased risk of developing other autoimmune disorders is found with:
  - increased age
  - female sex
  - longer duration of diabetes
  - other organ-specific autoantibodies
  - positive family history.

## Coeliac disease

- This occurs worldwide in ~3–16% (average 8%) of patients with T1DM; ~8× the background rate in the general population.
- The difference in incidence may reflect differing levels of the HLA markers DR3 and DQ2.
- It can precede, occur concurrently, or occur subsequent to T1DM. There is a threefold higher risk in children diagnosed with T1DM at <4 years of age compared with those <9 years.
- It is more commonly seen in girls.

Reasons for screening for and treating coeliac disease can be divided into three groups.

**Table 5.3** *IDDM* loci for which susceptibility loci for other autoimmune diseases have been mapped to the same region

| Locus | Other autoimmune disease |
|---|---|
| *IDDM1* | All autoimmune diseases |
| *IDDM2* | Multiple sclerosis |
| *IDDM3* | Coeliac disease |
| *IDDM6* | Rheumatoid arthritis |
| *IDDM9* | Rheumatoid arthritis |
| *IDDM12* | Rheumatoid arthritis, multiple sclerosis, autoimmune thyroid disease, Addison disease |
| *IDDM13* | Rheumatoid arthritis |
| 16q22–q24 | Psoriasis, asthma, Crohn disease |
| 12p; CD4 | Multiple sclerosis |
| GCK | Crohn disease/ulcerative colitis, multiple sclerosis |
| DXS998 | Multiple sclerosis |

Reproduced from Wass JAH, Shalet SM (eds) (2002). *Oxford Textbook of Endocrinology and Diabetes*. Oxford University Press. Copyright © 2002 OUP.

1. Intestinal symptoms: abdominal distention and pain, diarrhoea, vomiting, weight loss
2. Extra-intestinal symptoms: poor growth and short stature, pubertal delay, anaemia, osteopenia
3. T1DM: poor control with unexplained hypoglycaemia and raised HbA1c. A progressive reduction in insulin requirements may also occur.

As many patients (25–50%) may be asymptomatic, the following recommendations are made:

- All T1DM patients should be screened for coeliac antibodies at onset and at least biannually until age 10 or if symptomatic.
- Based on detection of autoantibodies, IgA endomysial antibodies and antibodies against tissue transglutaminase (anti-TTG) are commonly measured. The latter tends to have a greater sensitivity, and the former a greater specificity.
- Even in *asymptomatic* cases, intestinal biopsy should be recommended in patients with positive coeliac antibodies.
- Patients with positive serology should be advised to continue with a diet containing gluten until the results of the biopsy are available. Any biopsy should be done after at least 1–2 weeks on a high-wheat diet. Samples must be properly orientated and read by a trained pathologist.

The UK NICE guidance for screening for suspected coeliac disease (2015)[1] recommends:

'When healthcare professionals request serological tests to investigate suspected coeliac disease in young people and adults, laboratories should:

- test for total immunoglobulin A (IgA) and IgA tissue transglutaminase (tTG) as the first choice
- use IgA endomysial antibodies (EMA) if IgA tTG is weakly positive
- consider using IgG EMA, IgG deamidated gliadin peptide (DGP) or IgG tTG if IgA is deficient.

When healthcare professionals request serological tests to investigate suspected coeliac disease in children, laboratories should:

- test for total IgA and IgA tTG, as the first choice
- consider using IgG EMA, IgG DGP or IgG tTG if IgA is deficient'

and in addition

- 'Only consider using HLA DQ2 (DQ2.2 and DQ2.5)/DQ8 testing in the diagnosis of coeliac disease in specialist settings (for example, in children who are not having a biopsy, or in people who already have limited gluten ingestion and choose not to have a gluten challenge).'

NB: a persistent TG IgA and also HLA-DQA1*0501/B1*0201 are predictive of progression to coeliac disease, even if the initial biopsy is negative.

A gluten-free diet involves restriction of:

- wheat
- barley
- rye
- (oats)

although rice and maize (corn) are still allowed.

In the last England and Wales paediatric diabetes audit from 2017–2018,[2] 5.6% of patients were receiving a gluten-free diet.

While this inevitably produces further restriction within an already restricted diet, despite this, and in the absence of clear supportive evidence, it is recommended that even asymptomatic patients with a positive intestinal biopsy should adopt a gluten-free diet to protect against subsequent GI malignancy (adenocarcinoma and lymphoma) and conditions associated with subclinical malabsorption such as iron deficiency and osteoporosis.

NB: the insulin dose often needs to be increased in T1DM patients with coeliac disease following a gluten-free diet.

## Thyroid disease: hypothyroidism

- Thyroid autoantibodies, (specifically thyroid microsomal antibodies) are found in ~20–30% of children with T1DM and:
  - are more commonly seen in girls
  - commonly emerge during puberty
  - are associated with presence of GAD antibodies.
- Although thyroid antibodies are predictive (risk ratio = 25) for development of hypothyroidism (compensated or clinical), their absence does not exclude later development of thyroid disease.
- Either a visible or a palpable goitre may be found in up to 20%.
- Hypothyroidism (1°) occurs in 3–8% of children with T1DM, and is usually due to Hashimoto's thyroiditis. Degrees of compensated hypothyroidism may be seen in a further 1–10%.
- The symptomatology is not affected by underlying T1DM, and the development of hypothyroidism does not appear to have significant overall metabolic consequences apart from an increased risk of hypoglycaemia.
- Current recommendations are for annual (NICE)[1] and alternate-year (ISPAD)[3] thyroid function tests (with additional confirmatory thyroid antibodies). Guidelines also recommend thyroid antibody screening at diagnosis.

## Hyperthyroidism

- Although diagnosed much less frequently than 1° hypothyroidism, hyperthyroidism occurs more commonly in T1DM (0.5–6% of patients) than the background rate in the general population.
- Hyperthyroidism may precede T1DM, and vice versa, as well as present concurrently.
- May be due to Graves' disease or be the hyperthyroid phase of Hashimoto's thyroiditis.
- Hyperthyroidism may occasionally be transient.
- Thyroid hormone excess may precipitate hyperglycaemia and DKA by increasing glucose absorption, gluconeogenesis, and peripheral insulin resistance. It also increases lipolysis (thereby increasing circulating free fatty acids).
- The clinical features (weight loss, tachycardia) may mimic clinical features of diabetes and DKA. Unlike hypothyroidism, hyperthyroidism will often have metabolic consequences on diabetic control.

## Adrenal insufficiency (Addison disease)

(⊖ See also Chapter 8.)

- Although antibodies to the adrenal cortex are detected in ~2% of children with T1DM, and various HLA genotypes define high-risk patients, clinical adrenal insufficiency occurs rarely, and routine screening for adrenal dysfunction is not recommended.
- May also be associated with T1DM as part of the autoimmune polyglandular syndromes (APS-1 and -2) (⊖ see Chapter 8).
- It is worth considering when a diabetic patient has:
  - unexplained decreased insulin requirements or hypoglycaemia
  - unexplained weight loss
  - lethargy
  - increased skin pigmentation.

## Vitiligo

- Seen in ~1–7% of children with T1DM
- Patches of depigmentation (leucoderma) occur due to loss of melanocytes.
- Apart from cosmetic camouflage to disguise depigmentation, local (corticosteroids and calcineurin inhibitor) or generalized (ultraviolet B) therapies are rarely effective.
- As vitamin D deficiency commonly occurs as a result of vitiligo it is recommended to check levels in affected patients.
- Occurs in 0.06–1.6%.
- Commonly seen in the pre-tibial area, and consists of well-circumscribed red lesions often with central ulceration occurring in up to 1/3.
- May be associated with underlying microangiopathy such as retinopathy and nephropathy.
- A number of treatments have been tried, with limited benefit.

## References

1. National Institute for Health and Care Excellence (NICE). Coeliac disease: recognition, assessment and management. NG20. NICE, 2015. ℘ https://www.nice.org.uk/guidance/ng20
2. National Paediatric Diabetes Audit (NPDA). Annual report 2017–18. NPDA, 2019. ℘ https://www.rcpch.ac.uk/resources/npda-annual-reports#downloadBox
3. International Society for Pediatric and Adolescent Diabetes (ISPAD). Clinical Practice Consensus Guidelines 2018. Chapter 19: Other complications and associated conditions in children and adolescents with type 1 diabetes. *Pediatr Diabetes* 2018;19 (Suppl. 27):275–286. ℘ https://www.ispad.org/page/ISPADGuidelines2018

# Social problems and diabetes

## Alcohol

- Adolescents with T1DM almost certainly (ab)use alcohol to the same extent as their non-diabetic counterparts.
- While in theory alcohol should produce hypoglycaemia through reduced hepatic gluconeogenesis and depletion of hepatic glycogen stores, in practice the effects are quite variable.
  - Alcohol excess is now considered to be the most common identifiable cause of DKA in male (and female?) teenagers.
  - It is also a major cause of hypoglycaemia and has been implicated in sudden unexplained nocturnal death—the 'dead in bed' syndrome. In addition, when alcohol contributes to hypoglycaemia, glucagon may be ineffective.

For diabetics it is recommended to:

- refrain from binge drinking
- consume carbohydrate both before and after drinking alcohol
- monitor blood sugars regularly and maintain normoglycaemia by consuming carbohydrate-containing foods.
  - Alcohol consumption in adolescents and adults is associated with poorer adherence to insulin.
  - Long-term alcohol excess can lead to weight gain and worsening glycaemic control.

## Drug abuse

Although recent evidence (from 2016)[1] suggests that illicit or recreational drug use is less than in the background population, specific drugs can cause interactions with diabetes:

- Appetite-stimulating effects of marijuana can lead to binge eating and variations in blood glucose.
- Ecstasy is associated with symptoms in teenagers mimicking DKA: dehydration, hypotension, acidosis, and hyperglycaemia.

Moreover, by altering brain function these may increase the risks of mistakes in diabetes self-management.

Drug misuse is more likely in those with psychological disturbance, who are also at higher risk of brittle diabetes. This combination may be lethal.

## Smoking

Smoking is an independent risk factor for nephropathy, neuropathy, retinopathy, and cardiovascular disease. Specifically:

- it increases the risk of urine albumin excretion (both micro- and macroalbuminuria)
- it has an additive effect with diabetes on cardiovascular morbidity and mortality.

Although again recent evidence (from 2014)[1] indicates that diabetic youths smoke less commonly than their peers, those who do smoke should be given assistance with smoking cessation (e.g. nicotine patches, drugs, cognitive behavioural therapy).

### Eating disorders

- Adolescents with T2DM have a higher incidence of disordered eating problems (39.3%) and eating disorders (7.0%) than their non-diabetic peers (32.5% and 2.8% respectively).
- These are associated with poor diabetic control, and increased risk of microvascular disorders, especially retinopathy.
- Diabulimia is a term increasingly being used to describe intentional omission of insulin in order to induce weight loss. This is associated with increased risk of DKA, microvascular complications, and premature mortality.

Early identification (using one of a number of screening questionnaires) is important to enable appropriate support and intervention to be provided.

### References

1. International Society for Pediatric and Adolescent Diabetes (ISPAD). Clinical Practice Consensus Guidelines 2018. Chapter 17: Diabetes in adolescence. *Pediatr Diabetes* 2018;19(Suppl. 27):250–261. ℘ https://www.ispad.org/page/ISPADGuidelines2018
2. Candler T, Murphy R, Pigott A, Gregory JW. Fifteen-minute consultation: diabulimia and disordered eating in childhood diabetes. *Arch Dis Child Educ Pract Ed* 2018;103:118–123.

# Psychiatric problems and diabetes

There is now clear evidence of the importance of the interaction of psychological factors in diabetes control:

- increased risk of psychiatric disorders in children with diabetes (girls more so than boys)
- ~50% of poorly controlled patients, including those with recurrent DKA, have a psychiatric diagnosis, especially anxiety and depression.

Conversely, psychiatric problems are associated with less frequent glucose monitoring and poor glycaemic control. This increased risk is primarily associated with major depression and generalized anxiety disorder.

## Family interactions

These are important in diabetic control. Factors such as:

- close family cohesion
- agreement of management responsibilities
- supportive behaviours

are associated with better diabetes adherence and improved glycaemic control, while factors such as:

- single parent
- lower income
- ethnic minority

are associated with poor diabetic control.

Conversely, development of diabetes can be associated with psychological problems within the family with:

- clinical depression described in ~1/3 of parents of children diagnosed with diabetes in the preceding year
- symptoms of post-traumatic stress disorder recognized in ~1/4 of parents in the 6 weeks after diagnosis of diabetes.

Levels of diabetes-related family support are inversely related to age, with older children and adolescents reporting the lowest levels.

### Interventions
#### Family based

Better adherence with therapy along with improved glycaemic control have been shown following family-based behavioural interventions including goal setting, behavioural contracts, and taking shared responsibility for diabetes care. This is best delivered just after diagnosis, with intervention later showing no improvement in glycaemic control.

#### Individual based

In adolescents, motivational interviewing appears to be beneficial, with improvement demonstrated in QoL and also glycaemic control. This is also shown in group interventions targeting stress management and coping, along with treatment adherence.

Peer-group support has also shown to be beneficial in terms of improving short-term glycaemic control.

NB: there is increasing evidence of the benefit of Internet-based interventions.

*Interactions*

There is evidence that:
- adolescents whose parents are involved in guidance and supervision in their diabetes care have better metabolic control
- parent–child conflict is associated with poorer diabetes outcomes.

NB: patients who do not receive educational input are more likely to suffer diabetes-related complications. In previous studies, such as the DCCT,[1,2] improvement in glycaemic control was gained by both intensification of therapy and frequent, intensive, and continuous educational input.

## References

1. DCCT Research Group. The effect of intensive treatment of diabetes on the development and progression of long-term complications of insulin-dependent diabetes mellitus. *N Engl J Med* 1993;329:977–986.
2. International Society for Pediatric and Adolescent Diabetes (ISPAD). Clinical Practice Consensus Guidelines 2018. Chapter 16: Psychological care of children and adolescents with type 1 diabetes. *Pediatr Diabetes* 2018;19(Suppl. 27):237–249. https://www.ispad.org/page/ISPADGuidelines2018

# Diabetes education

- There is little doubt that the key to successful diabetes care is structured education with a view to self-management.
- Education needs to be provided in a consistent fashion by a multidisciplinary team, with understanding of the changing needs with age, and at post-diagnosis.
- An additional challenge is to find the level of parental involvement which is acceptable to all, and which does not risk deterioration in glycaemic control from over- or under-involvement.

International consensus guidelines[1] have made the following recommendations, with the level and depth of education varying according to age.

## Infants and toddlers

- These are totally dependent on others for all aspects of diabetes care: injections, food, monitoring.
- Parents may feel increased stress, depression, and reduced bonding, which is common in chronic diseases.
- Injections and blood glucose testing may be perceived as giving pain.
- May be erratic feeding and activity levels.
- May be difficulty distinguishing normal infant behaviour from diabetes-related mood swings.
- Hypoglycaemia, especially if severe, can be damaging.
- Care may also be provided outside of the home, e.g. nursery.

## School-age children

- Adjusting from home to school care requires increasing self-efficacy.
- Children start to do their own injections and monitoring (including within the school setting).
- Increasing recognition of hypoglycaemic symptoms.
- Adapting diabetic control/care to school timetable, meals, and exercise (including sport).
- Stepwise handover of parental responsibility to child.

## Adolescence

- Recognizing the importance of continuing some parental involvement, while promoting age-appropriate independence and diabetes self-management.
- Negotiating tasks, goals, and priorities which are understood, achievable, and also acceptable.
- Recognizing that knowledge of diabetes predicts better self-care and metabolic control, although the association is weak.
- Recognition that insulin omission is common.
- Dealing with personal and interpersonal emotional conflicts.
- Teaching strategies for dealing with changes from normal routine, e.g. inappropriate dietary intake, intercurrent illness, hypoglycaemia, alcohol and smoking, drugs, exercise and sport, and sexual health.
- Developing strategies to deal with the transition to adult care.
- Utilizing technology to augment diabetes management.

## Reference

1. International Society for Pediatric and Adolescent Diabetes (ISPAD). Clinical Practice Consensus Guidelines 2018. Chapter 6: Diabetes education in children and adolescents. *Pediatr Diabetes* 2018;19(Suppl. 27):75–83. ℘ https://www.ispad.org/page/ISPADGuidelines2018

# Diabetic complications

## Necrobiosis lipoidica diabeticorum

- An uncommon (occurring in 0.06–1.6%) necrotizing skin condition with well-circumscribed, raised lesions, often red, and with central ulceration.
- Lesions usually occur in the pretibial region.
- The aetiology is poorly understood, but does not appear to be associated with poor diabetic control, although there does appear to be an association with underlying microvascular complications including nephropathy and retinopathy.
- Several different therapies have been tried, often with limited response, including steroids given topically, systemically, or intra-lesionally.

## Hyperglycaemia

- Apart from increasing long-term complications, chronic hyperglycaemia, especially in young males, may produce adverse neurocognitive outcomes.
- Acute hyperglycaemia >15 mmol/L in experimental studies also reduces motor cognitive performance.

## Microvascular and macrovascular complications

There are a number of long-term vascular complications of diabetes, including:

- retinopathy: visual impairment and blindness
- nephropathy: renal failure and hypertension
- neuropathy: pain, muscle weakness, paraesthesia, and autonomic dysfunction
- macrovascular disease, cardiac disease, peripheral vascular disease, and cerebrovascular disease.

## Diabetes Control and Complications Trial

Over recent years there has been a move to improve diabetic control, reducing the incidence of complications. The key trial demonstrating the importance of diabetic control in the development and progression of diabetic complications was the DCCT,[1] which:

- included ~2000 patients with T1DM (~200 adolescents) treated for a mean of 7.4 years
- divided patients into those:
  - without complications (control group)
  - with diabetic complications (background retinopathy)
- randomized patients to treatment with either conventional insulin or intensive therapy (MDI or CSII).

### Key points

- At the end of the DCCT, adolescents treated with an intensive regimen had a mean HbA1c of 8.1% compared with 9.8% in the conventionally treated group, although both were ~1% higher than that seen in equivalent adult groups.
- Risk and progression: reduction in:
  - background retinopathy by 53%

- clinical neuropathy by 60%
- microalbuminuria by 54%.
- Reduction in retinopathy was related to improvement in HbA1c applied across the whole range (Fig. 5.6). A 10% reduction in HbA1c gave a 39% decrease in retinopathy risk, whether the reduction was from 9.0% to 8.1% or from 8.0 to 7.2%.

Compared with the conventional group, the intensively treated group had an:
- increased risk of severe hypoglycaemia (85.7 vs 56.9 per 100 patient-years)
- increased (2.9×) relative risk of obesity.

The trial provided clear evidence of the benefit of intensive insulin treatment, and good control in prevention of development and progression of diabetic complications. Although the control achieved within the DCCT was unachievable for many patients at that time, it also showed that any improvement in diabetic control was beneficial and also that, even after a period of poor glycaemic control, it was worth 'turning things round' although tight control throughout was less (but see following paragraph).

Even though all patients were subsequently transferred to intensive therapy, with subsequent equivalent HbA1c levels between the two groups, the follow-up EDIC study[2] demonstrated there was a metabolic memory for previous intensive therapy, although the benefits of initial intensive therapy on retinopathy had disappeared in adolescents but not adults,[3] emphasizing the importance of maintaining good glycaemic control from diagnosis.

## References

1. DCCT Research Group. The effect of intensive treatment of diabetes on the development and progression of long-term complications of insulin-dependent diabetes mellitus. *N Engl J Med* 1993;329:977–986.
2. White NH, Cleary PA, Dahms W, et al. Beneficial effects of intensive therapy of diabetes during adolescence: outcomes after the conclusion of the Diabetes Control and Complications Trial (DCCT). *J Pediatr* 2001;139:804–812.
3. White NH, Sun W, Cleary PA, et al. Effect of prior intensive therapy in type 1 diabetes on 10-year progression of retinopathy in the DCCT/EDIC: comparison of adults and adolescents. *Diabetes* 2010;59:1244–1253.

# Factors implicated in diabetic complications

Predominantly related to:
- overall diabetic control (⊝ see 'Diabetic complications', p. 200)
- duration of diabetes

although other factors such as
- older age
- puberty

also have an impact.

NB: the prepubertal years of diabetes have relatively less impact on development of complications than post-pubertal years, as for the same duration of diabetes, age and puberty increase the risk of retinopathy and increased albumin excretion (microalbuminuria).

## Diabetic retinopathy

A leading cause of acquired blindness. It may be asymptomatic, especially initially. The onset is related to:
- metabolic control
- age at onset of diabetes
- duration of diabetes.

Adolescents are at increased risk of rapid progression to sight-threatening retinopathy compared with adult diabetic patients. They should therefore be screened for signs of diabetic retinopathy in an attempt to modify any potential risk factors.

### Retinopathy types

Background retinopathy itself is not sight threatening and progression to proliferative retinopathy is not inevitable, especially for milder forms.

*Features of non-proliferative (previously called background) retinopathy*
- Microaneurysms (specific for diabetic retinopathy)
- Haemorrhages (pre-retinal and also intra-retinal)
- Soft exudates (cotton wool spots) involving micro-infarction
- Hard exudates (protein and lipid leakages)
- Intra-retinal microvascular abnormalities
- Constriction and tortuosity of vessels.

May also be subdivided into mild, moderate, and severe based on numbers of microaneurysms and additional features.

*Features of severe non-proliferative retinopathy (previously known as pre-proliferative retinopathy)*
- Vascular obstruction
- Progression of intra-retinal microvascular abnormalities
- Retinal nerve fibre infarction causing cotton wool spots.

*Features of proliferative retinopathy*
- Neovascularization of the retina and/or posterior vitreous
- These vessels may bleed into the vitreoretinal space, producing sight-threatening visual loss
- Adhesions can cause retinal detachment and produce haemorrhage.

Visual loss depends on:
- the extent and location of neovascularization
- signs of vitreous or pre-retinal haemorrhage.

*Diabetic maculopathy/macular oedema* may also occur.

### Assessment of retinopathy

Ideally done on dilated pupils using bimicroscopic fundus slit fundoscopy or stereoscopic fundal photography.

Retinopathy rates are falling from historical levels, ~50% in adolescence and almost 100% in adulthood; in England and Wales in 2018 the rate for abnormal retinopathy screening was 12.8% in diabetics aged 12 years and older.[1]

### Treatment

Macula-sparing laser photocoagulation to the retinal periphery reduces progression of visual loss by >50% in patients with proliferative retinopathy. It is not, however, indicated for mild/moderate non-proliferative retinopathy.

Anti-VEGF (anti-vascular endothelial growth factor) drugs are now increasingly used and show improved outcomes compared to laser photocoagulation; a recent Cochrane review (2018) indicated that one of the three drugs currently used (aflibercept) may be superior to the other two after 1 year.

### Cataracts

Occur in 0.7–3.4% of patients with T1DM, and are seen more commonly in:
- those who present late (especially with high HbA1c at diagnosis)
- females
- adolescents
- those with poor control.

The aetiology is unclear but may reflect increased induction of aldose reductase within the lens.

## Diabetic nephropathy

Renal changes in diabetes occur in five stages:
1. Glomerular hyper-
    a. filtration
    b. trophy
    c. perfusion
2. Increased albumin excretion but within normal range
3. (Micro)albuminuria
4. (Macro)albuminurua
5. End-stage renal disease (ESRD).

(Micro)albuminuria is assessed on a 24-hour or timed urine collection as:
- albumin excretion ratio (AER) 20–200 mcg/minute
- AER 30–300 mg/24 hours.

Pragmatically for screening purposes, early-morning urines for albumin:creatinine ratio (ACR) are used (⟳ see 'Screening for diabetic complications' p. 206).

(Macro)albuminuria is assessed as:
- AER >200 mcg/minute or >300 mg/24 hours

- Early detection of nephropathy and also treatment of hypertension are important in preventing ESRD.

As microalbuminuria can regress and exercise alone can increase AER, repeated samples (e.g. two of three abnormal samples over 3–6 months) are needed to confirm its persistence. Persistent microalbuminuria predicts progression to ESRD and development of macrovascular disease.

In England and Wales in 2017–2018, micro- and macro-albuminuria was found in 10.2% of diabetics aged 12 years and older.[1]

It is also recommended to investigate further if proteinuria is present (ACR ratio >30 mg/mmol).

### Treatment

- Antihypertensive therapy prolongs the time to ESRD. Angiotensin-converting enzyme (ACE) inhibitors are recommended for children and adolescents with hypertension, and have been shown to be both safe and effective. Hypertension tends to have an increased effect in diabetics compared with non-diabetics, and treatment is effective in reducing both cardiovascular morbidity and mortality.
- The protective effect of ACE inhibitors in diabetic patients without hypertension is less well defined, although recent trials such as AdDIT show it to be safe over 2–4 years, albeit with non-significant improvement in outcome measures. There are also concerns regarding potential teratogenic effects.

### Diabetic neuropathy

Both the somatic and autonomic nervous systems can be affected by T1DM, with rates ranging from <10% to 27% in adolescents.

- Somatic neuropathies can be focal or generalized.
- Focal neuropathies include mononeuropathies.
- Polyneuropathy (sensorimotor) is the most common form of generalized neuropathy, involving all types of peripheral nerve fibres (motor, sensory, and autonomic). This form of neuropathy usually presents with sensory loss (stocking and glove), and subsequently motor abnormalities.

Autonomic neuropathy can affect a number of systems (GI, urogenital, and cardiovascular), and presents with:

- hypotension
- vomiting and diarrhoea
- bladder abnormalities
- sweating abnormalities
- heart rate irregularities and prolonged QT interval, which have been implicated in sudden death.

Risk factors include:

- poor diabetic control
- long duration of diabetes
- raised BMI.

### Assessment

Initially involves history taking, with special attention to:

- numbness
- pain

- paraesthesia.

Physical examination should include assessment of:

- tendon reflexes
- vibration sense
- light touch sensation (most easily done using a monofilament).

There are a number of autonomic function tests.

- Assessment at rest:
  - variations in heart rate
  - variations in blood pressure
- Assessment in response to various manoeuvres:
  - standing
  - lying
  - straining (Valsalva)
- Pupillary responses to light and dark may also be used.

Peripheral nerve assessment uses quantification of vibration and temperature senses, together with nerve conduction studies. These are, however, only usually used in a research setting.

While overt signs are uncommon in childhood and adolescence, subclinical signs can be found even shortly after diagnosis.

## Macrovascular disease

- Both morbidity and mortality of cardiovascular disease are substantially increased in patients with diabetes compared with the normal population.
- High blood pressure is also recognized to have a greater impact on diabetic patients than on the normal population.
- Antihypertensive therapy has been shown to reduce both morbidity and mortality in diabetic patients.
- Adverse factors include:
  - a family history of early cardiovascular disease
  - T2DM
  - hyperlipidaemia
  - hypertension
  - smoking.
- The origins of atheroma are in childhood and adolescence, and in diabetic patients coronary atherosclerosis and cardiovascular events are associated with poor diabetic control.
- While well-controlled diabetes is not associated with lipid abnormalities, poor diabetic control is associated with a potentially atherogenic lipoprotein profile.
- Prevalence of raised non-high-density lipoprotein was 25% in diabetics under 21 years of age in one study, with another showing hypercholesterolaemia in almost half of young adults with T1DM.
- In adults, intervention studies in T1DM have shown that statins have a protective effect in terms of major cardiovascular events, stroke, and limb revascularization.
- Long-term data are lacking, although statins appear to be both safe and effective in children and adolescents.

## Reference

1. National Paediatric Diabetes Audit (NPDA). Annual report 2017–18. NPDA, 2019. https://www.rcpch.ac.uk/resources/npda-annual-reports#downloadBox

# Screening for diabetic complications

The aim of screening is to detect complications at a subclinical level, so that therapy can be instituted at an early stage to prevent progression. Guidance for both England and Wales[1] and also internationally (ISPAD)[2] is available

## Recommendations for diabetic screening

### Eye screening

- Initial eye assessment should be performed after diagnosis.
- Screening for retinopathy should also be performed: minimum assessment should be dilated fundoscopy by a trained observer, although digital fundal photography is increasingly being used.
- Retinopathy screening should be performed from 11 years of age with diabetes duration of 2–5 years (ISPAD). If diabetes duration <10 years with good glycaemic control and (at most) non-proliferative retinopathy, then screening can be 2-yearly.
  - In England and Wales, annual screening is recommended from 12 years of age.
- This strategy will capture most patients at risk.
- After institution of retinopathy screening, follow-up should be performed annually.

### Microalbumin

- Screening involves early morning urine or timed urine collections.
- As there is considerable day-to-day variation, at least two of three consecutive collections need to be abnormal to provide evidence.
- ISPAD recommends that screening is performed from 11 years of age with diabetes duration of 2–5 years, i.e. the same ages and durations as for diabetic retinopathy screening. Cut-offs are an ACR on spot urine of 2.5–25 mg/mmol (or 30–300 mg/g) in males, and 3.5–25 mg/mmol (42–300 mg/g) in females.
- In England and Wales, an ACR of >3–30 mg/mmol on three early morning urines is recommended, with annual screening recommended from 12 years of age. Further investigation is recommended if the ACR exceeds 30 mg/mmol.

This will capture most patients at risk of evolving microalbuminuria.

- If microalbuminuria is detected, there should be screening for other diabetic complications.

### Blood pressure monitoring

- ISPAD recommends that screening is performed from 11 years of age with diabetes duration of 2–5 years.
- In England and Wales, annual screening is recommended from 12 years of age.
- Blood pressure should be measured at least annually and compared with age-appropriate centile charts.
- 24-hour ambulatory blood pressure monitoring may be required to confirm the diagnosis.

*Lipids*
- ISPAD recommends that screening is performed from 11 years of age with diabetes duration of 2–5 years, and repeated every 5 years if normal.
- Fasting lipids are the gold standard but not always practical. Non-fasting lipids can be initially obtained, with a subsequent fasting sample if triglycerides and/or low-density lipoprotein levels are raised.

*Foot care*
- Children <12 years of age should be given basic foot care advice.
- From 12 to 17 years of age, NICE guidelines[3] recommend an annual foot care review. If a diabetic foot problem is found, then the patient should be referred to an appropriate specialist.

References

1. National Institute for Health and Care Excellence (NICE). Diabetes (type 1 and type 2) in children and young people: diagnosis and management. NG18. NICE, 2015. ℘ https://www.nice.org.uk/guidance/ng18
2. International Society for Pediatric and Adolescent Diabetes (ISPAD). Clinical Practice Consensus Guidelines 2018. Chapter 18: Microvascular and macrovascular complications in children and adolescents. *Pediatr Diabetes* 2018;19(Suppl. 27):262–274. ℘ https://www.ispad.org/page/ISPADGuidelines2018
3. National Institute for Health and Care Excellence (NICE). Diabetic foot problems: prevention and management. NG19. NICE, 2015. ℘ https://www.nice.org.uk/guidance/ng19

# Type 2 diabetes

WHO defines T2DM as 'characterized by disorders of insulin action and in-sulin secretion, either of which may be the predominant feature'. Previously known as:
- non-insulin-dependent diabetes (NIDDM)
- adult-onset diabetes.

## Epidemiology
- T2DM is the most common form of diabetes in adults, affecting 85–95% of all people with diabetes in the UK.
- There are currently estimated to be 415 million people aged 20–70 years worldwide with diabetes, including 3.6 million people (90% of whom have T2DM) in the UK, with a further 1 million people undiagnosed.
- T2DM usually presents over the age of 40.
- Increased incidence in people of South Asian and African-Caribbean origin, where it often appears after the age of 25 years.

### Children with T2DM
- Initially described in the USA, especially in ethnic minorities.
- Now represents 8–45% of newly diagnosed cases of diabetes in children and adolescents in the USA.
- The first cases of childhood T2DM in the UK were described in 2000. Recent data (2019)[1] indicate 745 affected children in England and Wales.
- There is over-representation of children from ethnic minorities: those of black and Asian origin represented 13.0% and 37.3% of the total, whereas these groups represent 7.5% and 2.2% of the population respectively.
- 9.5% were overweight and 84.6% obese according to International Obesity Task Force (IOTF) guidelines.
- 84% had a family history of T2DM.

## Genetics
There is a strong genetic element:
- almost 100% concordance between monozygotic twins (cf. 30–70% in T1DM)
- increased risk in siblings (~10% compared with ~3% in the general population).
As with T1DM, the rapid rise in T2DM is unlikely to reflect any genetic shift, and environmental factors are implicated.
Investigation of genetic causes of T2DM has involved several approaches.
- Genome-wide scans have identified at least 250 genomic regions predisposing to T2DM, with several of these containing potential causal variants and genes.
- Most of these act by inhibiting insulin secretion, although some have an effect on insulin sensitivity.
- These genes appear to account for only 5–10% of the total genetic susceptibility to T2DM.

An individual polymorphism tends to increase the odds ratio by 1–1.45, although the presence of multiple polymorphisms substantially increases the risk.

## Presentation

- Affected children are usually:
  - overweight or obese
  - female
  - pubertal
  - ethnic minority (usually South Asian in UK) origin
  - with a family history of T2DM.
- Approximately 1/3 have ketonuria at diagnosis, and 5–25% of children subsequently diagnosed as T2DM have DKA at presentation. HHS may also occur.
- NB: given that T2DM commonly presents during puberty, both growth hormone and sex steroids, which increase during puberty and exacerbate insulin resistance, have been implicated. In addition, hyperglycaemia itself may be toxic to the β-cell and cause further pancreatic damage. Insulin resistance means that hypoglycaemia is less common than in T1DM.

It is important to consider the possibility of T2DM in children and young people with suspected diabetes with:

- obesity
- a strong family history of T2DM
- evidence of insulin resistance, e.g. acanthosis nigricans
- high-risk racial/ethnic group (e.g. South Asian or African-Caribbean in the UK)
- no insulin requirement, or an insulin requirement of <0.5 U/kg bodyweight/day after the partial remission phase (honeymoon period).

### Other features

- Normal or high C-peptide levels
- Absent pancreatic autoantibodies.

It is now recognized that T2DM forms part of the metabolic syndrome:

- T2DM/insulin resistance
- hypertension
- hyperlipidaemia
- cardiovascular disease
- adrenarche/PCOS.

## Biochemical features

- Insulin resistance with hyperinsulinaemia is present in the pre-diabetic normoglycaemic state. Evolution of normal to IGT is associated with increasing insulin resistance.
- Insulin secretory failure: failure of the β-cell to continue hypersecreting insulin underlies the transition from insulin resistance to frank diabetes.
- Reduction in food-induced insulin secretion through first-phase insulin release. As a result, postprandial hyperglycaemia is one of the earliest features of T2DM.

Adult data indicate that:

- ~50% of β-cell function has to be lost in T2DM before diabetes supervenes
- fasting hyperglycaemia contributes predominantly to HbA1c as it rises above 7.3%

but

- postprandial glucose levels are more important at lower HbA1c levels.

Frank T2DM is diagnosed using the ADA criteria as for T1DM, although these tests have not been specifically validated in children and adolescents.

NB:

- The OGTT has poor concordance (<30%) between tests performed several weeks apart.
- There is dispute whether an HbA1c of ≥6.5% as used in adults is also applicable to children, although it does appear to be predictive of retinopathy risk as well as glucose abnormalities.

## Management

Complications may already be present at diagnosis due to:

- the insidious onset of T2DM
- a (potentially) prolonged asymptomatic period before diagnosis
- implication of insulin resistance in micro- and macrovascular complications.

In a large adolescent T2DM study in India, at presentation 26.7% had retinopathy, 14.7% microalbuminuria, 14.2% neuropathy, and 8.4% nephropathy.

Glycaemic control should be even tighter in T2DM than in T1DM. In a prospective study of T2DM in adults (UK Prospective Diabetes Study (UKPDS)[2]) reduction in HbA1c from 7.9% to 7.0% produced a 25% reduction in microvascular complications.

### Principles of management of T2DM

- Lifestyle change is central, including promotion of:
  - healthy eating
  - exercise (including 60 minutes of at least moderate exercise daily).
- Diagnosis and treatment of comorbidities.
- An HbA1c level of 6.5% (48 mmol/mol) should be aimed for, with avoidance of severe hypoglycaemia.

### Therapy

Lifestyle changes in adults (including exercise and weight reduction) are unlikely to reduce HbA1c levels by >1%. A number of algorithms for therapy have been produced:

- those from the American Academy of Paediatrics indicate that lifestyle changes should be initiated first, and medical therapy only instituted if HbA1c remains >7%.[3]
- those from ISPAD indicate medical therapy (metformin and/or insulin) along with lifestyles changes dependent on symptomatology, acidosis, and initial HbA1c level.[4]

In the 2018 ISPAD guidelines,[4] if at diagnosis the patient is:

1. asymptomatic, metabolically stable, HbA1c is <8.5% (69.4 mmol/mol), and there is no acidosis then metformin and lifestyle change should be instituted

2. ketotic/ketoacidotic and HbA1c is >8.5%, then insulin (potentially once daily) should be instituted, along with metformin if there is no acidosis. If appropriate, the insulin can be tapered over 2–6 weeks.

The English and Welsh guidelines (NICE, 2015)[5] recommend standard-release metformin to all new patients with T2DM.

The goal of initial treatment is to attain an HbA1c of <7.0% (53 mmol/mol) and even <6.5% 47.5 mmol/mol). If this is not achieved on:

- metformin alone then basal insulin should be added
- combination metformin and basal insulin then prandial insulin should be added.

The optimal insulin regimen is probably MDI using insulin analogues. It is recommended that both pre- and postprandial blood sugars are checked, with a target fasting blood sugar <7.0 mmol/L and postprandial blood sugar <7.5 mmol/L (International Diabetes Foundation (IDF)) or <10 mmol/L (American Diabetes Association (ADA)[6]).

### Oral hypoglycaemic agents

#### Biguanide

Metformin is the first-line drug, as it:

- is an insulin sensitizer, reducing hepatic gluconeogenesis, increasing insulin-stimulated glucose uptake in muscle and adipose tissue, and reducing appetite
- has a low risk of hypoglycaemia
- is cardioprotective
- may normalize ovulatory abnormalities in PCOS.

*Dose of metformin*: starting at 500 mg a day, increasing over 3–4 weeks to 1000 mg twice daily or 2000 mg of extended-release metformin daily is achieved.

Trials have shown reductions of 1–2% in HbA1c during treatment with metformin, although side effects include:

- GI symptoms (nausea, abdominal pain, bloating, diarrhoea), which are unpleasant but self-limiting
- renal and hepatic dysfunction
- lactic acidosis (rarely).

These side effects (especially GI) mean that non-adherence is very high, although gradual increase in dose and slow-release/liquid preparations may reduce this.

Although not licensed in children <18 years of age in some countries, other potential drugs include (with reduction of HbA1c in adult trials in parentheses):

- sulphonylureas (1.5–2.0%)
- glitazones (0.5–1.3%)
- meglitinide analogues
- α-glucosidase inhibitors (0.5–1.0%)
- Incretin mimetics (GLP receptor analogues) (0.5–0.8%)
- (DPP-IV inhibitors)
- (Sodium-glucose co-transporter-2 (SGLT-2) inhibitors)

although there is little evidence of benefit in children.

Current (2017–18) treatments for T2DM in England and Wales are:

- no insulin: 16.9%
- one to three insulin injections a day: 2.6%
- four insulin injections a day: 9.8%
- insulin pump therapy: 0.8%
- oral hypoglycaemic agents: 38.5%
- oral hypoglycaemic agents and insulin: 18.5%
- (missing data: 8.8%).

Gastric surgery is also being increasingly used in obese (>35 kg/m²) children with T2DM and comorbidities, especially where lifestyle and medical therapy has failed. Trials indicate that bariatric surgery can remit T2DM in most children, and achieve better HbA1c levels than that seen with medical management alone.

### Screening for complications

The UK NICE guidance (2015)[5] and also ISPAD (2018)[4] recommend offering children and young people with T2DM annual monitoring:

From diagnosis for:

- hypertension
- dyslipidaemia
- microalbuminuria

and the NICE guidelines[5] recommend screening from 12 years of age for diabetic retinopathy.

### References

1. National Paediatric Diabetes Audit (NPDA). Annual report 2017–18. NPDA, 2019. ℅ https://www.rcpch.ac.uk/resources/npda-annual-reports#downloadBox
2. UK Prospective Diabetes Study (UKPDS) Group. Intensive blood-glucose control with sulphonylureas or insulin compared with conventional treatment and risk of complications in patients with type 2 diabetes (UKPDS 33). *Lancet* 1998;352:837–853.
3. Springer SC, Silverstein J, Copeland K, et al. Management of type 2 diabetes mellitus in children and adolescents. *Pediatrics* 2013;131:e648–e664.
4. International Society for Pediatric and Adolescent Diabetes (ISPAD). Clinical Practice Consensus Guidelines 2018. Chapter 3: Type 2 diabetes in youth. *Pediatr Diabetes* 2018;19(Suppl. 27):28–46. ℅ https://www.ispad.org/page/ISPADGuidelines2018
5. National Institute for Health and Care Excellence (NICE). Diabetes (type 1 and type 2) in children and young people: diagnosis and management. NG18. NICE, 2015. ℅ https://www.nice.org.uk/guidance/ng18
6. American Diabetes Association. 12. Children and adolescents: standards of medical care in diabetes—2018. *Diabetes Care* 2018;41(Suppl. 1):S126–S136.

# Other forms of diabetes

Uncommon. Includes monogenic diabetes, which accounts for 1–6% of diabetes cases in children.

Types

- Genetic defects of insulin secretion: MODY
- Genetic defects of insulin action: leprechaunism, Rabson–Mendenhall syndrome
- Uncommon forms of immune-mediated disease:
  • syndromic: Down syndrome, Klinefelter syndrome, Turner syndrome, Wolfram syndrome (DIDMOAD)
- Diseases of the exocrine pancreas: cystic fibrosis, pancreatitis
- Endocrinopathies: Cushing syndrome, hyperthyroidism
- Drug-induced: thyroxine, steroids, tacrolimus
- Infections: rubella, cytomegalovirus, Coxsackie B.

The possibility of other forms of diabetes should be considered if there is:
- in 'T1DM':
  • diagnosis of diabetes <6 months of age (<12 months if absent ICA)
  • a family history of diabetes which appears to have autosomal dominant inheritance
  • marked insulin resistance
  • substantially reduced insulin requirement outside the 'honeymoon phase', i.e. after 3 years post-diagnosis, especially if confirmed by detectable C-peptide levels
  • absence of islet autoantibodies in T1DM (especially at diagnosis)
- in 'T2DM':
  • patient or family members diagnosed with T2DM who are not markedly obese
  • ethnic background with a low incidence of T2DM (e.g. Caucasian)
  • no evidence of insulin resistance, e.g. clinically no acanthosis nigricans, and biochemically fasting C-peptide within the normal range
- others:
  • associated features suggestive of a syndrome, e.g. deafness, optic atrophy
  • history of exposure to drugs/infections known to be toxic to $\beta$-cells, or which produce insulin resistance.

MODY

A group of monogenic autosomal dominant inherited diabetic disorders, initially described in the 1970s in the UK and USA (Table 5.4).

### Clinical features
- Early-onset disease (usually in the second or third decade)
- Lean body mass
- Impaired glucose secretion.

### Genetics
The first MODY gene was identified in 1992, and there are now at least 14 identified genes producing a MODY-like phenotype, with 3–4 accounting for the majority of cases: 1 for a glucose sensor (glucokinase), and 2–3

**Table 5.4** Differentiation between the main forms of MODY

| | |
|---|---|
| MODY1 (HNF4A) | Rare form of MODY, accounting for 3–5% of cases |
| | Gene located on chromosome 20q |
| | Onset often at puberty or young adulthood |
| | 50% of carriers show macrosomia at birth, and 15% have neonatal hyperinsulinaemic hypoglycaemia which is diazoxide responsive and remits in infancy |
| | Due to β-cell dysfunction |
| | Similar features to MODY3, although lowered renal threshold does not occur and patients tend to present later |
| | Microvascular complications are frequent |
| MODY2 (glucokinase) | Accounts for 10–15% of cases |
| | Gene located on chromosome 7p |
| | Pathophysiology is 2° to β-cell dysfunction and abnormal glucose sensing |
| | Often diagnosed in childhood, or even during pregnancy, with fasting hyperglycaemia (blood sugar 5.5–8.5 mmol/L) which is often stable for months or years. HbA1c often just below or above the upper limit of normal (5.5–5.7%) |
| | Patients do not need to be treated in the paediatric age range, and even in adults can often be treated with meal planning alone |
| | Micro- and macrovascular complications are rare even without treatment |
| MODY3 (HNF1A) | Causes up to 65% of MODY |
| | Gene located on chromosome 12q |
| | Onset often at puberty or young adulthood |
| | Due to β-cell dysfunction |
| | Ketosis does not occur |
| | Similar features to MODY1 although patients may also demonstrate glycosuria at relatively normal blood glucose levels, with a lowered renal glucose threshold. Oral glucose tests at early stages may show a very large glucose increment (often >5 mmol/L), with glucose rising into the diabetic range at 2 hours despite normal fasting values |
| | Marked sensitivity to sulphonylureas, resulting in hypoglycaemia despite previous poor glycaemic control |
| | Micro and macrovascular complications are frequent, with complications occurring at a similar frequency to that seen in T1DM and T2DM |
| MODY4 (IPF1) | Rare form of MODY |
| | Produces relatively mild diabetes |
| MODY5 (HNF1B) | Rare, accounting for <1% of cases of monogenic diabetes |
| | Associated with kidney disease which is often diagnosed first, resulting in renal failure <45 years in half, and diabetes itself rarely occurs. Other abnormalities include uterine and genital developmental abnormalities, subclinical pancreatic exocrine deficiency, hyperuricaemia, and abnormalities in LFTs |
| | Patients are not sensitive to sulphonylureas, and hence require treatment with insulin |
| MODY6 (NEUROD1) | Extremely rare form of MODY |
| | Severity of diabetes unknown as yet |

Further details are available at ℑ http://www.diabetesgenes.org

for transcription factors controlling insulin production from the pancreatic β-cells (*HNF1A, HNF1B, HNF4A*).

MODY accounts for 1.8% of children with non-T1DM, although it is estimated that 80% of cases are misdiagnosed as type 1 or 2 diabetes.

MODY should be considered if:
- diabetes presenting <25 years of age
- apparent monogenic autosomal inheritance, i.e. evidence of diabetes in one parent and ideally that parent's parent
- off insulin or measurable C-peptide 3 years after diagnosis
- absence of severe ketosis.

Other causes of monogenic diabetes have been also described, including insulin promoter factor 1 (*IPF1*), carboxyl ester lipase (*CEL*), ATP-sensitive potassium channel (*KCNJ11, ABCC8*) and neurogenic differentiation 1 (*NEUROD1*).[1]

An online probability calculator is available at ℛ https://www.diabetesgenes.org/mody-probability-calculator/.

In monogenic diabetes, a molecular genetic diagnosis can be made in >80%.

## Neonatal diabetes
- A rare disorder, occurring in around 1 in 100,000–500,000 births.
- May be associated with intrauterine growth retardation (IUGR).
- Pancreatic autoantibodies are rarely found, and HLA antigens are usually protective.

Two different clinical forms are recognized, although initially it may be impossible to distinguish between them.

### Transient neonatal diabetes mellitus (TNDM)
- Occurs in ~50–60% of patients, and resolves at a median age of 12 weeks.
- Macroglossia (enlargement of tongue) may occur.
- Permanent diabetes mellitus later in life may occur in up to 50–60% of this group, usually at puberty although can occur at younger ages.
- ~70% of these patients have abnormalities in an imprinted area within 6q24; in these patients severe IUGR is characteristic.
- Most remaining cases are due to activating mutations in *KCNJ11* or *ABCC8* encoding the two subunits of the ATP-sensitive potassium (KATP) channel of the β-cell membrane, although these are both more associated with permanent forms (see later in topic).
- A small number are also due to mutations in *HNF1B*, which is known to cause MODY5.

### Permanent neonatal diabetes mellitus (PNDM)
- Unlike TNDM, IUGR is less common, occurring in ~1/3 of patients.
- ~20% have neurological features with:
  - developmental delay
  - muscle weakness
  - epilepsy.
- The most severe end of this spectrum is referred to as DEND (Developmental delay, Epilepsy, Neonatal Diabetes).

Around a dozen genes have been implicated, involved in pancreatic development (aplasia of the pancreas may be found), β-cell apoptosis, or development number of different genes:

- In PNDM the most common identified cause are mutations in the *KCNJ11* gene (encoding the Kir 6.2 subunit of the β-cell K$_{ATP}$ channel) and *ABCC8* gene (encoding the sulphonyurea receptor (SUR1)).
- Heterozygous mutations in the insulin gene (*INS*) account for 15–20% of cases; these mutations are not associated with extra-pancreatic features apart from IUGR.
- Homozygous mutations in glucokinase and *IPF1* produce PNDM, (whereas heterozygous mutations produce MODY).

### Management

- As autoimmune T1DM is exceedingly rare at this age, and even in the presence of autoantibodies, all patients should have genetic testing.
- Despite this, all neonates presenting with diabetes should be treated initially with insulin.
- A continuous insulin infusion is often required initially to normalize blood sugars and metabolic decompensation.
- Subsequent treatment using an MDI regimen or CSII is commonly used.
- ~90% of patients with *KCNJ11* mutations can be successfully transferred from insulin to an oral sulphonylurea.
- Although genotype is not always predictive, those with neurological features are less likely to have a good response.

### IPEX

- In this autoimmune condition (*I*mmune dysregulation, *P*olyendocrinopathy, *E*nteropathy, *X*-linked syndrome) diabetes presents <6 months of age.
- Due to mutations in *FOXP3* gene.
- T1DM autoantibodies (GAD, IAA, ICA) may be found as well as those against the thyroid and other organs.

Treatment with immunosuppressive agents (steroids or sirolimus) or allogeneic bone marrow transplant is recommended.

### Other monogenic diabetes conditions

#### Wolfram syndrome

Also known as DIDMOAD: *D*iabetes *I*nsipidus, *D*iabetes *M*ellitus, *O*ptic *A*trophy, and *D*eafness.

- Prevalence is 1 in 500,000, with ~120 patients in the UK.
- Inheritance: autosomal recessive.
- Gene: *WFS1* located on 4p16.1 encodes wolframin protein, which localizes to the endoplasmic reticulum.
- Mutations found in >85% if diabetes mellitus and optic atrophy present <15 years of age.
- Diabetes is non-autoimmune and insulin deficient, is usually the first presenting feature at a mean age of 6 years. Lifelong insulin therapy is required from onset.
- Early death at a mean age of 30 years is usually 2° to neurodegenerative disease.

*Wolcott–Rallison syndrome*
- Autosomal recessive disorder.
- Mutations in the gene *EIF2AK3*, which encodes a protein involved in endoplasmic reticulum stress response, have been identified in families with this condition.
- Diabetes usually presents in infancy and may be the first clinical feature, by presentation may be delayed until as late as 4 years of age.
- Other features include:
  - skeletal dysplasia (spondyloepiphyseal dysplasia)
  - hepatic dysfunction
  - renal dysfunction
  - (mental retardation).

NB: consider in early-onset diabetes in patient groups with high levels of consanguinity.

*Thiamine-responsive megaloblastic anaemia (TRMA) (Roger syndrome)*
- A rare diabetic syndrome associated with:
  - early-onset megaloblastic anaemia (responsive to thiamine)
  - sensorineural deafness.
- Diabetes presents from infancy to adolescence, is insulin deficient and responsive to thiamine in some patients, although all become insulin-dependent long term.
- Deafness does not respond to thiamine.
- Arises from mutations in the thiamine transporter SLC19A2.

Ciliopathy related

*Bardet–Biedl syndrome (BBS)*
( See also Chapter 6, p. 235.)
 Diabetes resembling T2DM occurs in up to 6% in one study, presents in adolescence and adulthood, and appears to be related to the level of obesity.

*Alström syndrome (ALMS)*
( See also Chapter 6, p. 218.)
 Features of insulin resistance plus IGT occur early in childhood, with T2DM developing at a mean age of 16 years.

Others

*Prader–Willi syndrome (PWS)*
( See also Chapter 6, p. 234.)
- Diabetes is increasingly recognized, occurring in 7–20% of adults with PWS.
- The diabetes, which resembles T2DM, is probably due to the gross obesity in these patients, although PWS patients tend not to have the same degree of insulin resistance.
- Insulin release in response to a glucose load is impaired, with increased hepatic insulin extraction.
- No evidence of adverse effects of GH therapy on glucose metabolism.
- Treatment of diabetes is similar to that in T2DM. Glucagon-like peptide-1 (GLP1) agonists/analogues are also increasingly being advocated.

### Mitochondrial diabetes

- Maternal transmission of abnormal mitochondrial DNA can lead to maternally inherited diabetes, although this rarely occurs in the paediatric age range. This form of diabetes is commonly associated with:
  - deafness (sensorineural)
  - short stature.
- The most common mutation is at position 3243 in the tRNA leucine gene, which leads to an A-to-G transition.
- One mutation is identical to that seen in MELAS (Mitochondrial myopathy, Encephalopathy, Lactic Acidosis and Stroke-like syndrome).
- Has a variable phenotype, ranging from an acute onset with/without ketoacidosis, to a more T2DM phenotype with gradual onset.
- Patients have progressive non-autoimmune β-cell failure, and may progress to requiring insulin therapy. Metformin should be avoided as it impacts on mitochondrial function.

### Insulin resistance syndromes: type A insulin resistance, Donohue syndrome (leprechaunism), Rabson–Mendenhall syndrome

Often due to gene mutations within the insulin receptor gene (*INSR*) (homozygous in the latter two conditions) are all characterized by:
- acanthosis nigricans
- hyperandrogenism
- hyperinsulinism, even in the absence of obesity.

The more severe the insulin resistance, and the earlier the onset, the more likely is diabetes to occur.

Treatment of severe insulin resistance is challenging, as insulin requirements are often substantial, with poor glycaemic control and development of long-term complications.
- Insulin sensitizers (e.g. metformin and glitazones) have also been used.
- IGF-1 therapy may also reduce both fasting and postprandial blood sugars.

### Lipodystrophy

Characterized by selective loss of adipose tissue.
- Congenital generalized lipodystrophy (Berardinelli–Seip syndrome) is a recessive disorder due to mutations in either AGPAT2 or BSCL in ~80% of patients. Diabetes usually occurs in early adolescence.
- Familial partial lipodystrophy usually presents post-puberty, and around half of cases are due to heterozygous mutations in *LMNA* or *PPARG*. Diabetes usually occurs in late adolescence or early adulthood, and may respond to insulin sensitizers and glitazones, at least initially.

### Cystic fibrosis-related diabetes (CFRD)

CFRD is associated with:
- increasing age of cystic fibrosis patients, e.g.:
  - <5% in patients aged <10 years
  - ~13% aged 15–19 years
  - >50% aged >40 years.
- female gender.

*Diabetes in CFRD*
- Not autoimmune in origin.
- It is predominantly insulin (and also glucagon) deficient due to scarring and destruction of the pancreatic islets and β-cells, possibly due to thickened exocrine secretions.
- There may also be a degree of insulin resistance, which may be stress (illness) related, or 2° to drugs, e.g. glucocorticoids and $β_2$-agonists (bronchodilators).
- Glucose homeostasis may also be affected by high caloric intake, gut motility including delayed gastric emptying, and liver disease.

*Development of CFRD*
1. Usually postprandial hyperglycaemia (demonstrated on CGM, and also as indeterminate glycaemia during OGTT), followed by:
2. IGT, then
3. overt diabetes.

NB: in the early stages of diabetes fasting blood glucose levels may be normal.

*Presentation*
- Patients may be symptomatic of hyperglycaemia, although many are asymptomatic.
- Poor weight gain, growth, or pubertal failure are also seen.
- Fasting or reactive hypoglycaemia (following OGTT) may occur in up to 15%.
- DKA is rare, as there is usually residual insulin secretion, glucagon is also deficient and there is poor fatty acid metabolism.

*Screening*
- Updated diagnostic criteria were established by the CFRD Guidelines Committee in 2010.[2] This uses the diagnostic criteria of the standard OGTT, with the addition of indeterminate glycaemia (INDET: glucose >11.1 mmol/L mid-OGTT).
- The guidance is that yearly screening should be performed by 10 years of age who have not already developed CFRD.
- HbA1c is not recommended as a screening test, but a raised level may be diagnostic in the presence of hyperglycaemic symptoms. A low or normal level does not exclude diabetes as HbA1c can be spuriously low, due to increased RBC turnover
- CGM may be useful in the management of CFRD, but is not sufficiently accurate enough to be able to make the diagnosis.

*Treatment*
- Although the diabetes is in many ways similar to T2DM, it cannot be treated with diet or oral hypoglycaemics as:
  - calorie intake needs to be maintained to meet the increased metabolic demands of cystic fibrosis; energy levels are characteristically 120–150% of recommended dietary allowances, with 30–40% from fats
  - there is little evidence of the efficacy of oral hypoglycaemics, and they are not currently recommended. Moreover they can exacerbate liver dysfunction, and sulphonylureas interfere with the chloride transporter.

- Treatment is therefore with insulin, although relatively low doses are required (~0.5–0.8 U/kg/day). Whereas 2014 guidance recommended that basal insulin alone may be sufficient if there is no fasting hyperglycaemia, the 2018 guidance indicates that this has now been superseded by frequent short-acting analogue.[3]

*Monitoring*

- Patients should perform SMBG at least three times a day (although for many four to eight is more appropriate).
- Patients should be ideally reviewed every 3 months by a specialist multidisciplinary team with expertise in cystic fibrosis and also diabetes. As microvascular complications have been described in CFRD, it would seem logical to aim for similar glycaemic targets as in T1DM.
- HbA1c should be performed 3-monthly, with a target of <7%.

## Other forms of diabetes

### Stress hyperglycaemia

- Found in up to 5% of children attending A&E departments.
- Acute illness, injury (including traumatic), burns, febrile seizures, and pyrexia >39°C are the most common associated features.
- Progression occurs in 0–32%, with ICA and IAA having a good predictive value for who will and will not develop subsequent T1DM.

### Drug-induced hyperglycaemia

May produce hyperglycaemia through insulin secretion and/or action, or through permanent β-cell damage.

*Steroid related*

- Steroids such as dexamethasone used in neurosurgery (to prevent cerebral oedema) may exacerbate surgical stress. This may be exacerbated by dextrose infusion, especially if large volumes are given for diabetes insipidus.
- High-dose steroids along with L-asparaginase in oncology/haematology patients may produce hyperglycaemia. Often occurs cyclically along with the courses of chemotherapy.
- In transplant patients steroids are often given alongside tacrolimus or ciclosporin. The latter two may also produce permanent diabetes due to islet cell destruction, with the risk greater in patients with pre-existing obesity.

*Others*

- Antipsychotics (e.g. olanzapine, risperidone, quetiapine, ziprasidone), often in association with weight gain.

### References

1. McDonald TJ, Ellard S. Maturity onset diabetes of the young: identification and diagnosis. *Ann Clin Biochem* 2013;50:403–415.
2. Moran A, Brunzell C, Cohen RC, et al. Clinical care guidelines for cystic fibrosis-related diabetes. *Diabetes Care* 2010;33:2697–2708.
3. International Society for Pediatric and Adolescent Diabetes (ISPAD). Clinical Practice Consensus Guidelines 2018. Chapter 5: Management of cystic fibrosis-related diabetes in children and adolescents. *Pediatr Diabetes* 2018;19(Suppl. 27):64–74. ℘ https://www.ispad.org/page/ISPADGuidelines2018

# Further reading

Atkinson MA. The pathogenesis and natural history of type 1 diabetes. *Cold Spring Harb Perspect Med* 2012;2:pii: a007641.

Atkinson MA, Bluestone JA, Eisenbarth GS, et al. How does type 1 diabetes develop? The notion of homicide or β-cell suicide revisited. *Diabetes* 2011;60:1370–1379.

Barbetti F, D'Annunzio G. Genetic causes and treatment of neonatal diabetes and early childhood diabetes. *Best Pract Res Clin Endocrinol Metab* 2018;32:575–591.

International Society for Pediatric and Adolescent Diabetes (ISPAD). Clinical Practice Consensus Guidelines 2018. Chapter 1: Definition, epidemiology, diagnosis and classification of diabetes in children and adolescents. *Pediatr Diabetes* 2018;19(Suppl. 27):7–19. ♫ https://www.ispad.org/page/ISPADGuidelines2018

International Society for Pediatric and Adolescent Diabetes (ISPAD). Clinical Practice Consensus Guidelines 2018. Chapter 2: Stages of type 1 diabetes in children and adolescents *Pediatr Diabetes* 2018;19(Suppl. 27):20–27. ♫ https://www.ispad.org/page/ISPADGuidelines2018

International Society for Pediatric and Adolescent Diabetes (ISPAD). Clinical Practice Consensus Guidelines 2018. Chapter 3: Type 2 diabetes in youth. *Pediatr Diabetes* 2018;19(Suppl. 27):28–46. ♫ https://www.ispad.org/page/ISPADGuidelines2018

International Society for Pediatric and Adolescent Diabetes (ISPAD). Clinical Practice Consensus Guidelines 2018. Chapter 4: The diagnosis and management of monogenic diabetes in children and adolescents. *Pediatr Diabetes* 2018;19(Suppl. 27):47–63. ♫ https://www.ispad.org/page/ISPADGuidelines2018

International Society for Pediatric and Adolescent Diabetes (ISPAD). Clinical Practice Consensus Guidelines 2018. Chapter 5: Management of cystic fibrosis-related diabetes in children and adolescents. *Pediatr Diabetes* 2018;19(Suppl. 27):64–74. ♫ https://www.ispad.org/page/ISPADGuidelines2018

International Society for Pediatric and Adolescent Diabetes (ISPAD). Clinical Practice Consensus Guidelines 2018. Chapter 6: Diabetes education in children and adolescents. *Pediatr Diabetes* 2018;19(Suppl. 27):75–83. ♫ https://www.ispad.org/page/ISPADGuidelines2018

International Society for Pediatric and Adolescent Diabetes (ISPAD). Clinical Practice Consensus Guidelines 2018. Chapter 7: The delivery of ambulatory diabetes care to children and adolescents with diabetes. *Pediatr Diabetes* 2018;19(Suppl. 27):84–104. ♫ https://www.ispad.org/page/ISPADGuidelines2018

International Society for Pediatric and Adolescent Diabetes (ISPAD). Clinical Practice Consensus Guidelines 2018. Chapter 8: Glycemic control targets and glucose monitoring for children, adolescents, and young adults with diabetes *Pediatr Diabetes* 2018;19(Suppl. 27):105–114. ♫ https://www.ispad.org/page/ISPADGuidelines2018

International Society for Pediatric and Adolescent Diabetes (ISPAD). Clinical Practice Consensus Guidelines 2018. Chapter 9: Insulin treatment in children and adolescents with diabetes *Pediatr Diabetes* 2018;19(Suppl. 27):115–135. ♫ https://www.ispad.org/page/ISPADGuidelines2018

International Society for Pediatric and Adolescent Diabetes (ISPAD). Clinical Practice Consensus Guidelines 2018. Chapter 10: Nutritional management in children and adolescents with diabetes. *Pediatr Diabetes* 2018;19(Suppl. 27):136–154. ♫ https://www.ispad.org/page/ISPADGuidelines2018

International Society for Pediatric and Adolescent Diabetes (ISPAD). Clinical Practice Consensus Guidelines 2018. Chapter 11: Diabetic ketoacidosis and hyperglycemic hypersmolar state. *Pediatr Diabetes* 2018;19(Suppl. 27):155–177. ♫ https://www.ispad.org/page/ISPADGuidelines2018

International Society for Pediatric and Adolescent Diabetes (ISPAD). Clinical Practice Consensus Guidelines 2018. Chapter 12: Assessment and management of hypoglycemia in children and adolescents with diabetes. *Pediatr Diabetes* 2018;19 (Suppl. 27):178–192. ♫ https://www.ispad.org/page/ISPADGuidelines2018

International Society for Pediatric and Adolescent Diabetes (ISPAD). Clinical Practice Consensus Guidelines 2018. Chapter 13: Sick day management in children and adolescents with diabetes. *Pediatr Diabetes* 2018;19(Suppl. 27):193–204. ♫ https://www.ispad.org/page/ISPADGuidelines2018

International Society for Pediatric and Adolescent Diabetes (ISPAD). Clinical Practice Consensus Guidelines 2018. Chapter 14: Exercise in children and adolescents with diabetes. *Pediatr Diabetes* 2018;19(Suppl. 27):205–226. ♫ https://www.ispad.org/page/ISPADGuidelines2018

International Society for Pediatric and Adolescent Diabetes (ISPAD). Clinical Practice Consensus Guidelines 2018. Chapter 15: Management of children & adolescents with diabetes requiring surgery. *Pediatr Diabetes* 2018;19(Suppl. 27):227–236. ℘ https://www.ispad.org/page/ISPADGuidelines2018

International Society for Pediatric and Adolescent Diabetes (ISPAD). Clinical Practice Consensus Guidelines 2018. Chapter 16: Psychological care of children and adolescents with type 1 diabetes. *Pediatr Diabetes* 2018;19(Suppl. 27):237–249. ℘ https://www.ispad.org/page/ISPADGuidelines2018

International Society for Pediatric and Adolescent Diabetes (ISPAD). Clinical Practice Consensus Guidelines 2018. Chapter 17: Diabetes in adolescence. *Pediatr Diabetes* 2018;19(Suppl. 27):250–261. ℘ https://www.ispad.org/page/ISPADGuidelines2018

International Society for Pediatric and Adolescent Diabetes (ISPAD). Clinical Practice Consensus Guidelines 2018. Chapter 18: Microvascular and macrovascular complications in children and adolescents. *Pediatr Diabetes* 2018;19(Suppl. 27):262–274. ℘ https://www.ispad.org/page/ISPADGuidelines2018

International Society for Pediatric and Adolescent Diabetes (ISPAD). Clinical Practice Consensus Guidelines 2018. Chapter 19: Other complications and associated conditions in children and adolescents with type 1 diabetes. *Pediatr Diabetes* 2018;19(Suppl. 27):275–286. ℘ https://www.ispad.org/page/ISPADGuidelines2018

International Society for Pediatric and Adolescent Diabetes (ISPAD). Clinical Practice Consensus Guidelines 2018. Chapter 20: Management and support of children and adolescents with type 1 diabetes in school. *Pediatr Diabetes* 2018;19(Suppl. 27):287–301. ℘ https://www.ispad.org/page/ISPADGuidelines2018

International Society for Pediatric and Adolescent Diabetes (ISPAD). Clinical Practice Consensus Guidelines 2018. Chapter 21: Diabetes technologies. *Pediatr Diabetes* 2018;19(Suppl. 27):302–325. ℘ https://www.ispad.org/page/ISPADGuidelines2018

Noble JA, Ehrlich HA. Genetics of type 1 diabetes. *Cold Spring Harb Perspect Med* 2012;2:a007732.

Stančáková A, Laakso M. Genetics of type 2 diabetes. *Endocr Dev* 2016;31:203–220.

# Obesity

# Introduction

## Definition

Obesity is often defined as 'an excess of body fat frequently resulting in a significant impairment of health and longevity'.

## Background

Obesity in most cases is not a 1° endocrine condition. It may be a presenting feature of a disease state. However, the consequences of obesity produce endocrine morbidity such as T2DM.

The prevalence of overweight and obesity is increasing nationally and also worldwide for both adults and children. There is some evidence, however, that this is now starting to plateau.

Worldwide, obesity-related conditions account for 2–7% of total healthcare costs, with costs to the National Health Service (NHS) being:

- 2015: indirect costs of high BMI estimated at £6.4 billion/year
- 2025: £8.3 billion/year
- 2050: £9.7 billion/year.

Obesity is responsible for 9000 premature deaths/year in England, with a reduction in life expectancy by ~9 years, and in the UK it accounts for:

- 58% of T2DM
- 21% of heart disease (~28,000 myocardial infarctions, and ~750,000 cases of hypertension)
- 8–42% of certain malignancies (endometrial, breast, and colon).

## Key facts

In England, currently according to the National Child Measurement Programme:

- almost a quarter of children at primary school entry were overweight including obese. At age 10 years it was over a third
- the prevalence of obesity has increased at age 4 years but remained similar aged 10 years
- obesity prevalence was higher for boys than girls in both age groups.

The House of Commons Select Committee concluded (2004) that 'this will be the first generation where children die before their parents as a consequence of childhood obesity'.

## Assessment

Clinical assessment often tends to underestimate overweight and obesity, and an ideal measure needs to be a simple, low-cost, accurate, and reproducible assessment of fat mass. In terms of auxological criteria, a number of different indirect methods are used to assess adiposity, including:

- weight for height (WFH)
- ponderal index (PI)
- waist:hip ratio
- waist circumference
- skinfold thickness.

Using WFH, commonly used cut-offs are:

- >110% of ideal weight for overweight
- >120% of ideal weight for obesity.

BMI (weight (kg)/height (m)$^2$) is the most widely used assessment of adiposity. Classification defines overweight based on health risk, as a BMI in adults of 25–30 kg/m$^2$, and obesity as a BMI of ≥30 kg/m$^2$, with morbidity risk appearing to increase above the 95th centile.

BMI is affected by both age and sex, extrapolating these risks to children and adolescents (aged 2–19 years old) uses various cut-offs (Table 6.1).

*Practice tip*: to easily calculate BMI on a smartphone, divide weight in kilograms by height in metres and divide by height again.

Specific BMI charts have been produced for children (→ see Chapter 1). However, as it is the BMI *centile* that matters for clinical decision-making, the BMI look-up can be used as a quick reference.

- Measure height and weight
- Plot both on growth chart and read off the centiles
- Plot centiles on the BMI look-up
- At the intersection is the BMI centile for age.

For research purposes, the following are used to measure adiposity:

Direct methods:

- DXA
- CT/MRI scanning
- Densitometry.

Indirect methods:

- Bioelectrical impedance
- Air displacement plethysmography.

**Table 6.1** Cut-offs of BMI for age and sex

| Obesity | Overweight | Country/reference |
| --- | --- | --- |
| ≥95th centile | ≥85th centile | USA |
| ≥98th centile | ≥91st centile | UK |
| ~99th centile | ~91st centile | International Obesity Task Force (IOTF) |

# Classification of obesity

Obesity may be considered to be (Table 6.2):
- 1°, often known as 'exogenous or *simple* obesity'
- 2°, due to
  - identified genetic syndromes, e.g. Prader–Willi, Laurence–Moon–Bardet–Biedl, Alström syndromes, pseudohypoparathyroidism
  - monogenic disorders, e.g. leptin deficiency, leptin receptor abnormalities, melanocortin receptor (*MC4R*) defects
  - CNS disease, e.g. hypothalamic obesity
  - endocrine disorders, e.g. hypothyroidism, Cushing syndrome, GHD, precocious puberty
  - immobility, e.g. cerebral palsy, spina bifida
  - iatrogenic, e.g. steroids, anticonvulsants, antithyroid drugs.

**Table 6.2** Differences between primary and secondary obesity

|  | 1° obesity | 2° obesity |
|---|---|---|
| Incidence | Common | Rare |
| Family history | Very common | Uncommon |
| Height | Tall stature | Short stature |
| Dysmorphic features | None | Often present |
| Development | Normal | Developmental delay common |
| Bone age | Advanced/normal | Delayed |

# Exogenous obesity

An obesogenic environment arises from a multitude of factors: genetic, biological, psychological, sociocultural, and environmental factors (both intra- and extrauterine), which affect both sides of the energy balance equation.

## Factors

A number of factors have been implicated:

### Socioeconomic

• Obesity prevalence for children is a marker of poor socioeconomic status. The deprivation gap as measured by the differences in obesity prevalence between the most (13.5%) and least (4.8%) deprived areas has increased over time. It has increased more at age 10 years (29.2% and 11.3% respectively).

### Geography

• Obesity rates in adults are higher in Scotland and Northern England than the South of England.

### Ethnicity

• Afro-Caribbean, South Asian, Hispanic, and Native-American children have an increased risk of obesity compared with white children.

### Genetic factors

• Data from twin studies indicate that 40–70% of body weight variations are attributable to genetic factors.
• If both parents are obese then there is a 70% chance that their child will be obese.
• If one parents is obese then there is a 50% chance that their child will be obese.
• If neither parent is obese then there is only a 10% chance that their child will be obese.
• This is more likely to occur if the mother is overweight.

### Intrauterine environment

• Extreme maternal obesity in pregnancy
• Maternal gestational diabetes is associated with an increased risk of obesity in offspring.

There is also recognition that low birthweight and the subsequent pattern of growth has long lasting effects into adulthood. The fall in body fat and subsequent rise, the so-called *adiposity rebound*, is felt to be critical in the long-term development of metabolic syndrome.

### Behaviours

*Activity*

• Hours of television viewing and overweight are positively correlated, especially in older children and adolescents. In the UK, under 16s now watch an average of 17 hours of television a week.
• <1/3 of schoolchildren now participate in regular physical activity at school. Only ~25% of adolescents regularly exercise in the USA, and 14% don't exercise at all.

*Sleeping*
- Decreased sleep duration is implicated in obesity.

*Eating*
- Consumption of high-energy density snacks, high-sugar soft drinks.
- Missing or only eating a small breakfast, along with consuming more food in the latter half of the day (especially evening meal).
- Eating meals faster than usual, with no slowing down towards the end of the meal.

Breastfeeding is associated with a reduced risk of obesity.

Obesity arises as a result of a positive energy balance; i.e. either
1. an increased energy intake and/or
2. a reduced energy expenditure.

In practice, factors implicated in the rise in obesity have been very difficult to identify, as the imbalance is often only a few calories each day.

# Identified syndromes

## Prader–Willi syndrome (PWS)

(⊖ See also Chapter 5, p. 218.)

Incidence is 1 in 12,000–15,000.

Caused by deletion of paternal copies of imprinted genes (*SNRPN* and *NDN*) located in the region of chromosome 15q11–13, by mechanisms including:

- mutation (chance or sporadic)
- uniparental disomy
- chromosome translocation
- gene deletions.

A genetic disorder can be found in ~97%, with >70% having a deletion of the paternal copy, ~25% maternal uniparental disomy (MUPD) of chromosome 15, with other causes accounting for the remainder.

Diagnosis is made on clinical features, plus identification of a genetic defect.

### Clinical features

- Reduced fetal movements and postnatal hypotonia.
- Initial failure to thrive with poor feeding, followed by rapid weight gain and hyperphagia from ~2–4 years of age.
- Delayed milestones.
- Learning difficulties, with mild/borderline/low average intelligence range IQ in 50–65%.

### Dysmorphic features

- High, narrow forehead
- Almond-shaped eyes
- Prominent nasal bridge
- Thin, down-turned lips
- Small hands and feet
- Light skin and hair
- Skin lesions (from picking).

### Endocrine problems

- Biochemical GH deficiency in 40–100% of patients. Features supporting this are short stature, obesity, decreased fat free (muscle) mass, increased fat mass, decreased bone density, and reduced total energy expenditure.
- Hypogonadism (hypogonadotropic hypogonadism), producing undescended testes and/or micropenis in males, plus delayed and arrested puberty in both sexes.
- Premature adrenarche occurs more commonly in females.
- Increased incidence of diabetes mellitus (both T1DM and T2DM).
- Obesity in PWS is due to a combination of:
  - increased energy intake (hyperphagia with decreased satiety) and
  - decreased energy expenditure (hypotonia with decreased muscle tone).

Increased levels of the peptide ghrelin, which has central actions opposite to those of leptin and an orexigenic (appetite-stimulating) action have been demonstrated in PWS.

NB: early initiation of GH replacement can produce not only improved growth, but also a reduction in body fat especially central distribution. Thus the phenotype of a GH-treated older child or adolescent is now very different and becoming the norm. The hyperphagia persists despite the GH replacement.

## Bardet–Biedl syndrome (BBS)
(➲ See also Chapter 5, p. 218.)

Also known as Laurence–Moon–Biedl and Laurence–Moon–Biedl–Bardet syndrome, although some consider Laurence–Moon syndrome a separate entity.

Occurs in 1 in 160,000. Most cases are autosomal recessive. 21 BBS genes currently account for ~75% of cases.

### Features
- Obesity (in ~75%)
- Rod-cone dystrophy (including retinitis pigmentosa), leading to visual loss and blindness (in 90–100%)
- Post-axial polydactyly/syndactyly
- Hypogonadism, plus Müllerian abnormalities in females
- Retardation of growth and development
- Renal dysfunction (cystic renal dysplasia).

## Alström syndrome
(➲ See also Chapter 5, p. 218.)

A rare autosomal recessive disorder (1 in 500,000) caused by mutations in *ALMS* (found in 25–40% of affected individuals).
- Like BBS it is a ciliopathy.
- Shares similarities with BBS, although affected patients do not have intellectual disability and polydactyly.
  Features include:
- obesity (in 100%)
- endocrine dysfunction: insulin resistance, T2DM, hypothyroidism, hypogonadotropic hypogonadism
- visual: cone-rod dystrophy, with photophobia, nystagmus, and progressive visual impairment
- hearing: progressive sensorineural hearing impairment
- renal disease, interstitial fibrosis progressing to end-stage renal failure
- dilated cardiomyopathy and congestive heart failure in 2/3
- developmental delay.

## Pseudohypoparathyroidism
(➲ See also Chapter 10.)

Caused by parathyroid hormone resistance, due to dysfunctional G-proteins involved in cyclic AMP production. Several different forms (types 1a, 1b, and 2 and pseudopseudohypoparathyroidism) based on the presence/absence of physical and biochemical features are recognized.

*Clinical features*
- Short stature
- Round face
- Short fourth and fifth metacarpals
- Calcification of basal ganglia
- Developmental delay.

*Biochemical features*
- Low calcium
- High phosphate
- Raised parathyroid hormone.

## Leptin deficiency

Identified through animal studies, leptin is involved in the control of appetite, both stimulation and suppression. It was initially felt that leptin might represent 'the fat hormone', but it is now felt that the effect of leptin is to increase food intake when body weight is low.

Patients with leptin deficiency and leptin receptor abnormalities have:
- normal birthweight
- rapid weight gain in the first months of life
- increased fat distribution over the trunk and limbs
- marked hyperphagia, with increased energy intake
- delayed/absent pubertal development.

Biochemical findings include:
- hyperinsulinaemia, with T2DM in some patients
- abnormalities of T-cell number and function
- central hypothyroidism (low $T_4$ with high serum TSH that is bio-inactive)
- hypogonadotropic hypogonadism.

Administration of leptin to leptin-deficient individuals results in:
- normalization of hyperphagia.
- improvement/reversal of hypogonadotropic hypogonadism.
- improvement in thyroid function.

There is no evidence that administration of leptin to patients with simple obesity is of any effect, as these patients tend to have high levels of leptin.

## Other genes associated with obesity

A number of monogenic obesity syndromes have been described, several of which include the leptin–melanocortin regulation pathway. In addition, genes have been identified which contribute to increased risk of weight gain, without themselves producing obesity. With the advent of genome-wise association studies, many candidate genes for obesity are being recognized, and the relevance for diagnostic or therapeutic intervention will become clearer over time.
- Heterozygous mutations of the melanocortin receptor gene (*MC4R*) cause significant obesity, but are not associated with a distinctive phenotype. This is the most common identified cause of monogenic human obesity, found in up to 6% of early-onset and severe childhood obesity, and 0.5–1.0% of obese adults.

- Variable nucleotide tandem repeat (VNTR) polymorphisms upstream of the insulin gene are associated with increased fasting insulin levels and childhood obesity in individuals of European descent.
- Adults homozygous for the risk allele of the *FTO* (fat mass and obesity-associated) gene weigh ~3 kg more and have a ~1.7× increased odds of obesity.
- A polymorphism in the 11-beta hydroxysteroid dehydrogenase type 1 gene (*HSD11B1*) has also been associated with obesity.

Although some genetic variants are associated with extreme forms of obesity, changes in genes alone cannot account for the rapid change in obesity at a population level. An obesogenic environment exposes the biological vulnerability of individuals, and prevention therefore needs to be aimed at altering this environment.

## Hypothalamic obesity

This is a particularly severe form of obesity, which is often resistant to therapy with dietary and/or exercise. It occurs as a result of lesions of the hypothalamus (including tumours, surgery, and radiotherapy). In craniopharyngioma, hypothalamic obesity occurs in 50–80%, and correlates with structural damage to the hypothalamus on neuroimaging. Marked, uncontrollable hyperphagia is the key feature.

Hypothalamic dysfunction is also found in the following monogenic conditions:
- PWS
- BBS

plus mutations in:
- *MC4R*
- leptin
- leptin receptor
- proopiomelanocortin gene (*POMC*)
- prohormone convertase.

The obesity is multifactorial and includes abnormalities of:
- energy intake: hyperphagia with reduced satiety
- energy expenditure: reduced voluntary activity or possibly related to a disability, reduced basal metabolic rate
- endocrine dysfunction: vagally mediated hyperinsulinaemia, leptin resistance, hypopituitarism.

Endocrine causes of obesity are dealt with in the appropriate chapters.

# Complications of obesity

- Metabolic
- Cardiovascular
- Respiratory
- GI/hepatic
- Orthopaedic
- Neurological
- Dermatological
- Gynaecological
- Psychological.

## Metabolic

Recent studies indicate that in children with a BMI >95th centile:
- 58% have either hypertension, hyperlipidaemia, or insulin resistance
- 25% have two or more of these conditions.

In the USA, it is recommended that all overweight youngsters who have at least two other risk factors:
- family history of T2DM in first- or second-degree relatives; certain ethnic groups (i.e. Native American, African American, Hispanic, Japanese, or other Asian/Pacific Islander); in the UK this is likely to be Afro-Caribbean or South Asian
- signs associated with insulin resistance (hypertension, dyslipidaemia, acanthosis nigricans, or PCOS)

should be tested for T2DM beginning at 10 years of age or at the onset of puberty, and every 2 years thereafter.

### Metabolic syndrome

There is an association between the development of the metabolic syndrome and the development of T2DM and cardiovascular disease.

The International Diabetes Federation (IDF) definition for children and adolescents:
- Aged 6–9 years: waist circumference >90th percentile; suggestive. Further measurements should be made if there is a family history of metabolic syndrome, T2DM, dyslipidaemia, cardiovascular disease, hypertension, and/or obesity.
- Aged 10–15 years: waist circumference ≥90th percentile or adult cut-off if lower:
  - Triglycerides ≥1.7 mmol/L (≥150 mg/dL), high-density lipoprotein (HDL)-cholesterol <1.03 mmol/L (<40 mg/dL)
  - Systolic blood pressure ≥130 or diastolic blood pressure ≥85 mmHg
  - Fasting blood glucose ≥5.6 mmol/L (100 mg/dL).
- Aged 16+ years: use existing IDF criteria for adults.

The IDF and American Heart Association propose that any three (or more) of the following factors constitute a diagnosis of metabolic syndrome in adults:
- Increased waist circumference: ethnicity specific—e.g. Caucasian men ≥94 cm and women ≥80 cm; South Asian men ≥90 cm and women ≥80 cm.

- If BMI is >30 kg/m², central obesity can be assumed and waist circumference does not need to be measured.
- Raised triglycerides:
  - >150 mg/dL (1.7 mmol/L)
  - or specific treatment for this lipid abnormality.
- Reduced HDL-cholesterol:
  - <40 mg/dL (1.03 mmol/L) in men
  - <50 mg/dL (1.29 mmol/L) in women
  - or specific treatment for this lipid abnormality.
- Raised blood pressure:
  - systolic ≥130 mmHg.
  - diastolic ≥85 mmHg.
  - or treatment of previously diagnosed hypertension.
- Raised fasting plasma glucose:
  - fasting plasma glucose ≥100 mg/dL (5.6 mmol/L).
- Most people with T2DM will have metabolic syndrome based on these criteria.

### Impaired glucose tolerance (IGT)

This is also described in ⮞ Chapter 5, p. 137.

It is a pre-diabetic state, defined on an OGTT as a 2-hour blood sugar ≥ 7.8 mmol/L but <11.1 mmol/L. It is a predictor of T2DM and also cardiovascular disease.

- IGT occurs in ~20% of children with obesity.
- ~30% of obese adolescents with IGT progress to develop T2DM.
- Therapy with the biguanide metformin has been shown to reduce BMI, fasting glucose, insulin, and lipids.

### Respiratory

Obese children are 4–6× more likely to have obstructive sleep apnoea (OSA) compared to lean subjects. In adults, OSA has been implicated in hypertension, cardiovascular diseases, behavioural disorders, and reduced QoL.

Weight reduction is the preferred treatment, although some patients may require continuous positive airway pressure. Obesity may also exacerbate asthma.

### Cardiovascular

Obesity produces:
- increased blood volume and cardiac output, with increased left ventricular mass
- endothelial dysfunction, carotid intimal medial thickening, and development of early aortic and coronary arterial fatty streaks and fibrous plaques
- sleep apnoea and obesity-related hypoventilation may produce pulmonary arterial hypertension, leading in some cases to cardiomyopathy.

## Hypertension

Childhood obesity is the leading cause of hypertension in the paediatric age range, with systolic blood pressure in children and adolescents correlated with BMI, skinfold thickness, and waist:hip ratio. Hypertension has been linked to several obesity-related factors, including:

- hormonal factors: insulin resistance, raised aldosterone, and elevated leptin levels
- genetic factors.

*Practice point*: always use the largest cuff available when taking blood pressure in an overweight/obese child/adolescent.

## Gastrointestinal/hepatic

A spectrum of liver abnormalities including non-alcoholic fatty liver disease (NAFLD) have been described in association with obesity, in its most extreme form proceeding to hepatic fibrosis and even cirrhosis, so-called non-alcoholic steatohepatitis (NASH).

- Mean age of presentation is 12 years
- Boys more commonly affected than girls.

Although most patients are asymptomatic, the following may occur:

- diffuse abdominal discomfort or right upper quadrant pain (in 42–67%)
- weakness, fatigue, and malaise.

Later on in the disease the following are found:

- hepatomegaly
- stigmata of liver disease: palmar erythema, jaundice, spider naevi, muscle wasting, and hepatic encephalopathy.

### Investigations

*Biochemistry*

- Abnormal liver function tests: raised hepatic transaminases (alanine transaminase usually > aspartate transaminase), gamma-glutamyl transpeptidase and liver alkaline phosphatase
- Raised bilirubin, albumin, and also abnormal clotting (prothrombin time) may occur in advanced disease.

*Ultrasonography: key test for diagnosis*

- Hepatic ultrasound initially shows an echogenic liver of fatty infiltration.
- Cholelithiasis (gallstones) may also be noted coincidentally.

Diagnosis of NAFLD and NASH/cirrhosis is made histologically on liver biopsy.

Weight loss is beneficial. In some patients the biguanide metformin and also vitamin E have been used.

## Orthopaedic

As excess weight may damage epiphyses, a number of orthopaedic problems are associated with obesity, including:

- slipped capital femoral epiphysis (SUFE)
- genu valgum (knock knees)
- tibia vara (Blount disease)
- spondylolisthesis (low back pain)
- osteoarthritis long term.

## Dermatology

Features associated with obesity:
- Acanthosis nigricans. These are hyperpigmented (brown to black), hyperkeratotic, velvety plaques found on the dorsal surface of the neck, in the axillae, around the umbilicus, in the groin and over joints.
- Severe skin changes correlate with insulin resistance and can be improved by weight loss.
- Skin tags in the neck and axillae.

## Neurology

The risk of benign intracranial hypertension (aka pseudotumour cerebri) is increased even at 10% above ideal body weight; with increasing obesity the risk can be as high as 15-fold.

Features of benign intracranial hypertension include:
- Headache (characteristically on waking, worst on straining)
- Visual abnormalities (blurred vision or loss of peripheral vision)
- Tinnitus
- Cranial nerve abnormalities (sixth nerve palsy)
- Neuroimaging demonstrates no intracranial lesion, but reveals slit-like ventricles
- Lumbar puncture reveals increased opening pressure.

## Gynaecology

### Polycystic ovarian syndrome

( See also Chapter 2, p. 80.)

Although a number of diagnostic classifications exist, recent consensus guidelines diagnose PCOS if two out of the following three criteria are met:
1. irregular or absent periods (oligo/amenorrhoea)
2. excess androgen activity (hirsutism)
3. polycystic ovaries on pelvic ultrasound scan

with other endocrine disorders excluded.

There is an association with adiposity, insulin resistance, and hyperandrogenaemia in adolescents and women:
- Excess central or abdominal adiposity is associated with increased androgen levels, with ~50% of circulating testosterone derived from fat tissue.
- The degree of insulin resistance correlates with central adiposity.
- Hyperinsulinaemia and high androgen activity are also associated, with the former stimulating ovarian and adrenal androgen and also oestrogen production.

Low concentrations of sex hormone-binding globulin (SHBG) 2° to high androgen and insulin levels increase free sex hormones levels. Weight loss induces a decrease in insulin resistance and androgenic activity, particularly in adolescent girls.

# Investigation of obesity

This is to identify:
1. medical causes of obesity
2. medical consequences arising from obesity.

## Suggested points

### History

*Maternal health*
- Health/smoking during pregnancy (ask about gestational diabetes).

*Birth history*
- Birth order
- Singleton or multiple births
- Gestational age
- Birthweight.

*Previous history*
- Breastfeeding or bottle feeding (how long for)? Age at weaning?
- Any significant illnesses?
- Drug history: steroids (including inhaled, topical), antipsychotic drugs.

*Family history*
- Parental history: significant illnesses? Diabetes, heart disease? Are the parents obese?
- Are parents related, and if so, how?
- List siblings in order and any health problems
- Any illnesses in extended family members, e.g. grandparents?
- Social history.

*Other*
- How is child performing at school? Any teasing or bullying? Self-esteem?
- What opportunities for physical exercise? How much exercise?
- How many hours a day sedentary, e.g. watching television, computer?
- Systematic review: any evidence of symptomatology arising from obesity, e.g. snoring, OSA?
- Evidence of underlying condition.

*Dietary history*
- Assessment of caloric intake, including dietary quality (balance of nutrients and food groups). Food preferences and aversions.
- Family eating practices: eat with family or snack/grazing?
- Takeaways how often? Sweets/snacks? Fizzy drinks?

### Examination
- Accurate height and weight, calculation of BMI.
- Pattern of obesity: central or generalized.
- Dysmorphism suggestive of underlying syndrome.
- Blood pressure (relate to UK reference data): *use largest cuff.*
- Pubertal assessment.
- Signs of acanthosis nigricans, skin tags.
- Signs of endocrinopathy: striae, hirsutism, hypothyroidism.

The growth chart may be useful.

*Investigation*

Directed at identifying causes and also comorbidities of obesity include:
- electrolytes
- hepatic function including transaminases
- thyroid function
- lipid profile
- fasting glucose and insulin
- OGTT
- LH, FSH, oestradiol, androgens, SHBG in girls with suspected PCOS
- urinary/serum cortisol levels if Cushing syndrome is considered
- karyotype, plus genetic testing
- bone age.

## Screening

As preventative strategies and effective interventions are not currently available, and other criteria are not met, population screening for childhood obesity is not currently recommended by the UK National Screening Committee.

# Treatment

Management of obesity is aimed at modifiable factors, restoring the balance between energy intake and expenditure, and involves:
- dietary advice
- exercise advice, reduction of sedentary activity
- lifestyle changes
- behaviour modification
- (pharmacotherapy)
- (surgery).

## Points

- Benefits are most likely to be achieved with a combination of diet and exercise along with counselling and behaviour modification.
- Any lifestyle intervention is only likely to be successful if diet and exercise programmes are individualized, and coordinated both with the individual and family.
- Need to provide frequent assessment/monitoring.
- Long-term success requires continuous implementation, as stopping treatment results in rebound weight gain in most patients.

## Should the aim be weight reduction or stabilization?

- Stabilization of weight leads to a reduction in BMI; adult studies indicate that a 5–10% reduction in body weight at 0.5 kg/week increases insulin sensitivity.
- Short-term reduction in overweight by 10–20% is possible.
- Long term, the aim should be to reduce BMI score to <98%.

## Where should care be provided?

Although national and international guidelines exist, some consider that most of these children should be seen in 1° care, while others call for obese children to have access to specialist care. There are several community-based programmes such as MEND and WATCH IT which have provided promising initial results and are being rolled out nationally.

In the UK, children attending a residential 'fat camp' for a mean of 29 days:
- lost a mean of 6 kg in weight
- reduced BMI by a mean of 2.4 units, and BMI SDS by a mean of 0.28.

## Dietary

- Mild caloric restriction such as the 'Traffic Light Diet' is safe and effective especially when obese children and their families are motivated and encouraged to change longstanding feeding behaviours.
- Diets should not be scaled-down versions of usual diet, but consist of reductions in high-risk foods while maintaining recommended daily allowances of nutrients and vitamins.
- Aim for high-fibre/low-salt diet with five portions of fruit or vegetables/day.
- Severely restricted diets (including high-protein, very low-calorie diets), may produce dramatic short-term weight loss but are potentially dangerous and unsustainable.

- Substantial reductions in weight are unusual and are not sustained unless restriction of calories is also accompanied by increased energy expenditure.

### Exercise

- Reduce sedentary activities to <2 hours a day.
- Non-weight-bearing activities may be initially required for very obese children.
- Start with 30 minutes of exercise a day and build up.
- Exercise for 30–60 minutes per day that 'works up a sweat'; includes fast walking, housework.
- Must be enjoyable, congruent with family, and rewarding.
- Any benefits of exercise, however, are rapidly reversed if the increased activity is not maintained.

# Pharmacotherapy

## Anorectic agents

In the past, several drugs including stimulants, e.g. amphetamine, fenfluramine, dexfenfluramine, thyroid hormone, and more recently sibutramine have been used, but they are rarely used today in childhood obesity due to side effects, some of which are potentially life-threatening.

*Leptin* has produced significant reduction in appetite and weight in leptin-deficient children, but appears to have little effect in other obese children, who have elevated levels of leptin.

## Reduction in absorption

Lipid absorption: *orlistat* inhibits pancreatic lipase and therefore increases faecal fat loss. In adults it reduces:
- body weight
- total and low-density lipoprotein cholesterol
- risk of T2DM in patients with IGT.

Similar findings have been found in adolescents during short-term studies. Side effects include diarrhoea and flatulence which may limit tolerance, and also deficiencies of the fat-soluble vitamins A, D, E, and K. NICE only recommends orlistat as a second-line treatment in children >12 years.

## Insulin sensitizers

*Metformin*, a biguanide:
- increases hepatic glucose uptake
- reduces hepatic glucose production, and
- reduces gluconeogenesis.

In adults it:
- reduces food intake
- promotes weight loss
- improves lipids
- decreases subcutaneous fat
- reduces risk of T2DM in patients with IGT.

Several trials in obese adolescents have shown a small benefit.

*Octreotide*: this drug binds to the somatostatin receptor and blocks glucose-dependent insulin secretion. Trials in patients with hypothalamic obesity have shown benefit in some, although the need for SC injection, drug cost, and side effects, e.g. gallstones, GI symptoms, inhibition of other hormones such as GH, limit its use.

- Drug therapy should be considered in selected obese patients: NICE recommends that drug treatment should be considered only if dietary, exercise, and behavioural approaches have already been commenced and evaluated. Any drug therapy should be prescribed by an experienced specialist multidisciplinary team, and should be discontinued if there is no response to treatment.
- Children <12 years: drug treatment is not generally recommended, and should only be prescribed in exceptional circumstances such as severe life-threatening comorbidities.

- Children >12 years: drug treatment is recommended only if there are severe comorbidities.
- Orlistat: selective benefit in some patients but often short term.
- Metformin: there are few trials in children, although in adults drug therapy produces an additional 2–10 kg of weight loss within the first few months.

# Bariatric surgery

Given the poor response to lifestyle changes and also pharmacotherapy, surgical approaches such as:
• laparoscopic gastric banding procedure
• Roux-en-Y gastric bypass
have been considered.

## Who should have surgery?

• Severe obesity: BMI >40 kg/m$^2$ (>+3.5 SDS) with comorbidities
• Puberty completed
• >6 months' attempted weight loss
• Fully investigated
• Commitment to medical/psychological evaluations before and after surgery
• Agree not to become pregnant for at least 1 year after operation
• Adhere to postoperative nutritional guidelines
• Although studies of bariatric surgery in adolescents are limited, they appear to produce similar results to that seen in adults, although most weight loss is in the initial phase.

Published studies and reviews suggest improvement in QoL but careful selection of patients, psychological assessment, and support are key factors in success.

# Guidelines for management of obesity

Details of NICE guidance are summarized in Box 6.1.

Outcome

In adults, 10 kg of weight loss is associated with a fall of:
- 20–25% in total mortality
- 30–40% in diabetes-related deaths
- 40–50% in obesity-related cancer deaths.

20–30 kg weight loss following surgical banding gastroplasty resulted in resolution of hypertension and diabetes in 89% and 43% of patients respectively.

## Box 6.1 NICE recommendations for preventing obesity in children

*Recommendations for the public*
- Children and young people should have regular meals in a pleasant, sociable environment with no distractions (such as television); parents and carers should join them as often as possible.
- Gradually reduce the time children are sitting in front of a screen.
- Encourage games that involve running around, such as skipping, dancing, or ball games.
- Be more active as a family, by walking or cycling to school, going to the park, or swimming.
- Encourage children to take part in sport inside and outside school.

*Recommendations for health professionals*
- For families at high risk (e.g. those where one or both parents are obese), offer individual counselling and ongoing support. Consider family-based and individual interventions, depending on the age and maturity of the child.
- In preschool settings, use a range of components. For example, offer interactive cookery demonstrations, videos, and discussions on meal planning and shopping for food and drink; in addition, offer interactive demonstrations, videos, and group discussions on physical activities, opportunities for active play, safety, and local facilities.
- In family programmes to prevent obesity, provide ongoing tailored support and incorporate behaviour change techniques.

*Recommendations for preschool settings*
- Provide regular opportunities for enjoyable active play and structured physical activity sessions.
- Ensure that children eat regular healthy meals in a supervised, pleasant, sociable environment, free from distractions.

*Recommendations for schools*
- Ensure that school policies and the whole school environment encourage physical activity and a healthy diet.
- Train all staff in how to implement healthy school policies.
- Create links and partnerships between sports clubs and schools.
- Promote physical activities that children can enjoy outside school and into adulthood.
- Ensure that children and young people eat meals in a pleasant, sociable environment, free from distractions.

*Recommendations for local authorities and their partners*
- Work with the community to identify barriers to physical activity.
- Ensure that the design of buildings and open spaces encourages people to be more active.
- Encourage active travel, and promote and support physical activity schemes.
- Encourage local shops and caterers to promote healthy food choices.

# Further reading

Alberti KG, Eckel RH, Grundy SM, et al. Harmonizing the metabolic syndrome: a joint interim statement of the International Diabetes Federation Task Force on Epidemiology and Prevention National Heart, Lung, and Blood Institute. *Circulation* 2009;120:1640–1645.

Black JA, White B, Viner RM, Simmons RK. Bariatric surgery for obese children and adolescents: a systematic review and meta-analysis. *Obes Rev* 2013;14:634–644.

Chesi A, Grant SFA. The genetics of pediatric obesity. *Trends Endocrinol Metab* 2015;26:711–721.

Department of Health and Social Care. Childhood obesity: a plan for action, chapter 2. 2018. ⅋ https://www.gov.uk/government/publications/childhood-obesity-a-plan-for-action-chapter-2

Fried M, Yumuk V, Oppert JM, et al. International Federation for Surgery of Obesity and Metabolic Disorders-European Chapter (IFSO-EC); European Association for the Study of Obesity (EASO); European Association for the Study of Obesity Obesity Management Task Force (EASO OMTF). Interdisciplinary European guidelines on metabolic and bariatric surgery. *Obes Surg* 2014;24:42–55.

National Institute for Health and Care Excellence (NICE). Obesity prevention in adults, young people and children. NICE, 2006, updated 2015. ⅋ https://www.nice.org.uk/guidance/CG43

National Institute for Health and Care Excellence (NICE). Obesity: identification, assessment and management. CG189. NICE, 2014. ⅋ https://www.nice.org.uk/guidance/cg189

National Institute for Health and Care Excellence (NICE). Obesity in children and young people: pre-vention and lifestyle weight management programmes. QS94. NICE, 2015. ⅋ https://www.nice.org.uk/guidance/qs94

Wang Y, Cai L, Wu Y, et al. What childhood obesity prevention programmes work? A systematic review and meta-analysis. *Obes Rev* 2015;16:547–565.

Zimmet P, Alberti G, Kaufman F, et al. The metabolic syndrome in children and adolescents. *Lancet* 2007;369:2059–2061.

# Hypoglycaemia

# Physiology

Under normal circumstances, after the first few days of life blood glucose in children and adults is tightly maintained at ~3.5–6.5 mmol/L during fasting and following feeding and exercise.

After food ingestion, the glucose level starts rising after 15 minutes, and in response to this insulin is secreted from the pancreatic β-cells. Glucose levels peak after 30–60 minutes and then decrease back to fasting levels after 4–5 hours; this is also reflected by insulin secretion.

Insulin:
- increases glucose uptake into skeletal muscle and adipose tissue
- promotes glycogen synthesis
- inhibits glycogenolysis and hepatic gluconeogenesis.

Postprandially, the blood sugar is maintained in a stable state by a balance between glucose delivery and glucose removal. Tissue uptake into all tissues except the brain is under the influence of insulin.

Excess glucose is stored as glycogen in the liver under the influence of insulin, and released at times of need to maintain blood glucose in response to the counter-regulatory hormones:
- glucagon
- GH
- cortisol
- adrenaline (epinephrine).

Pathways involved in glucose homeostasis are:
- hormonal responses
- glycogen breakdown
- gluconeogenesis
- fatty acid oxidation
- ketone body synthesis
- ketone utilization.

In healthy children, after 12–16 hours of fasting the glycogen stores are depleted and then hepatic gluconeogenesis supervenes, along with fatty acids which are β oxidized to ketone bodies (acetoacetate and β hydroxybutyrate) as an alternative fuel source to glucose. Generally, the occurrence and intensity of ketonaemia is in proportion to the level of hypoglycaemia.

## Definition

- There is considerable debate as to what constitutes hypoglycaemia, with definitions based on:
  - normal ranges within epidemiological studies
  - thresholds for clinical symptoms and signs
  - thresholds for metabolic and endocrine counter-regulation
  - long-term neurological outcome.
- Clinical hypoglycaemia is defined as 'a plasma glucose concentration low enough to cause symptoms and/or signs of impaired brain function'.

Various cut-offs have been recommended:
- <3.5 mmol/L: based on normal blood glucose levels, and also used as the cut-off for hypoglycaemia in diabetic patients. In these patients, the threshold also depends on previous blood sugar concentrations.

- <3.0–3.3 mmol/L; the level at which treatment is recommend to asymptomatic children. 3.3 mmol/L is the same level indicated by recent USA guidelines (2015) for investigation in children who are unable to convey symptoms.
- <3.0 mmol/L.
- <2.4–2.6 mmol/L is accepted by some as more appropriate in children who are otherwise well.
- <2.0–2.2 mmol/L is suggested by international and national (2015) consensus as an 'action threshold' in neonates, both full term and premature.

Children and adults are obligate utilizers of glucose for brain metabolism which, apart from a small amount of glycogen stored within astrocytes, and limited gluconeogenesis, depends on a continuous supply of glucose.

However, infants and young children can also utilize ketone bodies from free fatty acids as an alternative brain fuel source. In situations of non-ketotic hypoglycaemia (such as hyperinsulinism) where ketone bodies cannot be utilized, the cut-offs for treating hypoglycaemia are set higher, i.e. <3.0 mmol/L in the first 48 hours of life and <3.5 mmol/L thereafter.

# Aetiology

As hypoglycaemia occurs when the supply of blood glucose is unable to keep up with utilization, causes of hypoglycaemia can be broadly divided into:

- decreased amount of glucose, due to:
  - failure in receiving or absorbing nutrients
  - decreased glycogen production or release from the liver
  - limited substrate for gluconeogenesis
  - decreased production of alternative fuels
- increased glucose utilization.

## Decreased glucose

### Neonate

- Prematurity
- IUGR
- Inborn errors of metabolism
- Hypopituitarism, including GH deficiency
- Adrenal insufficiency (1° or 2°)
- Prolonged fasting.

### Child

- Ketotic hypoglycaemia
- Drugs (e.g. β-blockers, alcohol).

## Increased glucose utilization

### Neonate: transient

- Infant of diabetic mother (insulin dependent or gestational)
- IUGR
- Perinatal asphyxia
- Hypothermia
- Sepsis
- Rhesus haemolytic disease (erythroblastosis fetalis)
- Beckwith–Wiedemann syndrome
- Other syndromes (e.g. Sotos, Costello, Kabuki, Usher).

### Neonate: persistent

- Congenital hyperinsulinaemia.

### Child

- Dumping syndrome
- Insulin excess
- Insulinoma.

# Decreased glucose

## Neonatal hypoglycaemia

This is common, especially in the first 24 hours of life during adaptation to extrauterine life. It depends on:
- definition of hypoglycaemia
- gestational age: more common in premature babies as a consequence of:
  - reduced reserves of liver glycogen and fat
  - reduced gluconeogenesis
  - relatively elevated insulin levels compared with full-term babies
- size for gestational age: more common in SGA neonates, who may also demonstrate increased glucose utilization 2° to transient hyperinsulinaemia and reduced glucagon levels
- feeding postnatally
- associated problems: e.g. neonatal asphyxia, hypothermia, illness.

## Metabolic and endocrine problems

Can be caused by abnormalities in counter-regulatory hormones, such as:
- cortisol deficiency due to hypopituitarism or adrenal insufficiency
- GHD
- inborn errors of metabolism
- (hypothyroidism).

### Metabolic diseases

These produce hypoglycaemia by impairment of:
- mobilization of glucose stores (e.g. glycogen metabolism defects)
- gluconeogenesis (e.g. gluconeogenic defects such as fructose-1,6-bisphosphatase and glucose-6-phosphatase deficiencies))
- utilization of alternative energy supplies such as fatty acids and ketones (e.g. impaired ketogenesis and ketone utilization):
  - *fatty acid oxidation defects*: medium, long, and very long chain acyl-CoA dehydrogenase deficiencies (MCADD, LCHADD, VLCADD), primary carnitine deficiency and carnitine cycle defects. NB: the commonest of these, MCADD, has an incidence of 1 in 10,000 births, and is part of the newborn screening programme in the UK (since 2009); fatty acid oxidation defects are also screened for in other countries
  - *ketone synthesis defects*: hydroxymethylglutaryl-CoA synthase (HMG-CoA synthase) and lyase defects
  - *ketone utilization defects*: monocarboxylase transporter1 (MCT1), succinyl-CoA oxoacid transferase (SCOT) and acetoacetyl-CoA thiolase (ACAT1) deficiencies
- liver function (e.g. acute liver failure, end-stage chronic liver disease).

## Glycogen storage diseases

These are inherited defects of either glycogen synthesis or breakdown. In glycogen synthase deficiency (GSD 0), ketotic hypoglycaemia occurs with fasting, with hyperglycaemia and raised lactate postprandially. Hypoglycaemia is also found in GSD types I and III (VI and IX may have only mild predisposition).

Other features are:
- persistent hepatomegaly
- elevated urate, triglycerides
- ketosis in type I, lactic acidosis in the remainder.

Other features are specific to the individual conditions.

Diagnosis is based on:
- enzyme analysis in liver and leucocytes
- mutation analysis.

## Idiopathic ketotic hypoglycaemia (IKH)

- The commonest cause of hypoglycaemia in young non-diabetic children.
- Onset 18 months to 5 years.
- More common in boys, children born SGA, and those with poor weight gain and thinness.
- Recurrent episodes of hypoglycaemia, especially during illnesses involving anorexia and vomiting.
- During fasting children are more hypoglycaemic and ketonaemic compared with controls, with low levels of alanine, the major gluconeogenic amino acid (cause or effect?).
- Aetiology is unclear but probably reflects underproduction rather than overutilization of glucose.
- May reflect end of normal range for fasting tolerance; polymorphisms or partial deficiencies of hormones involved in glucose homeostasis may be present.
- Neurological damage and other sequelae are rare.
- Treatment consists of avoidance of prolonged periods of fasting.
- Usually resolves spontaneously by 7 years.

# Increased glucose utilization

## Congenital hyperinsulinism
May be:
- transient or persistent.
- severe or mild.

## Transient hyperinsulinism
### Beckwith–Wiedemann syndrome
A rare condition, but the most common of the overgrowth syndromes, with an estimated incidence of 1 in 13,700.

The most common features (all with frequency >50%) are as follows:
- macroglossia (large tongue)
- excessive pre/postnatal growth (weight:length ratio at birth and subsequently >97th centile)
- abdominal wall defects (including omphalocoele)
- ear creases or pits
- neonatal hypoglycaemia due to hyperinsulinaemia, which is:
  - transient in ~50% and settles spontaneously in the first few days of life
  - persistent in ~5%, requiring continuous feeding, medical therapy, or occasionally surgery (near-total pancreatectomy).

Other features include:
  - naevus flammeus (port-wine stain) usually on the forehead or neck
  - renal abnormalities (enlargement, structural, nephrocalcinosis)
  - hemihypertrophy
  - malignancy (embryonal tumours), e.g. Wilms tumour, hepatoblastoma, neuroblastoma, rhabdomyosarcoma
  - cardiac defects, malrotation
  - intellectual disability.

Diagnosis is predominantly clinical, based on major (and minor) criteria.
- Although most cases are sporadic, ~15% are familial.
- Up to 70% of patients have abnormalities involving 11p15, including:
  - loss of DNA methylation (~50%)
  - paternal uniparental disomy (10–20%)
  - gain of DNA methylation (2–7%)
  - mutations (5–10%), but 40% in familial cases
  - maternal chromosomal rearrangements.

## Hyperinsulinaemia
### Hyperinsulinaemic hypoglycaemia (HH)
- Produced by unregulated production of insulin in relation to the blood glucose concentration.
- Most common cause of persistent hypoglycaemia in both the neonatal period and infancy.
- Can be transient or persistent.
- Can be sporadic (incidence ~1 in 40,000) or familial (incidence as high as 1 in 2500 in some populations).
- Typically presents shortly after birth with symptomatic hypoglycaemia.

- Babies may or may not be macrosomic; and absence does not exclude HH.
- May have mild facial dysmorphism.

*Diagnosis*
See Table 7.1.

*Genetics*
Currently 11 key genes involved in regulating insulin secretion from β-cells are implicated in monogenic HH (*ABCC8, KCNJ11, GLUD1, GCK, HADH1, UCP2, MCT1, HNF4A, HNF1A, HK1, PGM1*).

*Transient HH*
Mutations in the gene encoding the hepatic nuclear transcription factor-4α (*HNF4A*) have been reported.

*Persistent HH*
Mutations leading to dysregulated insulin secretion have been described in a number of different genes. These are further subdivided into:
- channelopathies, where β-cell K$_{ATP}$ channel defects within the pancreas lead to unregulated insulin secretion
- metabolopathies, with increased ATP formation within the β-cell or accumulation of intermediary metabolite accumulation, producing insulin secretion (Fig. 7.1).

**Table 7.1** Diagnostic biochemical features of hypoglycaemic hyperinsulinaemia

| |
|---|
| Glucose infusion rate >8 mg/kg/min |
| Laboratory blood glucose <3 mmol/L with: |
|     detectable serum insulin/C-peptide |
|     suppressed/low serum ketone bodies |
|     suppressed/low serum fatty acids |
|     suppressed branch-chain amino acids |
| Serum ammonia level may be raised (HI/HA syndrome) |
| Raised plasma hydroxybutyrylcarnitine and urinary 3-hydroxyglutarate (HADH deficiency) |
| Supportive evidence (when diagnosis is in doubt): |
|     positive glycaemic (>1.5 mmol/L) response to IM/IV glucagon |
|     positive glycaemic response to SC/IV dose of octreotide |
|     low levels of serum IGFBP1 |

HADH, hydroxyacyl-coenzyme A dehydrogenase; HI/HA, hyperinsulinism and hyperammonaemia; IGFBP1, insulin growth factor binding protein 1.

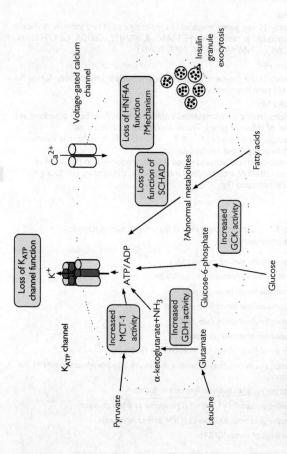

**Fig. 7.1** Summary of the known genetic causes of hypoglycaemic hyperinsulinaemia.

*Channelopathy defects*
Inactivating mutations in genes affecting the regulation of pancreatic $K_{ATP}$ channels, lead to unregulated release of insulin despite hypoglycaemia:

- *ABCC8* encoding the SUR1 subunit (150 mutations)
- *KCNJ11* encoding the KIR6.2 subunit (~24 mutations).

These are the most common causes of HH. Generally, recessive mutations cause severe HH which does not respond to diazoxide, while dominant mutations usually produce a milder clinical picture.

*Metabolopathy defects*
*Glutamate dehydrogenase (GDH)* is the second most common cause of HH. Activating mutations in GDH produce hyperinsulinism–hyperammonaemia (HI/HA).

- Autosomal dominant inheritance.
- Presents with hypoglycaemia in infancy, although hypoglycaemia is milder than other forms of CHI.
- Patients have more neurological issues including learning difficulties and epilepsy.
- Associated with hyperammonaemia (up to 200 mmol/L).
- Responds well to diazoxide, and also to protein restriction.

*Glukokinase*: this functions as a glucose sensor, and activating mutations causes inappropriate glucose-stimulated insulin release, causing hypoglycaemia. The presenting age can range from infancy to adulthood, with a variable clinical phenotype.

Other HH mutations occur in:

1. *3-hydroxyacyl-coenzyme A dehydrogenase*: most reported patients respond to diazoxide
2. *HNF4A and HNF1A*: these usually cause MODY types 1 and 3; both present with macrosomia and either can be managed with diet alone or diazoxide. Heterozygous mutations in *HNF4A* may produce both transient or persistent HH
3. *solute carrier family 16, member 1*: causes exercise-induced hyperinsulinism and hypoglycaemia 30–45 minutes post vigorous exercise
4. *uncoupling protein 2 gene*.

*Histology*
Three predominant abnormalities are noted within the pancreas:

1. Diffuse, affecting the whole pancreas, previously known as nesidioblastosis. Usually 2° to either dominant or recessive mutations in *ABCC8* or *KCNJ11*.
2. Focal, localized to a single region of the pancreas.
3. Intermediate atypical forms are occasionally noted, containing both large and shrunken islets; the former are confined to a few pancreatic lobules.

*Treatment*
(See Fig. 7.2.)

This is aimed at maintaining normoglycaemia (blood sugar 3.5–6 mmol/L). It is important to maintain the blood sugar above 3.5 mmol/L as there are no alternative brain energy substrates during HH. Management is challenging, and HH should ideally be managed in the UK in collaboration with specialist centres: currently London (Great Ormond Street) and Manchester Children's Hospital/Liverpool Alder Hey Hospital (NORCHI) within England.

*Glucose*
- Nasogastric feeds (if necessary with added glucose polymer) and IV fluids are often required to provide adequate carbohydrate.
- High concentrations of dextrose may require central venous access.

*Medication*
- Diazoxide (an agonist of the $K_{ATP}$ channel): 5–20 mg/kg/day in three divided doses. Patients with transient and syndromic forms of HI usually respond to diazoxide, while those with severe neonatal HH often show

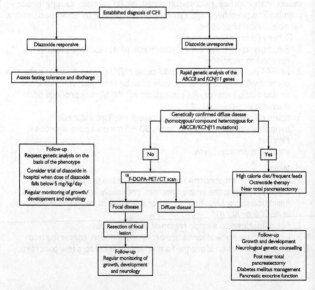

**Fig. 7.2** Flowchart for the diagnosis and management of congenital hyperinsulinism.

Reproduced with permission from Kapoor RR, Flanagan SE, James C, Shield J, Ellard S, Hussain K (2009). Hyperinsulinaemic hypoglycaemia. *Arch Dis Child* 2009; 94: 450–7. Copyright © 2009 BMJ Publishing Group Ltd.

no response. NB: genetic testing should be performed in patients who are unresponsive to diazoxide, as a genetic cause is found in ~80–90%, and will assist in determining future therapy.
- Chlorothiazide (activates $K_{ATP}$ channel, and also works synergistically with diazoxide): 7–10 mg/kg/day in two divided doses.
- Glucagon (increases glycogenolysis and gluconeogenesis): 1–10 mcg/kg/hour by SC/IV infusion or 0.5–1.0 mg IV or IM bolus.
- Somatostatin analogues, e.g. octreotide (stabilizes the $K_{ATP}$ channel and inhibits insulin secretion): 5–35 mcg/kg/day by SC/IV infusion or three or four SC injections/day. Often used short term together with glucagon. A long-acting formulation lanreotide/LAR-octreotide may also be used long term.
- Nifedipine (calcium channel blocker which inhibits β-cell membrane depolarization): 0.25–2.5 mg/kg/day in three divided doses.
- Glucagon-like peptide-1 (GLP-1) receptor antagonist. May benefit patients with $K_{ATP}$ HH.
- Rapamycin mTOR inhibitors (e.g. sirolimus) are also helpful in preventing the need for pancreatectomy in diffuse disease.

Although selective pancreatic venous sampling has been used historically, distinguishing between focal and diffuse disease is currently best done using [$^{18}$F]L-dopa positron emission tomography/CT (18F-DOPA-PET/CT) scanning. Sensitivity and specificity of distinguishing between focal and diffuse forms in meta-analysis is said to be 89% and 98% respectively.

This is important as:
- children with focal and also atypical forms of HH can be completely cured by selective surgical removal
- children with diffuse forms of HH who fail to respond to medical therapy require a near-total (95–98%) pancreatectomy.

NB: postoperatively patients may:
- have continued HH and remain dependent on medical therapy
- develop:
  - diabetes mellitus
  - exocrine pancreatic insufficiency.

# Symptoms

The symptoms of hypoglycaemia can be divided into:

- those due to counter-regulatory hormones:
  - adrenergic: epinephrine and norepinephrine
  - glucagon
- those due to neuroglycopenia.

Characteristically, as the blood sugar concentration decreases, there is activation of counter-regulatory hormones, followed by an autonomic sympathoadrenal response, followed by neuroglycopenia.

## Glucagon-related symptoms

- Hunger, nausea, abdominal discomfort
- Vomiting
- Headache.

## Adrenergic symptoms

- Sweating
- Pallor, coldness, clamminess
- Palpitations, tachycardia
- Shaking, tremor
- Anxiety.

## Neuroglycopenic symptoms

- Lethargy, fatigue, weakness, apathy
- Confusion, amnesia, dizziness
- Slurring of speech, blurred vision, ataxia
- Bizarre behaviour, tearfulness
- Anxiety, depression, mood swings
- Headache
- Aggression
- Coma, seizures (generalized or focal).

## Symptoms may also be dependent on

- age
- frequency of hypoglycaemia
- rate of onset and duration.

In infants, symptoms may be non-specific, and due to excitation or depression of the CNS (Table 7.2).

**Table 7.2** Infant symptoms of hypoglycaemia

| CNS excitation | CNS depression |
|---|---|
| • Jitteriness/tremor | • Poor feeding |
| • Irritability | • Apnoea, cyanotic episodes |
| • High-pitched cry | • Lethargy |
| • Tachypnoea | • Hypotonia |
| • Seizures | • Coma |

# Investigation

(➲ See also Chapters 13, p. 368 and Chapter 14, p. 422.)

Points

- Any child with unexplained hypoglycaemia should be investigated.
- Biochemical hypoglycaemia is common in the neonatal period, but in the majority is asymptomatic and transient. Prolonged (? and also pronounced) hypoglycaemia needs investigation in this age group.
- Hypoglycaemia due to a metabolic cause may be episodic in infants and older children, and be precipitated by either an intercurrent illness or a prolonged period of fasting.

Points in the history

- Pregnancy: maternal health (including diabetes), gestation (? prematurity), evidence of IUGR (serial scans)
- Delivery: birthweight/length, neonatal asphyxia
- Onset of hypoglycaemia: age, precipitating/relieving factors. Association with fasting or feeding
- Period of fasting tolerated
- Other associated symptoms.

Points in the examination

- Evidence of macrosomia.
- Dysmorphic features indicative of underlying syndrome.
- Features of hypopituitarism (e.g. midface hypoplasia, jaundice).
- Myopathy and cardiomyopathy in fatty acid oxidation defects.
- Hepatosplenomegaly: indicative of inborn errors of metabolism and glycogen storage disease, and suggestive of the following defects if associated with:
  - liver failure or hepatic necrosis: galactosaemia, tyrosinaemia, haemochromatosis, $\alpha_1$-antitrypsin deficiency, respiratory chain defects
  - cirrhosis: hereditary fructose intolerance, glycogen storage disease type IV
  - isolated hepatomegaly: glycogen storage diseases.

Initial investigation of hypoglycaemia

The most useful investigations are those done during a presenting episode.
▶ Important first to confirm hypoglycaemia with true lab blood glucose. Investigations at the time of hypoglycaemia and subsequently:

- At time of hypoglycaemia and prior to correction:
  - glucose, lactate, 3-hydroxybutyrate, free fatty acids, insulin/C-peptide, cortisol, GH
- Can be taken after correction of hypoglycaemia:
  - *blood*: U&E, LFTs, amino acids, ammonia, plasma/blood spot acylcarnitines
  - *first-passed urine*: organic acids, ketone bodies.

*Results*

- Blood gases: unexplained metabolic acidosis is suggestive of keto-acidosis/lactic acidosis or organic acidaemia. Ketoacidosis occurs in:

- maple syrup urine disease (MSUD)
- ketolytic defects
- glycerol kinase deficiency
- fructose-1, 6-bisphosphatase deficiency
- adrenal insufficiency.
- Acidosis without ketosis occurs in:
  - ketogenesis disorders
  - fatty acid oxidation disorders.
- Ammonia: increased in hepatic dysfunction and hyperinsulinism with hyperammonaemia.
- Lactate: increased in metabolic liver disease, glycogen storage disease, or prolonged convulsions.

### Metabolic

- Plasma non-esterified free fatty acids (NEFA) and 3-hydroxybutyrate: lipolysis suppressed in hyperinsulinism, while ketogenesis is defective in fatty acid oxidation defects (ratio of free fatty acids to 3-hydroxybutyrate usually <2; levels greater than this suggestive of fat oxidation defect).
- Plasma/urine amino acids: specific amino acid increases found in tyrosinaemia, maple syrup urine disease. Alanine is also raised if lactate is chronically raised.
- Blood spot and plasma acylcarnitines: abnormal species are found in fatty acid oxidation defects and organic acid disorders.
- Urine organic acids: pattern may indicate a specific organic acid or fatty acid defect.
- Urine ketones: absence is suggestive of a fatty acid oxidation defect, ketone body synthesis defect, or hyperinsulinaemia. Ketosis without acidosis occurs in adrenal insufficiency and ketotic hypoglycaemia.
- Urine reducing substances (non-glucose): presence suggests galactosaemia.
- Urine sugar chromatography: may indicate disorders such as galactosaemia or fructosaemia.

### Endocrine

- Insulin/C-peptide: raised levels indicative of hyperinsulinaemia. May not be demonstrated as insulin has a short half-life (~6 minutes) in the circulation. With raised insulin alone, indicative of exogenous insulin.
- GH: low levels indicate GHD, either isolated or as part of multiple pituitary hormone deficiencies.
- Cortisol: low levels may indicate hypoadrenalism (1° or 2°), although often poor cortisol response to hypoglycaemia if 2° to hyperinsulinaemia.

### Controlled fast

- If no diagnosis is established on baseline investigations, a controlled fast may be necessary. With improved diagnosis (including genetic panels) they are performed much less often. Some disorders may produce no metabolic abnormalities in 'unstressed' individuals, and the controlled fast assesses fasting tolerance under controlled conditions. The test

is potentially hazardous and requires an experienced unit and close monitoring. It should also be planned with the laboratory in advance.
- The controlled fast may be important both to exclude disorders and to establish normal fasting responses.

### Duration of controlled fast
( See also 'Prolonged fast', p. 422.)

If the patient becomes symptomatic or is hypoglycaemic (e.g. blood sugar ≤3mmol/L) then an urgent laboratory blood sugar should be performed along with the appropriate samples and the fast terminated. Post end-of-fast samples should be taken 60–90 minutes later; which may also provide important diagnostic information (Table 7.3).

### Measure at baseline, during fast, at end of fast, postprandially and after end of fast
- Bedside glucose (hourly)
- Glucose
- Lactate
- Free fatty acids
- Ketones.

### Measure at baseline, end of fast, and postprandially
- Carnitine and acyl carnitine profile.

### Measure at baseline and end of fast
- Cortisol
- Amino acids
- Organic acids
- Ammonia
- Total $CO_2$.

### Measure at end of fast and after end of fast
- GH.

### Measure at end of fast
- Insulin.

### Treatment
For management of HH and hypoglycaemia in diabetes, see 'Increased glucose utilization treatment', and 'Hypoglycaemia'. In emergencies, see p. 368.

Treatment is aimed at:

**Table 7.3** Duration of controlled fast

| Age | <6 months | 6–8 months | 8–12 months | 1–2 years | >2 years |
|-----|-----------|------------|-------------|-----------|----------|
| Duration (hours) | 8 | 12 | 16 | 18 | 20 |

- specific treatment of the underlying diagnosis
- maintenance of blood sugar above ~4.0 mmol/L; this may require:
  - regular feeding
  - glucose supplements to feeds
  - oral glucose 10–20 g, e.g. two teaspoons of sugar, 200 mL of milk, 100 mL of Lucozade®
  - buccal dextrose gel
  - IV 10% glucose, initial boluses (e.g. 10 mL/kg as IV bolus) and then by continuous infusion
  - IM glucagon (0.5 mg if <25 kg bodyweight, otherwise 1.0 mg).

Emergency regimen for use during illnesses:
- high-carbohydrate drinks
- presentation to hospital if not tolerated
- ◉ home blood glucose monitoring.

Specific management principles of glycogenoses, fatty acid oxidation defects (FAODs), gluconeogenic defects, and ketone defects.
- Avoidance of fasting with:
  - regular (2–4-hourly) daytime feeds
  - overnight nasogastric feeds (as in GSD 1 fasting tolerance may be as little as 1 hour)
  - uncooked corn starch (rarely tolerated <1 year of age due to lack of pancreatic amylase).
- Dietary manipulation:
  - low-fat diet and medium-chain triglyceride feeds in long-chain FAODs.
- Carnitine supplementation.
- Dietary management during intercurrent illnesses when fasting tolerance is reduced:
  - 'emergency regimen' of high-calorie supplement of glucose polymer
  - IV 10% glucose if feeds not tolerated (even if normoglycaemic).

# Further reading

Ghosh A, Banerjee I, Morris AAM. Recognition, assessment and management of hypoglycaemia in childhood. *Arch Dis Child* 2016;101:575–580.

Guemes M, Hussain K. Hyperinsulinemic hyperglycemia *Paediatr Clin N Amer* 2015;62:1017–1036.

Guemes M, Rahman SA, Hussain K. What is a normal blood glucose? *Arch Dis Child* 2016;101:569–574.

Senniappan S, Alexandrescu S, Tatevian N, et al. Sirolimus therapy in infants with severe hyperinsulinemic hypoglycemia. *N Engl J Med* 2014;370:1131–1137.

Shah P, Rahman SA, Demirbilek H, et al. Hyperinsulinaemic hypoglycaemia in children and adults. *Lancet Diabetes Endocrinol* 2017;5:729–742.

Sreekantam S, Preece AM, Vijay S, Raiman J, Santra S (2016). How to use a controlled fast to investigate hypoglycaemia. *Arch Dis Child Educ Pract Ed* 2017;102:28–36.

# Adrenal gland disorders

# Physiology

### Regulation of the adrenal cortex

The adrenal cortex which produces steroid hormones is under the control of both the HPA endocrine axis, regulating cortisol secretion, and the renin–angiotensin system regulating aldosterone secretion (Figs. 8.1 and 8.2). Adrenal androgens are also under ACTH control but some aspects of adrenal physiology, e.g. adrenarche, depend upon internal regulation.

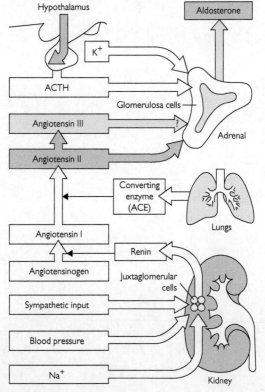

**Fig. 8.1** Physiology of the adrenal cortex.

Reproduced with permission from Besser M, Thorner GM (1994). *Clinical Endocrinology*. Mosby, St Louis, MO. With permission from Elsevier. Mosby-Wolfe, 1994.

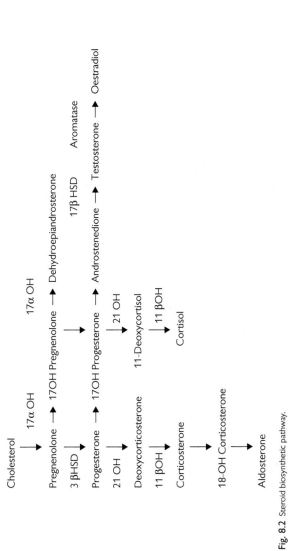

**Fig. 8.2** Steroid biosynthetic pathway.
Reproduced with permission from Turner HE, Wass JAH (2009). *Oxford Handbook of Endocrinology and Diabetes* (2nd edn), Oxford University Press, Oxford. Copyright © 2009 OUP.

## Development of the adrenal gland

During fetal life, the adrenal cortex develops an additional layer from 8 weeks' gestation under control of the gene *SF1*. The fetal adrenal zone is considerably thicker than the mature cortex and the steroid hormones produced including cortisol are thought to have a role in maintaining the pregnancy. The large fetal zone atrophies soon after birth. The mature adrenal cortex comprises of three layers:

- Outer layer:        zona glomerulosa—produces aldosterone
- Middle layer:      zona fasciculata—produces cortisol
- Inner layer:        zona reticularis—produces androgens
- Mnemonic:        G, glomerulosa; F, fasciculata; R, reticularis.

## Adrenarche

From 6 years of age in boys and girls there is a marked increase (5–10×) in adrenal androgen secretion, especially DHEA, DHEAS, and androstenedione. This is called adrenarche. There is also a concomitant rise in blood pressure but no alteration in growth velocity.

This rise in DHEA is thought to arise from the need to increase cortisol production as a child grows, and hence there is a greater pituitary ACTH drive to do this. The higher internal cortisol levels inhibit activity of the enzyme 3βHSD2 which consequently raises DHEA production. DHEA is sulphated to DHEAS by the enzyme SULT2A1 to become the most abundant hormone in the body.

In some children this process is more pronounced and may become noticeable on account of greasy skin and hair, the development of body odour, and light growth of pubic and axillary hair, occasionally as young as 4 years (➲ see Chapter 2). It is more common in children who are tall or overweight (for reasons previously mentioned) and those of southern Mediterranean, of central and south Asian, and of Afro/Caribbean descent. Although this may be a normal variant, often termed precocious (or exaggerated) adrenarche, exclusion of other forms of precocious sexual maturity may be necessary (➲ see Chapter 11).

## Cortisol metabolism

Cortisol is transported in the plasma:
- 75% bound to corticosteroid binding protein
- 15% bound to albumin
- 10% free.

The endogenous production rate is estimated at 6–10 mg/m$^2$/day. It is inactivated in the liver to the principal inactive metabolite cortisone, and 95% is excreted via the kidneys. Cortisol action is mediated via the glucocorticoid receptor found in the cell nucleus—the gene for the receptor is on chromosome 18p11.2

# Adrenal insufficiency

## Symptoms of primary adrenal failure

### Non-specific

- Tiredness, lethargy, and weakness
- Poor concentration, behaviour problems
- Craving of salt
- Frequent minor infections, more severe than usual and slow to recover
- Anorexia and weight loss
- Sickness, vomiting, diarrhoea
- Acute presentation: see later in topic.

## Clinical features

Hyperpigmentation is present, especially in the skin creases and mucosal surfaces. Beware apparent suntan below swimming costume area, as this can confirm true hyperpigmentation. This is caused by ACTH hyperstimulation of cutaneous melanocortin-1 receptors (MC1R). Note that 2° causes of adrenal insufficiency (ACTH deficiency) do not cause increased pigmentation (Box 8.1).

### Investigations for suspected adrenal insufficiency

- Low sodium
- High potassium

## Box 8.1 Causes of adrenal insufficiency

### Primary

#### Congenital

- Dysplasia, e.g. congenital adrenal hypoplasia (CAH)
- Enzyme blocks, e.g. 21-hydroxylase deficiency (21OHD) (70%)
- Adrenoleukodystrophy (4%).

#### Acquired (Addison's disease)

- Autoimmune adrenalitis (14%)
- Tuberculosis
- Waterhouse–Friedrichsen syndrome—meningococcal septicaemia
- (Total all others 12%).

### Secondary

- CRH receptor defect
- Isolated ACTH deficiency
- Panhypopituitarism (multiple pituitary hormone deficiency).

### Tertiary

- Pituitary tumours
- CNS malformations
- High-dose glucocorticoid therapy.

- Cortisol low/undetectable (8 am cortisol normally > 300 nmol/L (cortisol assay dependent))
- ACTH raised in 1° causes, low in 2°
- DHEAS low
- Synacthen test—low or absent cortisol rise.

## Acute adrenal crisis (Addisonian crisis)

- *Symptoms:* lethargy leading to coma, abdominal pain, vomiting
- *Signs:* dehydration, shock, tachycardia, acidotic breathing.

### Diagnosis of acute adrenal crisis

- Low sodium
- High potassium
- Hypoglycaemia
- Acidosis.

### Management

↪ See 'Adrenal insufficiency/adrenal crisis', p. 370.

## Autoimmune adrenalitis (classic Addison's disease)

This is the commonest cause of 1° adrenal insufficiency in children >3 years.

- *Isolated:* adrenal autoantibodies to 21-hydroxylase enzyme
- *Combined:* with other autoimmune diseases and mucocutaneous candidiasis—autoimmune polyglandular syndrome (APS) type 1 (*AIRE* gene mutation); and with Hashimoto's thyroiditis and T1DM—APS type 2 (associated with mutations in *CLTA4, HLA-DR3, HLA-DR4*).

## Congenital adrenal hypoplasia (adrenal hypoplasia congenita)

A rare form of 1° adrenal insufficiency. Severe forms (autosomal recessive, 1 in 70,000–600,000) present soon after birth with hyperpigmentation, hypoglycaemia, and acute adrenal crisis.

X-linked forms due to *DAX1* gene mutations on the X chromosome (1 in 12,000) may be combined with hypogonadotropic hypogonadism (HH), or Duchenne muscular dystrophy and glycerol kinase deficiency due to contiguous gene locations.

### Diagnosis

- Gonadotropin deficiency: GnRH test
- Duchenne muscular dystrophy: elevated creatine kinase
- Glycerol kinase deficiency: elevated triglycerides.

## Adrenoleukodystrophy

Males present aged 4–12 years with ataxia, spasticity, loss of cognitive function, and dementia due to progressive leukodystrophy. Associated features are red–green colour blindness, visual problems, and deafness.

### Cause

Mutations in *ALD* gene on chromosome Xq28, coding for ALD protein, an ABC (ATP-binding cassette) transporter.

*Diagnosis*

Elevated very long-chain fatty acids. Remember to check in all males with adrenal insufficiency (VLCFA).

## Familial glucocorticoid deficiency (FGD)

Cause of familial hyperpigmentation, hypoglycaemia, and frequent and severe infections. Salt wasting is absent.

*Causes*

- FGD type 1: inactivating mutations and polymorphisms in the ACTH receptor gene *MC2R* encoding the melanocortin-2 receptor protein on chromosome 18p11.2
- FGD type 2: no *MC2R* mutations, mutations in the *MRAP* gene encoding the melanocortin receptor-associated protein.
- FGD-DNA repair defect: associated with short stature and microcephaly—*MRM4* mutation.

*Diagnosis*

Low/absent cortisol levels and blunted/absent response to ACTH stimulation, with very raised ACTH levels. Electrolytes, plasma renin activity, and aldosterone levels are normal.

## Triple A syndrome (Allgrove syndrome)

This syndrome comprises Adrenal insufficiency, Alacrima, Achalasia, and neurological impairment in 60% (including neurogenic distal muscular atrophy, ataxia, intellectual disability, nasal speech, hyper-reflexia, optic atrophy, and autonomic dysfunction). Other clinical features include hyperkeratosis, deafness, caries, and impaired wound healing.

*Causes*

Mutations in the *AAAS* gene on chromosome 12q13 coding for a nucleoporin protein ALADIN, a gatekeeper for nucleocytoplasmic transport, regulator of the cell cycle, and regulator of gene expression.

*Other multisystem conditions affecting adrenal function*

- Zellweger syndrome (*PEX1*)
- Kearns-Sayre syndrome (mitochondrial DNA deletion).

## Congenital adrenal hyperplasia (CAH)

CAH is a group of adrenal enzyme disorders causing impaired cortisol secretion and subsequent raised ACTH secretion, which in turn causes hyperplasia of the adrenal glands. The commonest defect is 21-hydroxylase deficiency (21OHD) (1 in 10,000–16,000) which may also cause impaired aldosterone secretion, but the nature of the steroid block and its severity in this and all the forms of CAH mean that presentation can be very variable (Table 8.1).

Other forms of CAH are much rarer, the most often recognized of these is 11β-hydroxylase deficiency (1 in 100,000–200,000). This autosomal recessive condition is most likely to manifest with mild virilization of a female infant. Defects in 17α-hydroxylase prevent androgen formation, and consequently genetic males present with undervirilization (➲ see Chapter 11).

**Table 8.1** Principal enzymic defects causing adrenal dysfunction

| Enzyme defect | Gene | Effects in males | Effects in females | Diagnosis |
|---|---|---|---|---|
| 21-hydroxylase deficiency | CYP21A2 inactivating mutations | Classic: SW crisis Non-classic: late/mild virilization | Classic: variable virilization; SW crisis Non-classic: late/mild virilization | Serum: elevated 17OHP Urine: elevated androgens and metabolites |
| 11-hydroxylase deficiency | CYP11B1 inactivating mutations | Classic: virilization, adrenal insufficiency, hypertension Non-classic: late/mild virilization | Classic: virilization, adrenal insufficiency, hypertension Non-classic: late/mild virilization | Serum: elevated 11-deoxycortisol and 11-deoxycorticosterone Urine: elevated metabolites |
| 17-hydroxylase deficiency | CYP17A1 inactivating mutations | 46,XY DSD poor/absent virilization; cortisol insufficiency | Delayed puberty; cortisol insufficiency | Serum: elevated 11-deoxycorticosterone and corticosterone, low androgens Urine: elevated mineralocorticoid ratio |
| 3β-hydroxysteroid dehydrogenase deficiency | HSD3B2 inactivating mutations | Classic: DSD, SW crisis Non-classic: late/mild virilization, adrenal insufficiency | Classic: DSD, SW crisis Non-classic: late/mild virilization, adrenal insufficiency | Serum: increased androstenedione/testosterone ratio Urine: elevated DHEA/metabolites |

(Continued)

**Table 8.1** (Contd.)

| Enzyme defect | Gene | Effects in males | Effects in females | Diagnosis |
|---|---|---|---|---|
| Cytochrome P450 oxidoreductase deficiency | POR inactivating mutations | DSD in 75%; delayed puberty Cortisol deficiency Antley–Bixler skeletal abnormalities | DSD in 75%; delayed puberty Cortisol deficiency Antley–Bixler skeletal abnormalities | Serum: mild elevation 17OHP, pregnenolone Urine: impaired diagnostic ratios for CYP17A1 and CYP21A2 and raised pregnenolone |
| Congenital lipoid hyperplasia | STAR inactivating mutations | Classic: SW crisis Non-classic: variable | Classic: SW crisis Non-classic: variable | Absent/reduced steroids of all classes |

SW, salt-wasting.

### Causes of 21OHD

Autosomal recessive genetic inheritance, with the gene *CYP21A2* mapped to chromosome 6p21, in between the class III *HLA-B* and *HLA-D* loci. Within the gene there may be many different genetic lesions such as a deletion, or point mutation, or meiotic recombination.

Most affected subjects are compound heterozygotes. There is a good phenotype–genotype correlation. Molecular diagnosis is helpful, as well as for doubtful diagnosis and for prenatal diagnosis (⮡ see 'Prenatal diagnosis and treatment', p. 285).

### Classification

In 21OHD, presentation depends on gender and phenotype:
- *Classical*: presents at birth with adrenal crisis or ambiguous genitalia
- *Non-classical*: late-onset presentation
- *Salt wasting*: more severe defect affecting aldosterone secretion causing an adrenal crisis
- *Simple virilizing*: hyperandrogenism with reduced but adequate cortisol and aldosterone secretion and raised androgens.

### Presentation of different forms

#### Classical (75%)

Males often present with hyperpigmented scrotum and genitalia at birth, and poor feeding, weight loss, and failure to thrive. If CAH is not recognized, a severe Addisonian crisis may ensue and death is a possibility. Treatment requires hydrocortisone and fludrocortisone. Females will also develop a similar picture but the genitalia are usually virilized due to excess testosterone allowing earlier diagnosis. Virilization may range from mild clitoromegaly to full masculinization (classified according to Prader stages). ⮡ See Chapter 11 for further details.

#### Non-classical (25%)

More severe gene defects may cause androgen excess in early childhood with rapid growth and an advanced bone age, pubic hair development, penile growth in boys, and clitoromegaly in girls. Milder defects may present with only mild increases in androgen secretion causing minimal pubic hair growth, adult body odour, and skin greasiness which may be indistinguishable from normal adrenarche. The presence of acne in a prepubertal child may point to CAH. Treatment may require full hydrocortisone dosing or sometimes just emergency cover in acute illnesses. Fludrocortisone requirement is variable.

### Diagnosis

- Classical 21OHD is confirmed by a raised 17-hydroxyprogesterone (17OHP) level at birth if measured by tandem mass spectrometry or after day 3 of life by standard immunoassay.
- Salt wasting is confirmed by low plasma sodium, high potassium, and increased urinary sodium excretion.

#### Pitfalls in the diagnosis

- 17OHP levels are often falsely raised before postnatal day 3 due to fetal adrenal cortex metabolites interfering in an immunoassay.

- Levels are higher in preterm infants and sick/stressed neonates of all gestational ages due to the higher ACTH drive.
- Phenotypic males with undescended testes may be fully virilized genetic females with CAH. This should always be formally excluded to prevent an adrenal crisis.

### Initial management

Rehydration with normal saline and correction of hypoglycaemia are required urgently (➲ see Chapter 13). A bolus of hydrocortisone should be given and an infusion established.

When stable, regular maintenance treatment can be begun:

- Hydrocortisone 10–15 mg/m²/day
- Fludrocortisone 150 mcg/m²/day
- Sodium supplements may be needed for the first year, sometimes longer, pending maturation of renal tubular sodium resorption: 5 mmol/kg/day in divided doses.

### Follow-up

- Children with CAH require careful follow-up to ensure balanced steroid replacement.
- Girls with virilization require sensitive consideration of the need for surgical correction, its timing, and when to provide psychological support.

### Monitoring schedule

- 4–6-monthly clinic review, checking weight, height, height velocity, blood pressure, and observation of pubertal staging.
- 17OHP hormone profile 6–12-monthly (either in bloodspots, saliva, or 24-hour plasma profiling).
- Annual bone age estimation and measurement of plasma renin activity.

As with other children with adrenal insufficiency, emergency treatment plans should be put in place.

▶ *Special note*: in any established adrenal disease with patients on steroid replacement with glucocorticoid with or without mineralocorticoid, acute adrenal crises during intercurrent illnesses can be prevented by asking the patient or family to double or triple the dose of glucocorticoid at the onset of symptoms and continue until the condition has substantially improved.

Approximate emergency doses of IM hydrocortisone:

- 0–10 kg (1 year): 25 mg
- 10–30 kg (7 years): 50 mg
- >30 kg: 100 mg.

In predictable stressful situations such as routine or emergency surgery, the glucocorticoid (hydrocortisone) should be given IV at a dose of 2 mg/kg every 6 hours during induction of anaesthesia, during surgery, and in the immediate postoperative period, before returning to double the usual dose when oral intake is established.

It is always wise to seek expert help when managing patients in this situation.

## Complications of CAH

### Poor compliance with treatment

Causes initial overgrowth, rapid bone age acceleration, and therefore premature cessation of growth.

### Hyperandrogenism

Often associated with poor compliance, may cause clitoromegaly, penile growth, pubic hair development, and central gonadotropin-dependent precocious puberty due to hypothalamic activation ( see Chapter 2).

### Obesity

Common despite careful monitoring. The natural adiposity rebound occurs earlier than 6 years. The likely cause is the higher than physiological doses of glucocorticoid required to suppress androgen secretion.

### Testicular tumours

Tumours of adrenal rest cells in the testes more common in poorly compliant boys (testicular adrenal rest tumours (TARTs)). These benign tumours may cause disordered testicular architecture and impair fertility. Ultrasound examination may detect initial development more objectively than clinical examination which will only find well-established lesions.

### Treatment

Excess glucocorticoid causes excessive weight gain and impaired growth. Insufficient glucocorticoid allows increased androgen secretion which causes rapid growth, bone age acceleration, virilization of the genitalia, and can provoke central gonadotrophin-dependent precocious puberty.

Excess mineralocorticoid will cause hypertension, insufficient will put the child at risk of adrenal crisis.

Girls undergoing feminizing genitoplasty in infancy and early childhood may have a higher complication risk of vaginal stenosis and sexual dysfunction in adulthood ( see Chapter 11).

Infants with full masculinization registered and reared as male may develop a full and satisfactory male identity, but require careful counselling.

### Prenatal diagnosis and treatment

Virilization of a female fetus occurs just after sex differentiation in the embryo at 6–8 weeks post-conceptional age. Treatment of the mother with dexamethasone as soon as pregnancy is recognized may indirectly cause reduction in fetal adrenal androgen secretion and theoretically lessen the degree of virilization in a homozygous or compound heterozygous female. Previous studies where antenatal diagnosis was done by chorionic villus sampling at 11 weeks' gestation meant that targeting 1/8 affected fetuses resulted in unnecessary treatment of 7/8. There are reports of successes in reducing virilization, but potential adverse effects on neurological development in unaffected individuals. This treatment programme is still under review and may be better targeted with newer antenatal diagnostic techniques such as fetal DNA sampling.

# Adrenal steroid excess

## Exogenous glucocorticoids

This is the commonest cause of steroid excess in children and adolescents. Treatment courses with doses of glucocorticoids above the physiological cortisol secretion rate (10 mg/m$^2$/day) for >4 weeks will cause suppression of the HPA axis and slow recovery will ensue.

Children on inhaled corticosteroids for asthma in a total daily dose of >400 mcg/day may also be at risk of adrenal suppression and show clinical features of steroid excess in a dose-dependent fashion.

Relative glucocorticoid potencies:
- Hydrocortisone (cortisol) = 1
- Prednisolone = 4
- Dexamethasone = 27.

### Symptoms

Hyperphagia, weight gain, and slowing of growth.

### Management

The dose should be tapered to below physiological secretion levels before stopping. If the HPA axis is normal, morning (8 am) cortisol is >300 nmol/L (cortisol assay dependent). If uncertain, perform a standard short Synacthen test (➜ see Chapter 14). If the HPA axis remains suppressed, the patient should have additional (double or triple physiological) doses of glucocorticoid for 2–3 days during intercurrent illness and should seek emergency medical help if very unwell, especially with diarrhoea and vomiting. It is advisable to carry emergency parenteral hydrocortisone and a steroid card.

Approximate emergency doses of IM hydrocortisone:
- 0–10 kg (1 year): 25 mg
- 10–30 kg (7 years): 50 mg
- >30 kg: 100 mg

The HPA axis may take many months and maybe years to recover.

## Pathological adrenal steroid excess

### Features to alert concern
- Weight gain
- Hirsutism
- Acne
- Hypertension.

### Useful initial investigations
- 24-hour urine free cortisol
- Midnight/8 am plasma cortisol

### Second-line investigation
- Low-dose dexamethasone test.

### If adrenal lesion suspected
- High-dose dexamethasone test
- Abdominal ultrasound/MRI scans.

*If pituitary lesion suspected*
- Cranial high-resolution MRI scan
- Inferior petrosal sinus sampling with CRH stimulation.

For full investigation schedules, see Chapter 14.

## ACTH-independent Cushing syndrome

### Causes

The commonest cause of Cushing syndrome is iatrogenic due to excess exogenous glucocorticoids.

Other causes include an adrenal tumour (adenoma or adenocarcinoma), or adrenal dysplasia (primary pigmented nodular adrenal dysplasia)—both are rare.

### Diagnosis

Patients typically show rapid weight gain and slowing of growth often to minimal growth velocity, differentiating it from exogenous obesity. Often these are the only clinical signs. Patients may have a classic malar (cheek) flush. Other clinical symptoms (mood swings, fatigue) and signs (acne, central obesity, striae, hypertension, hirsutism) which may help to differentiate this clinical picture from exogenous obesity are less common in children and adolescents than adults with this condition.

## ACTH-dependent Cushing disease

### Cause

An ACTH-secreting pituitary adenoma. This is rare and differential diagnosis from other and adrenal causes of Cushing (syndrome) depends on a careful and precise investigation schedule.

### Treatment

If identifiable, surgical removal of the ACTH-secreting micro- or macroadenoma is required. Several attempts may be necessary with subsequent pituitary radiotherapy. Pituitary hormone replacement therapy may be required as well as hydrocortisone and follow-up is lifelong.

## Adrenal tumours

May present as Cushing syndrome (discussed earlier in this topic) or rapid-onset hirsutism and virilization in a young child.
- *Lesions <5 cm* usually benign and encapsulated and can be removed surgically. The remaining gland may be suppressed and take some years to recover. Physiological hydrocortisone (and fludrocortisone) may be needed with emergency cover.
- *Lesions >5 cm* are likely to be an adenocarcinoma and require careful co-management with the paediatric oncology team.

# Further reading

Flück CE. Update on pathogenesis of primary adrenal insufficiency: beyond steroid enzyme deficiency and autoimmune adrenal destruction. *Eur J Endocrinol* 2017;177:R99–R111.

Güemes M, Murray PG, Brain CE, et al. Management of Cushing syndrome in children and adolescents: experience of a single tertiary centre. *Eur J Pediatr* 2016;175:967–976.

Oberfield SE, Witchel SF (eds). The adrenal gland [special issue]. *Horm Res Paediatr* 2018;89:283–388.

Speiser PW, Azziz R, Baskin LS, et al. Congenital adrenal hyperplasia due to steroid 21-hydroxylase deficiency: an Endocrine Society clinical practice guideline. *J Clin Endocrinol Metab* 2010;95:4133–4160. [Erratum in: *J Clin Endocrinol Metab* 2010;95:5137.]

# Thyroid gland disorders

# Embryology, anatomy and physiology

## Embryology

- The thyroid gland develops from endoderm in the floor of the pharynx at 3–4 weeks' gestation, and travels caudally to leave the thyroglossal tract in the neck (which may persist as a thyroglossal cyst).
- The diverticulum becomes bi-lobed and fuses with the ventral aspect of the fourth pharyngeal pouch.

## Anatomy

- While in a neonate the thyroid weighs 2–3 g, in an adult it weighs 18–60 g, and consists of two lobes either side of the trachea ~4 cm long and ~2 cm thick, connected by the isthmus.
- The thyroid has more blood supply per gram of tissue than the kidney.
- The functional unit of the thyroid gland is the follicle, a roughly spherical group of cells around a protein-rich storage material, colloid.

## Physiology

### Hypothalamic–pituitary–thyroid axis
(See Fig. 9.1 and ➡ Chapter 3.)
- The hypothalamus secretes thyrotropin-releasing hormone (TRH).
- TRH stimulates the anterior pituitary to secrete thyroid-stimulating hormone (TSH).
- TSH binds to a specific receptor (TSH-R), activating thyroid metabolism via the G-stimulatory pathway.

### Synthesis of thyroid hormones requires
1. iodination of tyrosine molecules, and
2. combination of two iodinated tyrosine residues.

The thyroid has evolved to:
1. efficiently trap iodine from dietary sources. Of the average 150 mcg/day of dietary iodine, 125 mcg is taken up by the thyroid and concentrated 20–40×
2. produce thyroid hormones
3. store the hormones it produces within colloid.

### Steps in production of thyroid hormones
(See Fig. 9.2 and ➡ Chapter 3.)
- Dietary iodine is taken up by the thyroid follicular cells and oxidized to iodide.
- Tyrosine residues are iodinated to form mono- (MIT) and diiodo-tyrosine (DIT).
- These are coupled together to form iodothyronines.
- Cleavage of the residues produces MIT, DIT, $T_3$, and $T_4$.
- Tyrosine molecules then undergo deiodination to salvage the iodide.
- The thyroid gland is the sole producer of $T_4$ and produces ~20% of $T_3$, with the remainder produced by mono-deiodination of $T_4$ in peripheral tissues, such as liver, spleen, and kidneys.
- $T_3$ is about 10× more biologically active than $T_4$.

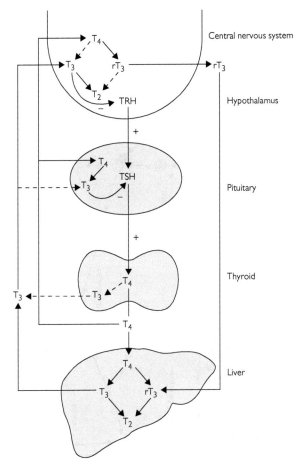

**Fig. 9.1** Schematic overview of the regulation of the production and metabolism of thyroid hormone in the hypothalamic–pituitary–thyroid periphery axis, showing the liver as a major $T_3$-producing tissue.

Reproduced from Wass JAH, Shalet SM (eds) (2002). *Oxford Textbook of Endocrinology and Diabetes*, Oxford University Press, Oxford. Copyright © 2002 OUP.

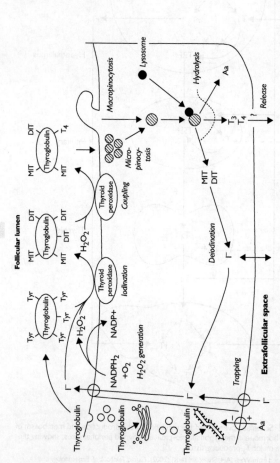

**Fig. 9.2** Schematic representation of a thyroid follicular cell and important steps in the synthesis of thyroid hormone (courtesy of Professor J. Dumont, Brussels). DIT, 3,5-diiodotyrosine; MIT, mono-iodotyrosine; Tyr, tyrosine.

- Only 0.03% of circulating $T_4$ and 0.3% of $T_3$ is unbound, the rest is bound to thyroxine-binding globulin (TBG) and other proteins, predominantly albumin.

## Actions

- The thyroid hormones have profound effects on growth, neurological development, metabolism, and cardiovascular function.
- Thyroid hormones bind to receptors in the pituitary/hypothalamus, liver, heart, and brain.
- This in turn results in increased oxygen consumption, altered protein, carbohydrate, and lipid metabolism, and also potentiation of the effects of catecholamines.

## Fetus

- The fetal thyroid produces little thyroid hormone until the 12th week of gestation, and the fetus is dependent on the small amounts of thyroid hormone that cross the placenta.
- TSH levels rise in the fetus during the second trimester, along with thyroid hormones $T_3$ and $T_4$, although these remain low.
- Unlike TRH, maternal TSH, $T_4$, and $T_3$ do not readily cross the placenta, hence thyroid levels at birth are a reflection of fetal thyroid hormone production. Babies with a total absence of endogenous thyroid hormone production have umbilical cord thyroid hormone levels ~40% of normal.
- Maturation of HP–thyroid feedback system occurs in the third trimester.

## Neonatal

- At birth there is an acute release of TSH, with this surge resulting in high $T_4$ and $T_3$ levels. These levels of $T_4$ and $T_3$ peak at 7 days, and then decrease to normal infant levels by 14 days of age.

# Congenital hypothyroidism

Congenital hypothyroidism (CH) is the commonest congenital endocrine disorder and also the commonest treatable cause of intellectual disability worldwide, with an incidence of 1 in 1800–2000 births, although in highly consanguineous group the incidence can be as high as 1 in 800.

Females are affected twice as commonly as males, and there is also an increased risk in infants with Down syndrome.

## Symptoms and signs
- Poor feeding and weight gain
- Decreased activity
- Prolonged jaundice (mixed conjugated/unconjugated)
- Constipation
- Hoarse cry (late).

### Signs
- Bradycardia
- Umbilical hernia
- Hypotonia
- Large/wide fontanelle
- Myxoedema
- Protruberant tongue
- Goitre (with dyshormonogenesis).

NB: Symptoms and signs may be highly variable, and whilst they may be present at birth in many cases develop weeks or months after birth.

## Causes
- Anatomical abnormality (dysgenesis) (80–85%), due to thyroid gland
  - Agenesis, dysgenesis
  - Ectopic
  - Sublingual
- Inborn error of thyroid hormone metabolism (dyshormonogenesis) (15–20%)
- Secondary/tertiary hypothyroidism (pituitary TSH, hypothalamic TRH deficiency (see Chapter 3) (<0.01%)
- Iodine deficiency

## Dyshormogenetic forms of CH
In these forms of CH, the thyroid is of normal size, or enlarged, and sited in a normal position.

These are often inherited in an autosomal recessive fashion.

In addition, up to 2% of thyroid dysgenesis is also familial.

Several genes are identified which are involved in the normal development and hormone production within the HP–thyroid axis (Table 9.1).

Genes associated with thyroid gland dysgenesis include:
- those with non-syndromic CH: TSHR
- those with syndromic CH: TTF1, TTF2, PAX8, and GNAS (encoding Gs-alpha).

Genes associated with dyshormonogenesis:
- thyroid peroxidase (TPO), thyroglobulin (TG), the sodium iodide symporter (NIS/SLC5A5), and pendrin (PDS).

**Table 9.1** Genetic diagnosis to detect the individual molecular basis of congenital hypothyroidism

|  | Thyroid morphology, as assessed by ultrasonography and/or scintigraphy | Family history | |
|---|---|---|---|
|  |  | Consanguinity or siblings/cousins with CH | Parents with CH |
| Isolated CH | Normally located thyroid with normal perchlorate discharge test | TSH-R (if hypoplasia), TG (if goitre low TG level) | PAX8 |
|  | Normally located thyroid with abnormal perchlorate discharge test (i.e. iodide organification defects) | TPO, DUOX2/DUOXA2 ± TG |  |
|  | Normally located thyroid on ultrasonography, with no iodide uptake on scintigraphy | SCL5A5/NIS, TSH-R (if hypoplasia) |  |
| Syndromic CH |  |  |  |
| Deafness | Normally located thyroid | SCL26A4/PDS |  |
| Short stature, obesity, hypocalcaemia | Normally located thyroid |  | GNAS |
| Cleft palate, 'spiky' hair | Athyreosis (hypoplasia) | FOXE1 (no mutations described in patients with ectopic or normally sized and sited thyroid gland to date) |  |
| Kidney agenesis or any malformation of the genitourinary tract | Athyreosis, ectopic thyroid gland, normally located thyroid ± hypoplasia | PAX8 | PAX8 |
| Choreoathetosis or neurological disease | Normally located thyroid, hypoplasia (athyreosis) | NKX2-1 (no mutations described in ectopic cases so far) | NKX2-1 |
| Lung disorders (surfactant deficiency syndrome at term, interstitial lung disease) | Normally located thyroid, hypoplasia (athyreosis) | NKX2-1 (no mutations described in ectopic cases so far) | NKX2-1 |
| Cardiac defects | Ectopy (athyreosis) | NKX2-5 | NKX2-5 |

*Pendred syndrome*

The incidence is 7.5–10 in 100,000 and is thought to account for up to 10% of hereditary deafness.

Pendred syndrome is associated with:
- congenital sensorineural deafness
- goitre (in 75%)
- congenital hypothyroidism.

Inheritance is autosomal recessive and linked to mutations in the *PDS* gene on chromosome 7q22.3, which codes for the pendrin protein, an iodide/chloride transporter. Patients with Pendred syndrome show reduced organification of iodine and a reduced/slow result on a perchlorate discharge test.

*Iodine deficiency*
- Although the commonest cause worldwide of hypothyroidism, patients are usually euthyroid.
- Very rare in the UK, more common in other European countries such as Germany and Poland.
- Iodine is relatively abundant in seawater and seafood. Areas of iodine deficiency tend to be inland, at high altitude, where daily iodine intake may be <25 mcg.
- In 1994, ~30% of the world was at risk of iodine deficiency, but the WHO commitment to iodide supplementation of salt has now reduced this risk to <15%. Iodine deficiency with goitre was estimated to affect 187 million people (2.7% of the population) globally in 2010.

## Screening for CH

As clinical detection of CH often occurs late, by which time neurological damage has already occurred, screening for CH has been instituted in many developed countries over the last decades.

The screening varies from country to country:
- *Sample:* cord blood, heel prick for filter paper, or whole blood.
- *Assay:* although some countries still use 1° measurement of $T_4$, most national programmes now screen using 1° TSH measurements, with $T_4$ determination for infants with elevated TSH values.

Using 1° TSH measurement, the following are missed:
- Delayed TSH elevation in TBG deficiency: 1 in 5000 births.
- Central hypothyroidism (TSH/TRH deficiency): 1 in 25,000–50,000 births.
- Hypothyroxinaemia with delayed TSH rise: 1 in 100,000 births.

*CH screening in UK*

Now ideally done on day 2–3 (day of birth being day 0), and certainly by day 5–8 on all babies regardless of prematurity and/or milk feeding. Premature babies should have a repeat screen at 36 weeks' gestation. Permanent CH incidence is 5.3 per 10,000 infants. Compared to children of white ethnicity (incidence rate 4.5; 95% confidence interval 4.0–5.1), children of Asian and Chinese ethnicity have a significantly higher incidence of permanent CH (incidence rate ratios: Asian 2.5, Chinese 4.2, respectively), while children of black ethnicity have lower incidence (incidence rate ratio 0.4).

*NB: ESPE suggests that the best 'window' for testing is 48–72 hours. It also* recommends repeat testing after 2 weeks in:
- preterm neonates (gestational age (GA) <37 weeks)
- low-birthweight and very low birthweight LBW neonates;
- ill neonates admitted to NICU
- specimens collected within the first 24 hours of life
- multiple births, particularly if same-sex twins.

### TSH level on initial screening
Babies with an initial TSH concentration
- <8 mU/L whole blood on the initial screening sample are considered to have a negative screening result for CH.
- ≥8 mU/L should be retested in duplicate from a different bloodspot on the same card.
- those with an initial TSH concentration ≥20 mU/L whole blood on the initial screening sample should be considered to have a positive screening result for CH.

*NB: The ESPE guidelines indicate that levels >40 mU/L should start treatment as soon as a venous blood sample has been taken, but before the results are available. They also state that at TSH levels >20 mU/L that treatment should be stared even if FT4 levels are normal.*
- Babies with an initial TSH concentration ≥8–<20 mU/L whole blood on the initial screening sample should be considered to have a borderline screening result for CH.

### For borderline tests
*Borderline results*
A repeat blood spot sample should be taken after 7–10 days and assayed in duplicate. On the second test:
- if TSH <8mU/L, the baby should be considered to have a negative screening result for CH
- if the TSH result on the second sample is ≥8mU/L, this is considered to be a positive screening result for CH.

Babies with a positive screening test should be referred to a specialist paediatrician either the same or next working day.

*NB: The ESPE guidelines recommend that when venous TSH levels are 6–20 mU/L in an otherwise well baby that diagnostic imaging should be performed, but that if they remain at this level for 3–4 weeks that treatment may be considered, with, if necessary a trial off treatment at a later stage.*

Essential diagnostic tests on babies
- Total or free $T_4$ (plasma or serum)
- TSH (plasma or serum)

- Thyroglobulin taken prior to institution of treatment may demonstrate if there is any thyroid tissue present. An undetectable level is highly suggestive of thyroid agenesis or a complete thyroglobulin synthesis defect.
► It is important to use age-related ranges for T$_4$.
Additional maternal tests (desirable)
- Total or free T$_4$
- TSH
- Thyroid antibodies

## Imaging

It is recommended that a thyroid radioisotope and ultrasound scan are performed, as this gives information relevant to possible underlying diagnosis. The thyroid radioisotope scan can be performed up to 5 days after commencing L-thyroxine treatment, but should not be delayed if there are problems organizing a scan. A thyroid ultrasound scan can be performed at any time and may provide additional anatomical information.

The ESPE guidelines indicate that radioisotope scans can be performed up to 7 days. They also state the benefit of knee X-Ray to assess the femoral and tibial epiphyses (presence or absence). Absence of one or both knee epiphyses has been shown to be associated with T4 at diagnosis and also IQ outcome, reflecting intra-uterine hypothyroidism.

As babies with CH are more likely to have congenital heart disease (ventricular septal defect, atria septal defect, pulmonary stenosis) and sensorineural deafness (especially with Pendred syndrome and dyshormogenesis), and careful neonatal examination should be performed. *ESPE guidance also includes assessment of dysmorphic features.*

### Therapy

- Treatment is usually started with l-thyroxine (T4) at 11–15 days (as opposed to 23–30 days at the start of screening). Current UK guidelines are that it should be ideally started by 14 days (21 days if diagnosis made on repeat sample).
- Higher doses of T4 are now recommended (10–15 mcg/kg/day) with a maximum of 50 mcg/day for those with severe disease, as this is associated with improved outcomes.
- Dose is usually given as crushed tablets or suspension manufactured liquid.
- Aim initially to suppress TSH into the normal range in the 1st month and then maintain free T4 at the upper end of normal range, and TSH within normal range. Higher-dose regimes tend to normalize T4 and TSH much faster (often within a few weeks) than standard doses.
- *Blood tests should be checked at least 4 hours after thyroxine administration (ESPE, 2014).*
- If the permanence or persistence of CH is unclear, a trial off-thyroxine can be performed at 2–3 years, with thyroid function tests performed 4–6 weeks later. One third of patients with CH and normally sited thyroid glands have transient thyroid dysfunction.

*ESPE guidance also indicates that re-evaluation should be carried out after 3 years of age. It may be carried out by decreasing the dose of L-T$_4$ can be reduced by 30% for 2–3 weeks and rechecking thyroid function. If TSH increases ≥10 mU/L, this confirms CH. If this does not occur the L-T4 dose can be reduced further, with retesting after another 2–3 weeks.*

### Outcome

- The best predictor of outcome is the thyroid hormone level at birth, which indicates the degree of intra-uterine hypothyroidism.
- There is a threshold effect, with babies with a total T4 <40 nmol/L (free T4 ~2.5 pmol/L) having an IQ reduced by ~10 points compared with those with levels above this value. In addition severe CH (agenesis) have a reduction of 12–15 IQ points.
- There is evidence that early high-dose l-thyroxine (10–15 mcg/kg/day) will normalize IQ even in severely hypothyroid babies, although this improvement in IQ is obtained at the expense of poor memory, poor attention, and deterioration in social behaviour.

Up to 10% of patients with CH have residual problems, (learning deficits, plus specific cognitive defects in visuospatial tasks, attention, and (memory)), which may be related to:
- late diagnosis

Therapy

- Treatment is usually started with L-thyroxine (T$_4$) at 10–15 days immediately. Current guidelines are that it should be started by 18 days.
- ▶ We recommend starting treatment immediately after baseline serum TSH and free T$_4$ determination if whole blood spot TSH concentration is >40 mU/L.
- Highest doses of T$_4$ are now recommended (15 mcg/kg/day) for infants with severe disease as this is associated with improved outcomes (see following 'Outcome' section).
- Dose is usually given as crushed tablets, or manufactured liquid.
- *Blood tests should be checked at least 4 hours after thyroxine administration (ESPE, 2014).* Aim to maintain free T$_4$ at the upper end of normal range, and TSH within normal range. Higher-dose regimens tend to normalize T$_4$ and TSH much faster (often within a few weeks) than standard doses.
- Subsequent evaluation should take place every 2 weeks until a complete normalization of TSH concentration is reached; then every 1–3 months thereafter until the age of 12 months.
- Between the ages of 1 and 3 years, children should undergo frequent clinical and laboratory evaluations (every 2–4 months).
- Thereafter, evaluations should be carried out every 3–12 months until growth is completed.
- If the permanence or persistence of CH is unclear, a trial off- thyroxine can be performed at 2–3 years, with thyroid function tests performed 4–6 weeks later. One third of patients with CH and normally sited thyroid glands have transient thyroid dysfunction.
- ESPE guidance also indicates that re- evaluation should be carried out after 3 years of age. It may be carried out by decreasing the dose of L-T4 can be reduced by 30% for 2–3 weeks and rechecking thyroid function. If TSH increases ≥10 mU/ L, this confirms CH. If this does not occur the L-T4 dose can be reduced further, with retesting after another 2–3 weeks.

▶in borderline cases, start treatment and re-evaluation of the thyroid axis, off treatment, should normally take place after the age of 3 years.

Outcome

- The best predictor of outcome is the thyroid hormone level at birth, which indicates the degree of intrauterine hypothyroidism.
- There is a threshold effect, with babies with a total T$_4$ <40 nmol/L (free T$_4$ ~2.5 pmol/L) having an IQ reduced by ~10 points, compared to those with levels higher than this.
- There is evidence that early, high-dose L-thyroxine (10–15 mcg/kg/day) will normalize IQ even in severely hypothyroid babies, although this improvement in IQ is bought at the expense of poor memory, poor attention, and deterioration in social behaviour.

Up to 10% of patients with CH have residual problems, which may be related to:
- late diagnosis
- inadequate treatment
- socioeconomic status

- poor adherence with therapy
- severity of CH at diagnosis
- learning deficits, plus specific cognitive defects in visuospatial tasks, attention and (memory).

This compares to ~40% of those diagnosed on symptoms prior to screening.

- Psychomotor development and school progression should be monitored and recorded in all children with CH, and particularly in at-risk cases (absent knee epiphyses at term, very low total $T_4$ or free $T_4$, and very high TSH concentrations at diagnosis, athyreosis, delayed normalization of TSH, poor control during the first year, delayed milestones).
- A personalized educational plan is required if school progress is affected in cases of severe CH.

### Reference

Léger J, et al. ESPE-PES-SLEP-JSPE-APEG-APPES ISPAE; Congenital Hypothyroidism Consensus Conference Group. European Society for Paediatric Endocrinology consensus guidelines on screening, diagnosis, and management of congenital hypothyroidism. *J Clin Endocrinol Metab* 2014;99:363–384.

# Transient neonatal hypothyroidism

## Causes

- Iodine deficiency
- Iodine excess (Wolff–Chaikoff effect), as this inhibits organification of iodide
- 2° to maternal thyrotoxicosis
- Transplacental transfer of maternal antibodies
- Maternal drugs (e.g. carbimazole, propylthiouracil)
- Maternal radioiodine administration
- If there is any doubt, it is best to initiate treatment with thyroxine, and then have a trial off therapy at a later date.

## Neonatal hyperthyroidism

Rare; 1-in-4,000 to 40,000 normal deliveries. Occurs in 1-in-70 pregnancies with Graves' diseases (although up to 1-in-5 if requiring anti-thyroid medication in last trimester). Has a high morbidity and potential mortality. It is due to the following:

Group 1.    Placental passage of thyroid-receptor antibodies (TRAb) from mothers with hyperthyroidism (usually Graves' disease, but occasionally Hashimoto's disease). The TRAbs may persist even after definitive therapy with radioactive iodine or surgery. This is a transient phenomenon which resolves on clearing of maternal antibody from the fetal circulation.

Group 2.    Secondary to activating mutations in the TSH receptor, or activating mutations of Gsα protein in McCune–Albright syndrome. This occurs much more rarely, is often persistent, and can be inherited in autosomal dominant fashion.

## Features

Symptoms and signs may be present at birth or be delayed up to 10 days, due to either co-existing blocking antibodies or maternal antithyroid drugs.

- Goitre
- Cardiac: tachycardia, arrhythmia, hypertension, cardiac failure
- CNS: irritability, jitteriness, restlessness
- GIT: hepatosplenomegaly
- Eyes: exophthalmos, periorbital oedema, lid retraction (even in the absence of maternal eye signs)
- Hypermetabolism: weight loss despite increased appetite, diarrhoea, sweating, flushing
- Other: premature fusion of cranial sutures, advanced bone age

### Diagnosis

The American Thyroid Association (ATA) gudelines recommend measurement of maternal TRAb at 24–28 weeks of pregnancy: if the value is > 3x normal they recommend close follow-up for fetal hyperthyroidism.

In Group 1, hyperthyroidism usually remits spontaneously by 20 weeks. However, thyroid ablation may be required in the persistent forms (Group 2).

Clinical examination, cord blood, and bloods at 10–14 days (also at 2–7 days in high-risk babies) should be performed in all babies for:
- signs of neonatal hyperthyroidism
- free T4, TSH, and TRAbs (if available). Presence or absence of raised TRAb may help determine whether is high or low risk for developing hyperthyroidism.

### Treatment (see p. 306)

It is still debated whether asymptomatic patients who are biochemically thyrotoxic should be treated. Treatment is as for other patients with hyperthyroidism:
- thionamides (carbimazole and propylthiouracil)
- β-blockers
- steroids (e.g. prednisolone) which reduce deiodination of T4 to T3 can also be used in severely toxic babies

Babies usually require weekly review. The duration of treatment following transfer of TRAb in mothers with Graves' disease is usually 4–8 weeks. Mortality is reported to be as high as 12–20%, and is usually due to heart failure.

# Acquired hypothyroidism

## Autoimmune hypothyroidism

Acquired hypothyroidism in children and adolescents is predominantly caused by end-stage autoimmune disease arising from a lymphocytic infiltrative and destructive process of the thyroid gland (Hashimoto's disease/thyroiditis). This may also be an atrophic form, which unlike Hashimoto's doesn't produce a goitre.

May also occur secondary to various drugs (anticonvulsants, lithium, amiodarone, sertraline), irradiation, cystinosis and Langerhans cell histiocytosis.

The usual autoimmune process is modulated by the raising of antibodies to the thyroid peroxisomes quantified by TPO antibody titres. The aetiology is unclear, family history may be relevant. There is a 10× female preponderance. The onset is rare in infancy, less common in childhood, but most common in adolescence. Occurs in ~1-in-1250 children.

### Symptoms and signs of hypothyroidism
- Slowing of growth, along with
- Weight gain
- Late/delayed puberty
- 1° amenorrhoea
- Precocious puberty with ovarian cysts (Van Wyk-Grumbach syndrome)
- Tiredness
- Feeling cold
- BUT no impairment of school performance.

### Clinical signs of autoimmune hypothyroidism
- Myxoedema
- Generalized or discrete hair loss
- Firm often smooth goitre with palpable Delphian node on the isthmus
- Features of underlying chromosomal abnormality:
  - Turner syndrome
  - Down syndrome.

### Investigation of autoimmune hypothyroidism
- Raised TPO antibodies
- Elevated TSH (slight elevation, often with normal/low normal free $T_4$ in early/subclinical disease)
- Imaging (ultrasound or thyroid scintigraphy) usually not helpful and may be misleading as shows patchy heterogeneous inflammation only and only in prolonged disease may it help exclude malignant transformation.

Autoimmune hypothyroidism may be associated with other autoimmune diseases, most notably T1DM and APS, especially type 2.

## Other causes of acquired hypothyroidism

Other causes of acquired hypothyroidism may arise as a side effect of childhood cancer treatment. These include direct radiation as given in Hodgkin's disease or during TBI prior to bone marrow transplantation, or indirect when radiation scatter occurs, e.g. in CSI in the treatment of medulloblastoma (➡ see Chapter 4).

## Treatment

L-Thyroxine can be replaced at a starting dose of 3–4 mcg/kg/day, depending on the degree of hypothyroidism. There is no need to start with a low dose and titrate upwards (as in the elderly), as the risk of atrial fibrillation is negligible in children and adolescents. The aim should be to normalize TSH and free $T_4$ levels in 2–4 weeks. Treatment thereafter will be lifelong.

*Side effects of treatment*: hypothyroid individuals are often described as being very placid and compliant and on thyroxine replacement may regain their liveliness, which may be associated with an initial decrease in school performance and an increase in behavioural problems. Rare complications include raised intracranial pressure and slipped femoral epiphyses (similar to growth hormone replacement).

## Low $T_3$ syndrome (sick euthyroid syndrome)

Thyroid function tests may be difficult to interpret during acute illnesses and most especially in sick preterm infants. These include:

- metabolic upset—especially acidosis
- acute/chronic liver disease
- hypocaloric states
- treatment with steroids.

Characteristically the first changes are a reduction in Free T3 with an increase in reverse T3 (rT3), and a subsequent fallgeneralisec in Free T4 levels, but TSH levels are usually normal, but may be suppressed.

There is currently no evidence which supports the supplementation of thyroid hormones during acute illness. There may be increased morbidity from $T_4$ therapy in sick preterm infants.

## Generalized thyroid hormone resistance

Occurs in 1-in-40,000 live births. 85% are due to mutations in the thyroid receptor gene *TRB*, which causes reduced binding of T3. The clinical effect is loss of sensitivity to thyroid hormones. Patients may be clinically euthyroid or present with symptoms of hypothyroidism (usually) or hyperthyroidism and a small goitre. An association with ADHD (attention deficit hyperactivity disorder) has also been described. Despite non-suppressed TSH levels, paradoxically free T4, and in particular free T3 may be raised.

## Differential diagnosis of goitre

### True goitre

- Diffuse: usually autoimmune thyroid disease (Graves' or Hashimoto's disease).
- Multinodular: usually also auto-immune disease. Rarely, malignancy.
- Familial history of colloid-containing multinodular goitre may be due to mutation in *DICER1* gene
- Single nodule: 30–50% malignant.

### False goitre

- Physiological enlargement of the thyroid at puberty.
- Midline lesions associated with the thyroid, e.g. thyroglossal cyst.
- Midline lesions that are not thyroid associated, e.g. branchial cysts, histiocytosis of the thymus.

# Hyperthyroidism

## Causes in children and adolescents

- Graves' disease
- Hashimoto's disease (stimulatory phase—Hashitoxicosis)
- Toxic nodules
- Congenital hyperthyroidism (maternal transplacental IgG passage)—see p. 303.

## Clinical symptoms

- Weight loss
- Sweating
- Heat intolerance
- Agitation
- Rapid tiring and reduced exercise capacity
- Poor concentration (**and** impaired school performance).

## Clinical signs of hyperthyroidism

- Tachycardia
- Cardiac compromise or failure (rarely)
- Goitre
- Tall stature and rapid growth
- Precocious, early, or rapid puberty
- Advanced bone age.

## Graves' disease

- This is caused by the development of autoantibodies to the TSH receptor (variably known as thyroid stimulating immunoglobulin (TSI) or thyrotrophin receptor antibody (TRAb)).
- Incidence is 1-in-10,000 adolescents.
- There is a familial predisposition with 15% of patients having a family history, and it is estimated that ~80% of the susceptibility to the disease is due to genetic factors.
- There is a 7:1 female preponderance.

Ophthalmopathy (exophthalmos) is less common in children and adolescents than adults, and if it occurs, is usually self-limiting and fully or nearly completely regressive.

## Hashimoto's disease

- Most often presents silently with signs of hypothyroidism or with a euthyroid goitre.
- Frank hyperthyroidism may occur (signs and symptoms as Graves' disease).
- The goitre may significantly enlarge.
- Very rare complications include papillary cell carcinoma.

### Initial management

The first-line treatment of choice is an antithyroid drug (ATD) to reduce the production of thyroid hormones and β-blockers to control cardiac symptoms. Inorganic iodine is almost never needed (with the exception of a thyroid storm (see Chapter 13).

- Carbimazole initially 0.5–1.0 mg/kg/day, given as a once-daily dose:
  - Blocks iodine organification
  - Side effects uncommon: rash 8%, granulocytopenia 6%, arthritis 2%
  - Subsequent management as follows

- β-blockers, e.g. propranolol 0.5–1.0 mg/kg/day in three divided doses if signs and symptoms associated with tachycardia
- Propylthiouracil (PTU) 5–10 mg/kg/day in three divided doses:
  - Blocks $T_4$ to $T_3$ conversion.
  - ▶ NOT used as first-line ATD as risk of idiosyncratic hepatocellular failure.

### Subsequent management

Once symptoms have been controlled, β-blockers may be withdrawn. Ongoing medical management may follow one of two regimens, either of which seems equally effective.

- Dose titration—*preferred option*: treatment is continued with the ATD but the dose is gradually reduced to a maintenance level once free $T_3$ and free $T_4$ fall within the normal range. TSH levels may remain suppressed for many months, and serve as an indicator of autoimmune disease activity.
  - *Advantages*—fewer drug-related side effects. Monotherapy.
  - *Disadvantages*—more frequent monitoring and dosage adjustments initially, but frequency less when stable.
- Block and replace: suppression of endogenous thyroid activity is maintained with the starting doses or equivalent of carbimazole or PTU. Once the patient is biochemically or clinically euthyroid and becoming hypothyroid, thyroxine replacement is begun (50–100 mcg once daily).
  - *Advantages: supposedly* less frequent investigation or follow-up.
  - *Disadvantages*: higher dose of ATD needed and thus greater risk of drug reactions.

### Longer-term treatment options

The prognosis for remission in children and adolescents with Graves's disease is less good than with adult patients. Despite patients becoming euthyroid within 3 months of initial therapy, >50% will have persistent disease after 2 years of medical treatment. Eventually 20% remit after 4 years, rising to 49% after 10 years.

*Ongoing ATD*—now recognized as a safe option for several years with monitoring at a reduced frequency once stable. The inflammatory process may burn out in due course. However, adherence to treatment needs to be taken in to consideration.

*Total thyroidectomy*—the preferred choice in the very young child or if suspicion of malignancy or if there is a germline activating *TSHR* mutation. Complications include scarring, damage to the recurrent laryngeal nerve, and transient and permanent hypoparathyroidism due to accidental damage to or removal of some or all of the parathyroid glands—rare with a good surgeon. Lifelong thyroxine replacement will be required.

$^{131}I$ *radioiodine treatment*—indications for radioiodine treatment include failure of or side effects from medical treatment, and contraindications to surgery. In some centres, depending on experience, it is often preferred over surgery for definitive treatment for children >6 years of age. Complications include treatment failure necessitating repeating the radioiodine dose, and worsening of ophthalmopathy if it is present. No long-term side effects of the radioactivity, e.g. increased cancer risk, infertility in the patient, or congenital abnormalities in subsequent children are currently reported. Lifelong thyroxine replacement will also be required.

Trials of immune modulating therapies such as monoclonal **antibodies** against CD20, found on **B**-cell surfaces are **now** being considered.

# Thyroid cancer in childhood

This is a rare malignancy in childhood and adolescence.

## Causes of thyroid cancer

- Environmental irradiation (e.g. after the Chernobyl nuclear disaster)
- Arising as a second malignancy following radiotherapy for other 1° conditions (e.g. Hodgkin's disease, TBI prior to bone marrow transplantation, or CSI (e.g. for medulloblastoma))
- Genetic (either inherited as part of MEN type 2A or 2B or familial medullary thyroid cancer (MTC) syndromes or a new mutation)
- Sporadic, e.g. a single cold nodule.

## Single thyroid nodules

- Rare in childhood with a prevalence from 0.05 – 1.8%.
- Approximately ¼ are malignant so this should always be suspected in children or adolescents, especially in younger children with more rapidly growing nodules.
- Early diagnosis is important as, compared to adults, children are more likely to have regional lymph node and pulmonary metastases.

Take a full history, including drug and radiation exposure, and a family history of other predisposing genetic conditions (MTC, Gardner or Cowden syndromes). Both cold (non-functioning) and hot (hyper-functioning) nodules should be investigated for malignant change. The most common form in childhood is papillary cell carcinoma.

### Investigations

- Thyroid ultrasound may help distinguish single isolated from widespread disease, but is non-specific in its findings.
- Thyroid scintigraphy does not help in the differential diagnosis between benign and malignant nodules.
- Fine-needle aspiration (FNA) which has 90% accuracy is the investigation of choice.

Whilst most nodules are benign, malignancy may be missed, even by experienced operators and cytogeneticists, so careful follow-up is necessary and consideration given to partial thyroidectomy, with the degree depending on clinical and radiological findings.

### Treatment of a malignant thyroid nodule

Close liaison between paediatric surgeons, oncologists, and endocrinologists is important to determine the extent of disease and extent of surgery required (degree of thyroidectomy and lymph node dissection). Beware of postoperative hypocalcaemia due to parathyroid gland excision or damage. Follow-up radio-iodine ($^{131}$I) treatment may be required to treat residual disease. Thyroglobulin levels should be undetectable if treatment to remove all thyroid tissue is successful.

### Long term management

Initial $T_4$ replacement therapy should aim for clinical euthyroidism, but a suppressed TSH (<0.1 mU/L) even if free $T_4$ and $T_3$ levels are slightly high. In the longer term, TSH levels should be maintained at <0.5 mU/L with clinical and biochemical euthyroidism.

## Multiple endocrine neoplasia syndromes

### MEN-1

Rare onset in childhood but 94% by age 40 years. Autosomal dominant with high penetrance, but a high proportion are sporadic. The gene, a proto-oncogene, is on chromosome 11q13. This codes for a tumour-suppressive protein, MENIN.

### MEN-4

Similar to MEN-1 but mutation on chromosome 12p13 in *CDKN1B* gene, also causative of parathyroid and pituitary adenomas, reproductive organ tumours, and adrenal tumours.

The current guidelines recommend that MEN-1 mutation analysis should be undertaken in:
- an index case with two or more tumours
- first-degree relatives (symptomatic or not) of known MEN-1 carrier
- single-sporadic MEN-1 associated tumour; discussion on a case-by-case basis.

*Features of MEN-1 (Wermer syndrome)*
Parathyroid hyperplasia and adenomas (Table 9.2):
- Usual presenting feature: hypercalcaemia.
Pancreatic endocrine tumours:
- Gastrinoma:                40%
- Insulinoma:               10%
- VIPoma:                   rare
- Glucagonoma:              rare
- PPoma:                    rare
- Non-functioning:          55%
- Pituitary adenomas:       30–40%
- Adrenocortical tumours:   20–40%
- Phaeochromocytoma:        rare.

### MEN-2

*Diagnosis of MEN-2*
Genetic diagnosis now first-line investigation of all at-risk children as transmission is autosomal dominant. Mutations occur in the *RET* proto-oncogene on chromosome 10q11.2 (*RET* = *RE*arranged during *T*ransfection). The gene contains 21 exons and encodes for the transmembrane receptor of tyrosine kinase family. Point mutations in exons 10 and 11 (85%) produce a

**Table 9.2** Screening programme for genetically at risk (mutation positive or affected parent) asymptomatic children and adolescents

| | |
|---|---|
| Annual | Serum calcium and PTH |
| | Prolactin |
| | Fasting gastrin and gut hormone profile |
| 2–3-yearly | MRI pancreas |
| 3–5-yearly | MRI pituitary |

**Table 9.3** Subtypes of MEN-2

| | | |
|---|---|---|
| MEN-2A (Sipple syndrome)<br>*Also known as MEN-2* | MTC, phaeochromocytoma, and parathyroid hyperplasia<br>Usually presents with MTC—often strong family history | 60–90% |
| MEN-2B (Gorlin syndrome)<br>*Also known as MEN-3* | MTC and phaeochromocytoma only<br>Phenotype typical, with marfanoid body habitus, thickened lips, mucosal (tongue) neuromas and gastrointestinal neuromas (Hirschsprung's disease), cutaneous lichen amyloidosis | 5% |
| Familial MTC | | 5–35% |

gain of function of this receptor, causing MEN. Identification of the specific mutation is now the key to deciding age of thyroidectomy and beginning of the screening programme for other manifestations (Table 9.3).

MTC is multicentric in 90% of patients with lymph node metastases and in 70% of those with palpable tumours. Surgery is the 1° preventative or curative treatment. Chemotherapy, external radiotherapy, or $^{131}$I radiotherapy are of no proven value for local or metastatic disease.

*Treatment*
- Prophylactic thyroidectomy recommended for high-risk mutations <12 months of age (M918T, C634, A883F)
- Thyroidectomy as soon as feasible in patients with moderate-risk gene mutation
- Parathyroidectomy and autotransplantation into forearm; controversial.

*Follow-up in MEN-2*
- Post-thyroidectomy annual calcitonin levels for 2 years then frequency determined individually.
- Annual screening for hypercalcaemia (calcium profile and PTH levels)—not MEN-2B.
- Annual blood pressure measurement and urine/plasma metanephrines for phaeochromocytoma. Imaging (abdominal ultrasound/MRI if suspected).

# Further reading

Al-Salameh A, Baudry C, Cohen R. Update on multiple endocrine neoplasia type 1 and 2. *Presse Med* 2018;47:722–731.

Caimari F, Kumar AV, Kurzawinski T, et al. A novel DICER1 mutation in familial multinodular goitre. *Clin Endocrinol (Oxf)* 2018;89:110–112.

Knowles RL, Oerton J, Cheetham T, et al. Newborn screening for primary congenital hypothyroidism: estimating test performance of different TSH thresholds. *J Clin Endocrinol Metab* 2018;103:3720–3728.

Kourime M, McGowan S, Al Towati M, et al. Long-term outcome of thyrotoxicosis in childhood and adolescence in the west of Scotland: the case for long-term antithyroid treatment and the importance of initial counselling. *Arch Dis Child* 2018;103:637–642.

Leger J, Gelwane G, Kaguelidou F, et al. Positive impact of long-term antithyroid drug treatment on the outcome of children with Graves' disease: national long-term cohort study. *J Clin Endocrinol Metab* 2012;97:110–119.

Leger J, Olivieri A, Donaldson M, et al. European Society for Paediatric Endocrinology consensus guidelines on screening, diagnosis, and management of congenital hypothyroidism. *J Clin Endocrinol Metab* 2014;99:363–384/*Horm Res Paediatr* 2014;81:80–103.

Prete FP, Abdel-Aziz T, Morkane C, et al. Prophylactic thyroidectomy in children with multiple endocrine neoplasia type 2. *Br J Surg* 2018;105:1319–1327.

Sinha CK, Decoppi P, Pierro A, et al. Thyroid surgery in children: clinical outcomes. *Eur J Pediatr Surg* 2015;25:425–429.

Szinnai G (ed). Paediatric thyroidology [special issue]. *Endocr Dev* 2014;26:1–251.

Thakker RV. Multiple endocrine neoplasia type 1 (MEN1) and type 4 (MEN4). *Mol Cell Endocrinol* 2014;386:2–15.

West JD, Cheetham TD, Dane C, et al. Should radioiodine be the first-line treatment for paediatric Graves' disease? *J Pediatr Endocrinol Metab* 2015;28:797–804.

# Calcium, vitamin D, and bone disorders

# Physiology of calcium regulation

The control of calcium metabolism is complex and dependent upon several systems—PTH, calcitonin, and vitamin $D_3$—which have an as yet not fully understood interdependence. This often makes recognition of signs and symptoms, diagnosis, and management of calcium disorders tricky, especially as the physiology of calcium and phosphate regulation in childhood is intimately entwined with bone metabolism and growth (Table 10.1).

Major changes in the skeleton with age

- Mineralization is dependent on normal health, diet, growth, and puberty.
- The size of the head at birth is one-quarter of the length of the body—as an adult, it is one-eighth of the length.
- Differential growth occurs in the bones of the skull and face during development.
- Curvature of the spine changes from birth.
- Osteoporosis may develop in older people and during disease in childhood and adolescence.

Control of bone growth

- Osteoblasts—cause new bone formation.
- Osteoclasts—promote bone resorption and remodelling.
- The commonest form of new bone formation is endochondral ossification.
- Factors which regulate chondrocyte growth and maturation in lacunae and stimulate the chondrocytes to ossify:
  - Indian hedgehog (IHH) protein and PTH-related peptide (PTHrP) acting via the PTH receptor type 1 (PTHr1) stimulate chondrocyte activity.
  - Fibroblast growth factor type 3 (FGF3) via its receptor FGFR3 inhibits chondrocyte differentiation and hence slows growth.

**Table 10.1** Hormones and receptors involved in calcium and bone metabolism

| | |
|---|---|
| Parathyroid hormone (PTH) | • Increases intestinal absorption of calcium<br>• Increases urinary resorption of calcium<br>• Increases phosphaturia<br>• Stimulates osteoclastic activity (bone resorption) |
| Vitamin $D_3$ | • Similar actions to PTH<br>• Calcifies osteoid |
| Calcitonin | • Opposite in effect to PTH and vitamin $D_3$<br>• Lesser role in calcium regulation (not fully determined) |
| Calcium sensing receptor | • Modulates PTH action<br>• Present in parathyroid and kidney |

## Vitamin $D_3$ (cholecalciferol) metabolism

Vitamin $D_3$ is metabolized from dietary sources of cholecalciferol (fish, oil, etc.) and from plants as ergocalciferol (vitamin $D_2$) but 80% is derived from conversion of 7-dehydrocholesterol by UV light (sunlight) in the skin.

Cholecalciferol is hydroxylated in the liver at the 25- position to form 25-hydroxylase vitamin $D_3$ by the enzyme 25 hydroxylase. This compound is the principal storage form of vitamin $D_3$ in the liver and circulation and is what is usually measured when vitamin $D_3$ levels are requested from the biochemistry laboratory.

25OH vitamin $D_3$ is converted to the active form 1,25 OH vitamin $D_3$ in the kidney by 25 hydroxyvitamin D 1α-hydroxylase under control of PTH stimulated by hypocalcaemia.

1,25 dihydroxyvitamin $D_3$ acts via the specific vitamin D receptor.

## The structure of a bone

- The mineral content of bone is principally calcium hydroxyapatite crystals. Bone contains 99% of the body stores of calcium.
- Organic protein content of bone is principally collagen together with other proteins which add to the flexibility and strength of bone.

### Collagen: 85–90% (12 principal types)

- II: mainly in growth plate cartilage
- IX: mainly in hyaline cartilage
- X: mutations cause Schmid metaphyseal chondrodysplasia
- XI: three subchains—absence of any one cause spondyloepiphyseal dysplasia (SED).

### Other proteins: 10–15%

- Proteoglycans
- Gamma carboxylated proteins
- Glycoproteins:
  - These include the thrombospondins 1–5
  - Thrombospondin 5 is known as COMP (cartilage oligomeric matrix protein)
  - Mutations in the COMP gene cause:
    —pseudoachondroplasia
    —multiple epiphyseal dysplasia (MED).

# Bone mineralization

Acquisition of bone mass, most especially the bone mineral content (BMC), is dependent upon good health and diet, normal mobility, and normal functioning of calcium homeostasis.

## Important facts about peak bone mass development

- 25% is accrued during puberty in the 2 years either side of peak height velocity (average 12 years in girls, 14 years in boys).
- In girls, the rate of bone mass acquisition declines after the menarche.
- In boys, bone mass acquisition continues into late adolescence, hence teenage boys are more prone to fractures from physiological reasons as well as the greater level of activity and risk-taking in this age group.
- Every 10% increase in bone mass is equivalent to a 50% reduction in fracture rate.
- Dietary factors are important. A calcium intake <500 mg/day is deleterious for bone mass gain.

## Assessment of bone mineralization

*Osteoporosis* or *osteopenia* is a loss of total bone content which can be caused by
- decreased bone formation
- increased bone resorption.

*Osteomalacia* refers to a defect in bone mineralization in mature bone. The commonest form of inadequate bone mineralization in childhood is rickets and its subtypes.

Assessment of BMC and bone mineral density (BMD) can be performed by:
- DXA scan—the usual methodology; this uses a very low-dose radiation body scan
- quantitative ultrasound—dependent upon appropriate equipment and computer software
- quantitative CT (qCT)—again dependent upon appropriate software, but a high dose of radiation is used.

## DXA

- DXA (Dual-energy X-ray Absorptiometry) measures differential absorption of two different X-ray energies.
- Whole body or regions, e.g. hip/lumbar spine, can be measured.
- Results can be calculated as BMC and bone area (BA).
- BMD is derived from (BMAD—bone mineral apparent density) BMC/BA. This is a two-dimensional value ($g/m^2$) and is dependent on the subject's height and weight.
- Volumetric BMD corrects for bone size ($g/cm^3$) and reflects true BMD more accurately.

Low bone mineral density

BMD is usually reported as a standard deviation score (SDS) known as the Z-score.

*WHO definitions of low BMD*
- Osteopenia: Z-score −1.0 to −2.0 SDS
- Osteoporosis: Z-score less than −2.0 SDS
- Interpretation needs to be based on good standards for age/height/weight/puberty stage/ethnicity.
- 1.0 SDS reduction in BMD is equivalent to a 2–3× increased risk of fracture.

# Causes of a loss of bone mass

## Osteogenesis imperfecta (OI)

OI is the commonest cause of 1° osteoporosis. It should be suspected in anyone with low BMD and no biochemical or other cause. There are at least 18 subtypes of OI (table 10.3), the commonest forms which are of principal clinical significance are as follows:

### Types I (mildest) and IV
- Autosomal recessive
- Skeletal abnormalities often absent.

### Type II
- Lethal neonatal form, often due to a new mutation
- Caused by mutations in *COL1A1* and *COL1A2* genes which encode type 1a collagen synthesis.

### Type III (classic OI)
- Autosomal recessive
- Multiple fractures
- Skeletal deformity
- Blue sclerae
- Abnormal dentition.

## Treatment of OI
- Treatment is mostly supportive and palliative as there is no 1° cure.
- It requires a multidisciplinary team-based approach involving a community paediatrician, paediatric endocrinologist, orthopaedic surgeon, physiotherapist, occupational therapist, dentist, etc.
- Bisphosphonates (e.g. 3-monthly pamidronate, 6-monthly zoledronate or neridronate) can be used to reduce bone pain symptomatically, and help prevent further vertebral crush and long bone fractures.
- Growth hormone therapy has been shown to help augment BMD in less severe cases.

## Pamidronate treatment guidelines

This schedule is for guidance and may need modification depending on the response to treatment or side effects. There is now good evidence that cyclic administration of pamidronate will improve bone mineralization in chronic renal failure, pregnancy, and untreated vitamin D deficiency (correct before starting pamidronate).

### Dosage
- Each cycle consists of 1.0 mg/kg pamidronate daily for three consecutive days by IV infusion.
- Pamidronate should be diluted in at least 250 mL 0.9% saline and infused over 4 hours (the speed of infusion may be increased in subsequent doses if no side effects).
- Repeat cycles 3-monthly.

*Monitoring*

1. *Bone profile*: plasma calcium and phosphate and bone-specific alkaline phosphatase in serum should be recorded prior to each 3-monthly cycle and prior to the third dose of each cycle. If serum calcium is <2.1 mmol/L—give or increase calcium supplements.
2. *Markers of bone turnover*: prior to the first cycle of treatment—bone alkaline phosphatase, osteocalcin, P1NP.
3. *DXA scan*: should be repeated 1 year after commencement of therapy (i.e. after four cycles).
4. A decision about continuing therapy after 1 year will be made when the response to therapy over the first year has been evaluated.

*Side effects*

Flu-like symptoms associated with pyrexia and back and/or limb pain. These can be treated with paracetamol (not NSAIDs)

Occasional transient hypocalcaemia.

## Idiopathic juvenile osteoporosis

This is a rare cause of osteoporosis with sporadic occurrence. It presents 2–3 years before puberty with bone pain and unexpected fractures (mostly vertebral) and a marked reduction in BMD on assessment. The condition resolves spontaneously over 2–5 years. Treatment is symptomatic. Vitamin D analogues and bisphosphonates have been used to help control symptoms (Box 10.1 and Tables 10.2 and 10.3).

---

**Box 10.1  Causes of osteoporosis in childhood and adolescence**

*Osteogenesis imperfecta*

*Connective tissue disease*
- Marfan syndrome
- Ehlers–Danlos syndrome.

*Chronic disease*
- Juvenile idiopathic arthritis
- Inflammatory bowel disease
- Childhood cancers: disease (ALL) and treatment (radiotherapy and chemotherapy).

*Nutritional/mobility problems*
- Anorexia nervosa/eating disorders
- Cerebral palsy.

**Table 10.2** Endocrine causes of osteoporosis

| 1° conditions | • Thyrotoxicosis |
| | • GH deficiency |
| | • Cushing syndrome/disease |
| | • Delayed puberty/hypogonadism |
| Iatrogenic | • Supraphysiological glucocorticoid treatment |
| | • Inadequate GH/sex hormone replacement |

**Table 10.3** Osteogenesis imperfecta type based on the genetic classification

| Osteogenesis imperfecta type | Inheritance | Mutated gene | Encoded protein | Clinical features |
|---|---|---|---|---|
| Impairment of collagen synthesis and structure | | | | |
| I, II, III, or IV | AD | *COL1A1* or *COL1A2* | Collagen α1(I) (COL1A1) or α2(I) (COL1A2) | Classic phenotype (Sillence classification) |
| Compromised bone mineralization | | | | |
| V | AD | *IFITM5* | Bone-restricted interferon-induced transmembrane protein-like protein (BRIL; also known as IFM5) | Normal-to-severe skeletal deformity, intraosseous membrane ossifications, radiodense band and radial head dislocation, normal-to-blue sclerae, and sometimes hearing loss |
| VI | AR | *SERPINF1* | Pigment epithelium-derived factor (PEDF) | Moderate-to-severe skeletal deformity, the presence of osteoid, fishscale appearance of lamellar bone pattern, and childhood onset |
| Abnormal collagen post-translational modification | | | | |
| VII | AR | *CRTAP* | Cartilage-associated protein (CRTAP) | Severe rhizomelia with white sclerae |
| VIII | AR | *P3H1* (previously known as *LEPRE1*) | Prolyl 3-hydroxylase 1 (P3H1) | |

**Table 10.3** (Contd.)

| Osteogenesis imperfecta type | Inheritance | Mutated gene | Encoded protein | Clinical features |
|---|---|---|---|---|
| IX | AR | PPIB | Peptidyl-prolyl cis–trans isomerase B (PPIase B) | Severe bone deformity with grey sclerae |
| Compromised collagen processing and crosslinking | | | | |
| X | AR | SERPINH1 | Serpin H1 (also known as HSP47) | Severe skeletal deformity, blue sclerae, dentinogenesis imperfecta, skin abnormalities, and inguinal hernia |
| XI | AR | FKBP10 | 65 kDa FK506-binding protein (FKBP65) | Mild-to-severe skeletal deformity, normal-to-grey sclerae, and congenital contractures |
| No type | AR | PLOD2 | Lysyl hydroxylase 2 (LH2) | Moderate-to-severe skeletal deformities and progressive joint contractures |
| XII | AR | BMP1 | Bone morphogenetic protein 1 (BMP1) | Mild-to-severe skeletal deformity and umbilical hernia |
| Altered osteoblast differentiation and function | | | | |
| XIII | AR | SP7 | Transcription factor SP7 (also known as osterix) | Severe skeletal deformity with delayed tooth eruption and facial hypoplasia |
| XIV | AR | TMEM38B | Trimeric intracellular cation channel type B (TRIC-B; also known as TM38B) | Severe bone deformity with normal-to-blue sclerae |
| XV | AR AD | WNT1 | Proto-oncogene Wnt-1 (WNT1) | Severe skeletal abnormalities, white sclerae, and possible neurological defects |

*(Continued)*

**Table 10.3** (Contd.)

| Osteo-genesis imperfecta type | Inheri-tance | Mutated gene | Encoded protein | Clinical features |
|---|---|---|---|---|
| XVI | AR | CREB3L1 | Old astrocyte specifically induced substance (OASIS; also known as CR3L1) | Severe bone deformities |
| XVII | AR | SPARC | SPARC (also known as osteonectin) | Progressive severe bone fragility |
| XVIII | XLR | MBTPS2 | Membrane-bound transcription factor site-2 protease (S2P) | Moderate-to-severe skeletal deformity, light blue sclerae, scoliosis and pectoral deformities |

AD, autosomal dominant; autosomal recessive; XLR, X-linked recessive.

# Hypocalcaemia

## Calcium regulation

Serum calcium levels are usually tightly regulated between 2.2 and 2.6 mmol/L. Approximately half is in the ionized active form. This measurement is reported by some laboratories instead of or as well as total calcium. As calcium is albumin bound in the serum, low albumin/total protein levels may affect the total calcium levels. Many laboratories now report corrected calcium levels.

Corrected calcium = total calcium + (40 − measured albumin) × 0.02

## Symptomatic hypocalcaemia

Patients are often not symptomatic until calcium levels fall well below 2 mmol/L. Mild symptoms include weakness and muscle cramps, and tingling and numbness of the fingers, toes, or lips. More severe hypoparathyroidism may cause carpedal spasm, stridor due to laryngospasm, or generalized seizures. Hypocalcaemia should be immediately excluded in any infant or child presenting with convulsions of unknown cause. Treatment of acute hypocalcaemia is a medical emergency—➔ see Chapter 13, p. 372.

Less acute symptoms include mood changes or diarrhoea.

## Other clinical signs of hypocalcaemia

Examine the child for signs of other conditions which can cause hypocalcaemia—mucocutaneous candidiasis, dystrophic nails, and coarse hair associated with 1° hypoparathyroidism (*AIRE1* gene deletion).

- *Chvostek's sign:* tapping the facial nerve in front of the ear lightly with the index finger elicits twitching of the corner of the mouth.
- *Trousseau's sign:* a blood pressure cuff inflated above systolic pressure on the upper arm causes the development of carpopedal spasm with painful paraesthesiae.

## Neonatal hypocalcaemia

- *Transient*: this may be associated with prematurity per se, birth asphyxia, and also in the infant of a diabetic mother. Maternal causes also include vitamin $D_3$ or PTH deficiency in the mother—often hitherto unrecognized. Hypocalcaemia may arise from iatrogenic causes such as parenteral nutrition with inadequate calcium or magnesium supplements or immediately following exchange transfusions.
- *Permanent*: usually associated with hypoparathyroidism, either isolated or as part of the DiGeorge syndrome (associated thymic hypoplasia and cardiac defects) (Box 10.2).

## Hypoparathyroidism

- PTH resistance syndromes: Albright's hereditary osteodystrophy (AHO; see later in this topic).
- Isolated genetic causes: inactivating mutations of the *PTH* gene (can be autosomal dominant, recessive, or X-linked).
- Biochemical profile:
  - low: calcium, PTH, urinary calcium, 1,25-OH vitamin D
  - high: phosphate.

Box 10.2  Causes of childhood hypocalcaemia

- 1° hypoparathyroidism
- PTH resistance syndromes
- Hypomagnesaemia
- Vitamin D deficiency (rickets)
- Chronic renal failure
- Multisystem disorders, e.g. DiGeorge syndrome
- Autoimmune—isolated or APS type 1 (APECED).

*Activating mutations of CASR*

- Biochemical profile:
  - low: calcium, PTH (or normal)
  - normal: 1,25-OH vitamin D
  - high: phosphate, urinary calcium

*Autoimmune*

- Isolated PTH deficiency
- APS type 1—often the presenting feature, associated with autoimmune polyendocrinopathy–candidiasis–ectodermal dystrophy (APECED). Due to mutations in *AIRE1* gene.

*Metabolic disease*

- Mitochondrial gene defects, e.g. Kearns–Sayre syndrome
- Long-chain 3-hydroxyacyl-coenzyme A dehydrogenase (LCHAD)
- Iron and copper overload
- Post surgery (especially thyroid, or neck dissection).

*Multisystem syndromes*

- DiGeorge syndrome: 22q11 deletion
- 10p haploinsufficiency: hypoparathyroidism, deafness, renal dysplasia (HDR) syndrome
- Kenney–Caffey syndrome
- Sanjad–Sakati syndrome (also known as Richardson-Kirk syndrome)
- AIDS.

Albright's hereditary osteodystrophy (AHO)

This is a family of PTH and other hormone resistance syndromes primarily caused by abnormalities in function of the GS-α part of the G protein-coupled PTH receptor. The part of the receptor is encoded by the *GNAS1* gene on chromosome 20q13.

The most well-known phenotype is that of classical pseudohypoparathyroidism (PHP) type 1a. If of familial inheritance and in the presence of hypocalcaemia, the inactivating mutation is inherited from an affected mother (Boxes 10.3 and 10.4).

Box 10.3 Features of classical PHP-1a

- Typical rounded facies
- Skeletal dysplasia
- Short stature
- Brachydactyly—short fourth metacarpals
- Ectopic calcification
- Skin plaques
- Intracerebral—basal ganglia
- Obesity
- Moderate learning difficulties.

Box 10.4 Endocrine features of PHP-1a

- Hypocalcaemia
- Hyperparathyroidism
- Hyperphosphataemia
- High TSH, low free $T_4$
- Elevated FSH/LH.

Other types of PHP

### Pseudopseudohypoparathyroidism (PPHP)

This can occur within the same families as PHP1a. The features of AHO are present, but hypocalcaemia is not manifested. This occurs if the inactivating mutation of *GNAS1* is on the paternal allele, i.e. it is inherited from the patient's father.

### PHP-1b

Clinical features of AHO are absent in type 1b, but PTH resistance remains. Patients present with hypocalcaemia, often in mid childhood with raised PTH levels. This condition is caused by paternal imprinting defects on account of differential methylation of *GNAS1*.

### PHP-1c

The phenotype is similar to AHO and there are features of multiple hormone resistance. There are no defects in *GNAS1* and GS-α activity is normal. The defect has not yet been identified.

### PHP-2

This rare form of PHP does not have the AHO phenotype, but PTH resistance is present, although its effects are limited to the phosphaturic response as aspects of the adenyl cyclase function are normal. The precise gene defect is unknown.

### Treatment of hypoparathyroidism

In the absence of regular supplies and easily administered recombinant PTH, the mainstay of treatment of hypocalcaemia is with vitamin D analogues.

*Treatment*

The drug of choice is $1\alpha$-hydroxyvitamin $D_3$ (alfacalcidol) 25–50 ng/kg/day as a single dose to aid compliance. This analogue is immediately active via the vitamin D receptor and does not need hydrolysing. Calcitriol may also be used but usually needs 2–3× daily dosing.

Initially oral calcium supplements may be needed (Calcium-Sandoz® or Sandocal®), aiming to keep calcium levels low normal.

*Complications*

Treatment may induce calciuria which can eventually cause nephrocalcinosis, so the aim should be to keep the urinary calcium/creatinine ratio <1.0. If calciuria is high despite keeping serum calcium levels low/normal consider adding a diuretic (hydrochlorothiazide 1.25 mg/kg twice daily or chlorothiazide 12.5 mg/kg twice daily).

*Follow-up*

Patients should be seen frequently, 3–4-monthly, checking calcium/phosphate/magnesium balance and urinary calcium:creatinine ratio. An annual renal ultrasound scan should be performed to detect and monitor the development of nephrocalcinosis.

# Hypercalcaemia

This is rare in infancy and childhood. A raised serum calcium of >2.65 mmol/L is usually detected by chance.

## Causes of hypercalcaemia of infancy

- Neonatal 1° hyperparathyroidism—homozygous inactivating mutation of *CASR* gene resulting in hyperparathyroidism.
- If there is maternal hypocalcaemia, the fetus may mount a hyperparathyroid response raising calcium levels.
- Mild hypercalcaemia is a recognized feature of Williams syndrome but usually mild, asymptomatic, and self-limiting to the first year only. The precise cause is unknown. Abnormalities of vitamin D or calcitonin metabolism have been reported rarely.
- Idiopathic infantile hypercalcaemia may also be present during the first year of life, and may also be linked to vitamin D hypersensitivity, but the aetiology is uncertain.

## Hypercalcaemia in childhood

Symptoms of hypercalcaemia:
- anorexia
- polyuria and polydipsia
- mood changes
- abdominal pain
- constipation.

## Signs

Often none.

### Biochemistry

Raised calcium level >2.65 mmol/L together with suppressed plasma PTH, and appropriate calciuric response.

## Causes of hypercalcaemia in childhood

Vitamin D excess through over-replacement is probably the most frequent cause of raised calcium levels in childhood. Other 1° causes include:
- malignant disease in bone acting via PTH-related peptide
- 1° hyperparathyroidism:
  - isolated parathyroid adenoma
  - MEN types 1A and 2A
  - 3° hyperparathyroidism—autonomous dysregulated PTH secretion due to longstanding hypocalcaemia, e.g. chronic rickets
- familial hypocalciuric hypercalcaemia caused by a heterozygous inactivating mutation in the *CASR* gene
- prolonged immobilization
- sarcoidosis.

Management of hypercalcaemia

- Acute: administer saline infusion, furosemide, and glucocorticoids. Rapid resolution of symptoms may be obtained from a pamidronate infusion.
- Longer term: in overtreatment with vitamin D, stop treatment and restart after several days at a lower dose.
- Parathyroid adenomas usually require surgical excision.

# Rickets

Rickets is defined as a failure to calcify the matrix of the growth plate with excessive accumulation of uncalcified cartilage and osteoid (uncalcified bone matrix).

It is the commonest disorder of calcium and bone metabolism. Usually resulting directly from vitamin D deficiency as dietary intake and exposure to adequate sunlight are often reduced in the UK due to cultural and social factors.

Vitamin D status:
- Sufficiency, >50 nmol/L
- Insufficiency, 30–50 nmol/L
- Deficiency, <30 nmol/L

Malabsorption syndromes such as *coeliac disease* may also cause rickets, as may failure of hydroxylation of cholecalciferol in liver disease. Genetic causes of rickets are very rare.

Severe dietary calcium or phosphate deficiency, or distal renal tubular acidosis, can also cause rickets even in the presence of normal vitamin D stores (Box 10.5).

The biochemical features of rickets may present in three stages (Table 10.4).

## Treatment of rickets

Acute hypocalcaemia should be treated as an emergency (➔ see Chapter 13, p. 372).

As rickets is a 1° deficiency of vitamin D then the appropriate treatment is replacement of vitamin D either as ergocalciferol (vitamin $D_2$) or cholecalciferol (vitamin $D_3$). Hydroxylated analogues such as 1α-calcidol may assist with bone healing but do not correct the 1° deficiency.

Oral calcium supplements may be necessary if hypocalcaemia is among the presenting features.

### Doses of vitamin $D_3$

This does not seem crucial as long as replacement is given. For conversion from IU to mcg, divide by 40. Vitamin $D_2$ egocalciferol also can be used.
- Daily dosing for 2–3 months:
  - Infants <6 months: 3000 IU orally daily
  - ≥6 months and older children: 6000 IU orally daily
- Single oral dose: children >1 year 150,000 IU, >12 year 300,000 IU
- Prevention of deficiency: 400–600 IU daily
- Preparations available either as multivitamin drops, e.g. Abidec®, Dalivit®, or as tablets usually combined with calcium.

> **Box 10.5  Clinical features of rickets**
> - Symptoms and signs of hypocalcaemia
> - Muscle weakness
> - Metaphyseal flaring
> - Bowed legs especially tibiae
> - Rickety rosary (flaring of costochondral junctions)
> - Pelvic distortion

**Table 10.4** Biochemical features of stages of rickets

| Stage 1 | |
| --- | --- |
| Calcium | Low—severe and symptomatic |
| Phosphate | Normal/high |
| Alkaline phosphatase | High on account of increased bone turnover |
| PTH | Raised 2° to hypocalcaemia |
| Clinical rickets | Not present at this stage |
| 25-OH vitamin D | Low |
| Stage 2 | |
| Calcium | Slightly low/low normal—not symptomatic |
| Phosphate | Low |
| Alkaline phosphatase | High on account of increased bone turnover |
| PTH | Further raised |
| Clinical rickets | Early features |
| 25-OH vitamin D | Very low |
| Stage 3 | |
| Calcium | Low—severe and symptomatic |
| Phosphate | Low |
| Alkaline phosphatase | High on account of increased bone turnover |
| PTH | Very high |
| Clinical rickets | Severe disease |
| 25-OH vitamin D | Severely low |

## Other forms of rickets

### Failure of 1α hydroxylation

- Chronic renal failure
- Mutation in 1α hydroxylase CYP27B1 (vitamin D-dependent rickets type 1):
  - 25-OH vitamin D levels are normal, but 1,25 $(OH)_2$ levels are low
  - Treatment is with large doses of alfacalcidol (150–200 ng/kg/day).

### Vitamin D receptor defects

- Hereditary vitamin D-resistant rickets:
  - 25-OH and 1,25 $(OH)_2$ vitamin D levels are very high
  - Treatment principally with calcium infusion or very large doses of alfacalcidol in a partial defect.

### Post-vitamin D receptor defects

*X-linked hypophosphataemic rickets (Table 10.5)*

- Mutation in the *PHEX* gene (*PH*osphate regulating gene with homology to *E*ndopeptidases on the *X* chromosome) which encodes a protein which cleaves fibroblast growth factor 23 (FGF23) thus preventing phosphaturia.
- Inheritance X-linked dominant, females and males affected, although males more severely
- *PHEX* haploinsufficiency causes low phosphate due to phosphaturia, high alkaline phosphatase. Calcium, 25-OH vitamin D and PTH are usually normal.
- Clinical features, short stature, progressive femoral and tibial bowing.
- Treatment:
  - phosphate supplements
  - alfacalcidol
  - GH in selected cases.

**Table 10.5** Biochemical features of different types of rickets

|  | Stage 1 | Stage 2 | Stage 3 | XLH | VDDR1 | HVDRR |
|---|---|---|---|---|---|---|
| 25-OH vitamin D$_3$ | Low | Very low | Extremely low | Normal | Normal | High |
| Calcium | Low | Low normal | Low | Normal | Low | Low |
| PTH | Slightly high | High | Very high | Normal | High | High |
| Phosphate | Normal/high | Low | Low | Low | Low | Low |
| ALP | High | High | High | High | High | High |

ALP, alkaline phosphatase; HVDRR, hereditary vitamin D-resistant rickets; VDDR1, vitamin D-dependent rickets type 1; XLR, X-linked rickets.

# Further reading

Allgrove J, Shaw N (eds). *Calcium and Bone Disorders in Children and Adolescents* (2nd rev edn). Basel: Karger AG, 2015.

Dattani M, Brook CDG (eds). *Brook's Clinical Pediatric Endocrinology* (7th edn). Oxford: Wiley-Blackwell, 2019.

Munns CF, Shaw N, Kiely M, et al Global Consensus Recommendations on Prevention and Management of Nutritional Rickets. *J Clin Endocrinol Metab.* 2016 Feb;101(2):394-415. doi: 10.1210/jc.2015-2175. Epub 2016 Jan 8 **and** Horm Res Paediatr. 2016;85(2):83-106. doi: 10.1159/000443136. Epub 2016 Jan 8.

# Differences of sex development (DSD)

# Embryology of sex development

The gonad is bipotential until 6 weeks after the last menstrual period.

The testes develop under active control of the *SRY* gene which upregulates *SOX9* in combination with other genes in the male (Table 11.1).

Ovarian development is protected and enhanced by *WNT4*/beta-catenin genes in the female (Table 11.1).

## Time sequence of male sex differentiation

- 7th week: the testes (Sertoli cells) secrete anti-Müllerian hormone (AMH) (also known as Müllerian inhibiting substance, MIS) to cause regression of Müllerian structures.
- 8th week: Wolffian ducts develop with testosterone secreted by testicular Leydig cells under stimulation from placental hCG.

**Table 11.1** Known genes in human sex differentiation

| Gene | Loss of function | Gain of function |
|---|---|---|
| CBX2 | 46,XY DSD | |
| WT1 | 46,XY DSD, Denys–Drash and Frasier syndromes | |
| SRY | 46,XY gonadal dysgenesis | 46,XX testicular DSD |
| SOX9 | 46,XY gonadal dysgenesis with campomelic dysplasia | 46,XX testicular DSD |
| NR5A1 (SF1) | 46,XY gonadal dysgenesis with adrenal failure | |
| NR0B1 (DAX1) | Hypogonadotropic hypogonadism and congenital adrenal hypoplasia | 46,XY gonadal dysgenesis |
| DMRT1 | 46,XY gonadal dysgenesis | |
| ATRX | 46,XY DSD | |
| MAP3K1 | 46,XY gonadal dysgenesis | |
| GATA4 | 46,XY DSD | |
| FOG2 | 46,XY DSD | |
| DHH | 46,XY DSD | |
| FGF9 | | 46,XX testicular DSD |
| WNT4 | 46,XX testicular DSD | 46,XY gonadal dysgenesis |
| RSPO1 | 46,XX testicular DSD with hyperkeratosis | |

Source: data from Ohnesorg T, Vilain E, Sinclair AH. The genetics of disorders of sex development in humans. *Sex Dev* 2014;8(5):262–72. doi: 10.1159/000357956.

- 8th–13th weeks: testosterone is converted to dihydrotestosterone (DHT) in genital tissue acting via the androgen receptor allowing masculinization of external genitalia.
- 13th week onwards: sex differentiation is complete, but the growth of the phallus continues with testosterone secretion now under control of LH secreted from the fetal pituitary gland.

Figs. 11.1 and 11.2 show the development of internal and external genitalia.

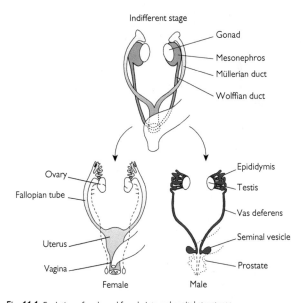

**Fig. 11.1** Evolution of male and female internal genital structures.

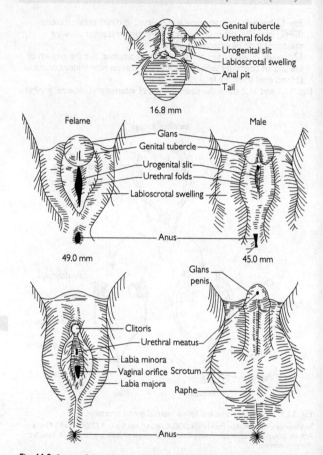

**Fig. 11.2** Stages of development of the external genitalia.

Reproduced with permission from Brook GGD, Clayton P, and Brown R (2005). *Brook's Clinical Pediatric Endocrinology* 5th edition, Wiley-Blackwell. Copyright © 2005 by John Wiley & Sons, Inc. All rights reserved.

# Definitions

The term difference of sex development (DSD) was formerly known as intersex and does not include transsexual or same-sex preference (homosexual) individuals.

Gender incongruence or dysphoria is not a difference of sex development. It is a combination of environmental, psychosocial, and possibly genetic components which affect an individual's gender role identification, independent of biological sex (⊖ see Chapter 12) (Table 11.2).

Different possible meanings of 'sex' include:
- prenatal ultrasound sex
- delivery suite sex: what is noticed initially
- phenotypic sex: male or female genitalia and 2° features
- chromosomal sex: 46,XY or 46,XX
- gonadal sex: presence of testes or ovaries or a combination.

Types of problems described as ambiguous genitalia are found in ~1 in 10,000 livebirths (but ~1 in 350 stillbirths) and include:
- hypospadias with one or no palpable gonads (1 in 250 livebirths)
- hypospadias with bifid scrotum
- micropenis with no palpable gonads
- bilateral undescended testes in a term infant
- clitoromegaly
- single female urogenital opening
- inguinal hernia in a girl containing a gonad.

Table 11.2 Current nomenclature for DSD

| Previous | Current |
|---|---|
| Intersex | Disorder (or difference) of sex development (DSD) |
| Male pseudohermaphrodite: Undervirilization of XY male Undermasculinization of XY male | 46,XY DSD |
| Female pseudohermaphrodite: Overvirilization of XX female Masculinization of XX female | 46,XX DSD |
| True hermaphrodite | Ovotesticular DSD |
| XX male or XX sex reversal | 46,XX testicular DSD |
| XY sex reversal (Swyer syndrome) | 46,XY complete gonadal dysgenesis |
| Sex chromosome abnormality | Sex chromosome DSD |

# 46,XY DSD (incomplete masculinization of a male fetus)

The commonest cause of DSD is androgen insensitivity syndrome (AIS)—resistance to testosterone action caused by mutations in the androgen receptor gene on X-chromosome in complete forms (CAIS) and alterations in androgen binding or post-receptor signalling defects (presumed) in partial forms (PAIS). Inheritance therefore is X-linked recessive, and frequency is ~1 in 50,000 livebirths.

## Partial androgen insensitivity syndrome

- There is a variable phenotype ranging from severe undervirilization to full normal male phenotype presenting with isolated male infertility.
- Gonads (testes) may be located in the scrotum, inguinal canal, or be intra-abdominal.
- No Müllerian structures are present as normally formed testes secrete AMH.
- Testosterone and LH are elevated due to receptor resistance.
- Peripheral aromatization of testosterone to oestradiol is unaffected, so gynaecomastia (breast development) occurs during puberty.
- As yet no single genetic cause has been identified.

## Complete androgen insensitivity syndrome (testicular feminization syndrome)

Technically a normal female external phenotype, so not 'ambiguous'.

### Modes of presentation

- Prenatal diagnosis 46,XY with phenotypic female infant at birth.
- Phenotypic girl with inguinal hernia containing a testis.
- 1° amenorrhoea in tall normal female, but absent pubic and axillary hair.

## Abnormalities in testosterone production and conversion

The phenotype is variable, dependent upon the degree of blockage of enzyme activity and build-up of precursor steroids. Most are autosomal recessive.

- Mutations of the LH (hCG) receptor
- Defects in steroid biosynthesis affecting testosterone production as well as other pathways.
- High-level blocks in steroid metabolism, e.g. steroidogenic acute regulatory protein (StAR), 3-beta hydroxysteroid dehydrogenase type 2 (3βHSD2), GYP17A1 mutations causing 17-alpha hydroxylase deficiency (17αOHD), and cytochrome P450 oxidoreductase deficiency also present with cortisol and aldosterone deficiency (such as congenital adrenal hyperplasia).

### Diagnosis

Absent/reduced steroid levels and their precursors in baseline samples and after Synacthen stimulation in serum or urine.

## Deficiencies in androgen pathway only

20,22 Desmolase deficiency, 17-beta hydroxysteroid dehydrogenase deficiency (17βHSD) present as undervirilized males of varying degree, sometimes with external female phenotype. Immature testes are usually present, and there are no Müllerian structures as the testes are able to secrete AMH.

### Diagnosis

Raised precursors to enzyme block, e.g. testosterone:androstenedione ratios at baseline and after hCG stimulation.

## Defects in testosterone action

5-Alpha reductase deficiency (5αRD) converts testosterone to DHT. Presentation is variable, but usually with severe hypospadias, bifid scrotum, and cryptorchidism. Subjects virilize spontaneously at puberty and do not develop gynaecomastia.

### Diagnosis

Raised testosterone:DHT ratio in basal and hCG stimulated samples.

## Gonadal dysgenesis

### Pure 46,XY gonadal dysgenesis (Swyer syndrome)

- Phenotype is unambiguously female; may present with delayed puberty.
- Müllerian structures are present but only streak gonads are seen.

### Mixed gonadal dysgenesis

- The most frequent situation with gonadal dysgenesis, usually asymmetrical, e.g. ovary on one side, streak gonad or ovotestis on the other
- Karyotype most frequently is 45,X/46,XY—may have a mild Turner syndrome phenotype with short stature; otherwise 46,XX/46,XY.
- Müllerian structures (often unicornuate uterus) are present on the side of the streak or ovary.
- No Müllerian structures are found and variably developed Wolffian structures are present on the side of the ovotestis/testis.
- Risk of gonadoblastoma in dysgenetic gonads is high so gonads should be removed surgically after biochemical diagnosis.

### Pure 46,XX gonadal dysgenesis

Presents with absent puberty in a phenotypically normal female, with intact Müllerian structures but streak ovaries. It does not cause ambiguity in the genitalia.

# 46,XX DSD (masculinization of a female fetus)

- The commonest cause is congenital adrenal hyperplasia (CAH) which accounts for half of all causes of 46,XX DSD (~1 in 30,000 live births).
- Inheritance is autosomal recessive.
- 90–95% are caused by 21-hydroxylase deficiency (21OHD).
- Other enzyme deficiencies include 11-beta hydroxylase, 3βHSD, cytochrome P450 oxidoreductase, and aromatase deficiency.

Gonadal causes (very rare)
- 46,XX pure gonadal dysgenesis—streak ovaries.

Maternal causes (very rare)
- Use of androgenic progestogens (e.g. danazol at time of conception)
- Virilizing ovarian or adrenal tumours.

# Ovotesticular DSD (true hermaphroditism)

- Rarest of all forms of DSD, aetiology unknown.
- Karyotype usually 46,XX despite anatomical variations.
- Asymmetrical gonad development, ovary and testis or ovotestis, with isosexual internal genital development, i.e. no Müllerian structures on the side with the testicular gonad.
- No increase in gonadoblastoma risk if gonad is not dysgenetic.

## Other conditions associated with DSD

- Trisomy 13
- Smith–Lemli–Opitz syndrome
- Antley–Bixler syndrome
- Campomelic dysplasia
- Cloacal dystrophy
- Ectopy of the bladder.

### Hypospadias

Isolated hypospadias (1 in 250 livebirths) is not usually considered within the DSD category unless very proximal (penoscrotal or perineal), especially if it also occurs with cryptorchidism. The aetiology is unclear but causes may include environmental agents acting as oestrogens preventing full masculinization (environmental disrupters).

# Management of the infant with DSD

- Usually unexpected and requires quick thinking.
- Need to involve most senior midwifery and medical staff available.
- Provide support and understanding to the parents and do not leave them alone initially until they request it.
- Examine the infant in the presence of the parents.
- Use neutral words for the explanation of the findings to colleagues, e.g. phallus, genital tubercle, urogenital opening, gonad, and simplify these terms for parental understanding such as sex organ, sex gland, genital opening, and urine opening.
- Advise that the sex of their baby is not immediately apparent, but that this will be able to be determined within a short period of time after expert evaluation and investigation and that we are used to seeing this problem.
- Explain that their baby has a variation of human development and that there is usually a reason for it.
- Do not refer to the infant as 'he' or 'she'. Either talk about 'baby' or perhaps ask the parents if they would like to use a neutral nickname while the diagnostic and evaluation processes are occurring to help bonding get underway.
- Advise them to keep the confidence of only close family initially.
- Involve an experienced multidisciplinary team including paediatric endocrinologists and specialist nurses, and if possible a paediatric urologist within the first day of life (see later in this topic)

## History

Ask about any previous occurrences, spontaneous abortions, stillbirths, or neonatal deaths; relatives with infertility or pubertal development problems; and consanguinity.

Enquire about maternal medications, and look for signs of virilization in the mother.

## Neonatal examination

### Important features

- General health, e.g. circulation, blood pressure, respiration, blood glucose levels
- Dysmorphic features
- General hyperpigmentation or specifically genital
- Chimerism and mosaicism (heterochromia of iris in 46,XX ovotesticular DSD).

### Careful documentation of external genitalia

- The Prader score system can be useful to describe the degree of virilization in an infant (Fig. 11.3). An External Masculinisation Score (EMS: from 0–12) is also used in males.
- Genital tubercle/phallus: presence of chordae, corpora cavernosa (erectile tissue), length, position, and size of urethral/genitourinary opening, nature of other genital swellings (labia or scrotum, bifid or rugose, etc.).

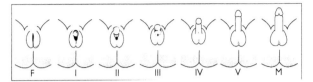

**Fig. 11.3** Prader score.

Reproduced with permission from Prader A (1958). Perfect male external genital development and salt-loss syndrome in girls with congenital adrenogenital syndrome. *Helvetica Paediatrica Acta* 13: 5–146. Copyright © 1958 Springer Science and Business Media.

**Table 11.3** Prader stages

| | |
|---|---|
| F | Normal female external phenotype |
| I | Labioscrotal fusion |
| II | Complete labioscrotal fusion, single introitus but with separate urethral and vaginal openings visible, clitoral enlargement |
| III | Scrotalized labia, single urogenital sinus, phallic enlargement often with chordee |
| IV | Further phallic enlargement, small perineal external urogenital opening |
| V | Near full male development, urinary meatus along penile shaft, towards distal end |
| M | Normal male development |

- Gonadal tissue: presence of gonads, position including the inguinal canal, size, symmetry, and consistency; retractile?
- Medical photographs may be helpful for later reference as spontaneous changes can occur, and for seeking external opinions.

Investigations
See Table 11.3.

*Day 1*
- Blood: serum/plasma sample for testosterone, FSH, and LH.
- Electrolytes and 17OHP levels are unhelpful at this stage as the infant is establishing its own physiology and there are many degradation products from the fetal adrenal cortex circulating to cause interference in immunometric steroid assays, but if tandem mass spectrometry is available, then day 1 sampling is possible.
- Karyotype: plasma sample in lithium heparin tube.
- Molecular genetics studies: EDTA tube sample for fluorescent *in situ* hybridization (FISH) studies or polymerase chain reaction (PCR) for *SRY* gene

- Pelvic ultrasonography (by experienced paediatric radiologist) to look for Müllerian structures (uterus); presence, size, consistency of any gonads present; adrenal hyperplasia.

*Day 3*
- Blood: electrolytes and 17OHP
- Urine: electrolytes; steroid profile.

Clinical differential diagnosis of DSD
- No gonads palpable—uterus present on US scan:
  - Phenotype otherwise normal female: 21OHD CAH
  - Other dysmorphic features: consider syndromic diagnosis or mixed gonadal dysgenesis
- Gonads palpable—uterus absent on US scan:
  - Phallic development minimal: 'high' steroid block, e.g. 3βHSD, 5αRD, 17βHSD, PAIS
  - Phallus developed with penoscrotal hypospadias: mild enzyme deficiencies, PAIS.

Considerations into 'sex of rearing'
This will depend on gonadal and genetic sex, on prior and future active androgen exposure, social and cultural context, parents, and medical opinion. This decision should be taken after careful evaluation by an experienced multidisciplinary specialist team and discussions with the parents. A temptation to guess should be avoided at all costs.

*DSD multidisciplinary management team*
- Neonatal paediatrician, nurses, and midwives
- Paediatric endocrinologist and specialist nurses
- Paediatric urologist/surgeon
- Paediatric radiologist
- Clinical biochemist
- Cytogenetics and molecular geneticist
- Psychologist
- General practitioner and health visitor.

Parental reaction to their baby with DSD
The birth of a baby with unclear sex is a traumatic enough event for the family as this is almost never expected. The other source of stress and anxiety is the way in which the initial situation is handled by the immediate staff, what is said, and how the parents are supported. Psychological feelings are very mixed. A sense of rejection and isolation are common. It is important therefore that all staff involved in maternity units and assisting with birthing are trained to handle such a situation with a sense of calm, knowledge what to do and whom to involve, and above all how best to support the parents immediately.

### Long-term outlook for infants born with DSD

This depends entirely on the nature of the diagnosis, severity of the virilization or undermasculinization, social and cultural elements, and on diagnostic and treatment approaches. Today's adults were managed under previous treatment regimens and the level of understanding at that time, so it will be some years before we can assess the outcome of current approaches. Decisions about sex of rearing should include a prediction of the likely psychosexual status as well, as early exposure of the developing brain to testosterone is likely to promote male-type patterns of behaviour. Satisfaction and psychosexual orientation are in part dependent on this.

The age at which decisions are made will depend upon local and cultural factors and the acceptability of a no-gender option. Follow-up studies also indicate that surgery to provide an individual with a definite unambiguous gender is generally associated with a more satisfactory outcome, untreated individuals living in areas where a surgical management is not available often being isolated in separate communities. Even in many developed societies, there is not yet a defined status for those individuals with neither classical male nor female gender.

However, surgical correction can result in scarring to the genital region. Physical complications of this include reduced sexual sensitivity and impaired functioning. A careful, sensitive, and considered approach to decision-making including all expert opinions, together with support for the family is therefore needed to result in the best outcome for each individual patient. There is increasingly a move away from early, destructive surgery, and where possible any consideration of surgery should be delayed until the patient can be involved in any discussions.

# Further reading

Ahmed SF, Khwaja O, Hughes IA. The role of a clinical score [external masculinisation score] in the assessment of ambiguous genitalia. *BJU Int.* 2000;85(1):120–4.

Brain CE, Creighton SM, Mushtaq I et al. Holistic management of DSD. *Best Pract Res Clin Endocrinol Metab.* 2010;24:335–354.

Crouch NS, Creighton SM. Transition of care for adolescents with disorders of sex development. *Nat Rev Endocrinol* 2014;10:436–442.

Hiort O, Birnbaum W, Marshall L, et al. Management of disorders of sex development. *Nat Rev Endocrinol* 2014;10:520–529.

Lee PA, Nordenström A, Houk CP, et al. Global disorders of sex development update since 2006: perceptions, approach and care. *Horm Res Paediatr* 2016;85:158–180. [Erratum in: *Horm Res Paediatr* 2016;85:180.]

Meyer-Bahlburg HF, Baratz Dalke K, Berenbaum SA, et al. Gender assignment, reassignment and outcome in disorders of sex development: update of the 2005 Consensus Conference. *Horm Res Paediatr* 2016;85:112–118.

Nordenström A. Psychosocial factors in disorders of sex development in a long-term perspective: what clinical opportunities are there to intervene? *Horm Metab Res* 2015;47:351–356.

Ohnesorg T, Vilain E, Sinclair AH. The genetics of disorders of sex development in humans. *Sex Dev* 2014;8:262–272.

Schober J, Nordenström A, Hoebeke P, et al. Disorders of sex development: summaries of long-term outcome studies. *J Pediatr Urol* 2012;8:616–623.

# Gender incongruence

# Gender incongruence

Gender incongruence (also known as dysphoria), a disassociation with birth gender or identification with the opposite gender may first appear either in childhood or in adolescence.

The diagnosis of gender incongruence is required to be made by an experienced mental health practitioner in accord with the Endocrine Society and World Professional Association for Transgender Health (WPATH) guidelines (see later in this topic).

Most young people presenting in childhood are less likely to go onto a physical treatment pathway (80%), whereas the majority (50–80%) of those presenting in adolescence may wish to socially and physically transition in their preferred gender.

Appropriate help and support should only be provided by an integrated paediatric medical and psychological/mental health team working in collaboration, with a psychosocial assessment preceding the medical review. Paediatric endocrinology provides a supportive rather than a diagnostic role. Gender incongruence is not associated with phenotypic, chromosomal, or endocrine abnormalities.

The initial medical assessment of a young person presenting with gender incongruence should be supportive only. A physical diagnostic approach is not required, and it is not considered similar to a DSD (→ see Chapter 11) (Box 12.1).

## Counselling about fertility loss

GnRH analogues will cause temporary suppression of the reproductive axis. Before this, counselling is needed about semen storage in transboys and oocyte harvesting in transgirls. Possibilities will depend on local facilities, funding level of maturity, stage of puberty attained, and the degree of dysphoria which may in itself preclude any consideration of this (Box 12.2).

## First-stage treatment: GnRH analogues

In those whose gender incongruence is clearly established and longstanding and who have participated fully in a multidisciplinary assessment process, GnRH analogues are the recommended first-stage medical intervention. According to the WPATH and the Endocrine Society guidelines, the GnRH analogues may be offered once an adolescent has demonstrated the first signs of physical puberty (Tanner stage 2 in either sex). Treatment is with standard regimen GnRH analogues for a minimum of a year before additional medical interventions can be considered. This is to allow further psychotherapeutic assessment to take place once the anxiety and distress related to the progression in puberty and processes such as menstruation, erections, and nocturnal emissions are reduced or stopped. All young people are counselled that GnRH analogue treatment does not convey contraceptive protection.

## Second-stage treatment: sex hormone replacement

Cross-sex hormone treatment, currently referred to as gender-affirming hormone treatment (namely the induction of the opposite-biological-sex puberty using testosterone in a phenotypic female and oestradiol in a phenotypic male) may be considered once full commitment to the

**Box 12.1  Criteria for the diagnosis of gender incongruence in children and adolescents**

1. A strong desire to be of the other gender or an insistence that one is the other gender.
2. A strong preference for wearing clothes typical of the opposite gender.
3. A strong preference for cross-gender roles in make-believe play or fantasy play.
4. A strong preference for the toys, games, or activities stereotypically used or engaged in by the other gender.
5. A strong preference for playmates of the other gender.
6. A strong rejection of toys, games, and activities typical of one's assigned gender.
7. A strong dislike of one's sexual anatomy.

**Box 12.2  Investigations in a child or adolescent with gender incongruence**

*First line*
- FBC
- Iron/ferritin
- U&E, LFT
- Bone profile
- Vitamin D
- Testosterone
- Oestradiol
- FSH/LH
- Prolactin
- Bone age in pre-menarchal female-to-male or pre-/in-puberty male-to-female individual
- DXA scan

*Second line*
   Only if abnormal results of for clarification.
- Androstenedione, 17OHP
- Karyotype
- Pelvic ultrasound.

preferred gender has been confirmed, and further detailed psychological exploration of the gender identity has been conducted, and fully informed consent given. This is usually over the age of 15 years.

The dose should be increased more slowly in those who have never completed puberty in their birth sex to allow emotional and social maturation as well as the completion of the adolescent growth spurt in height.

The GnRH analogue is continued in transmales until adult levels of testosterone are achieved. In transfemales, it is continued until gonadectomy is performed to prevent androgenic counter-effects on breast development.

## Surgical treatment

### Female-to-male

This can include:

- chest reconstruction, i.e. bilateral mastectomy (known as top surgery)
- metoidioplasty where the testosterone-enhanced clitoris is tubularized and a scrotum is constructed from the labia
- full male genital reconstruction using arm or abdominal skin flaps
- both known as bottom surgery.

### Male-to-female

- Feminizing genitoplasty with the penoscrotal skin refashioned to produce the vagina and labia, and preservation of the glans and neurovascular bundle to form a clitoris (also known as bottom surgery).

## Endocrine support for a non-binary identifying young person

Gender incongruence has typically been associated with a full identification with the opposite gender. However, a significant number of young people are unsure of their eventual gender status or may retain feelings related to their birth sex/gender as well as to their preferred gender or a mixture of both.

### Female-to-male

- Suppression of menstruation using continuous combined oral contraceptive pill with a break once or twice a year
- Progestogen-only mini-pill
- Progestogen-containing intrauterine device.

### Male-to-female

- Antiandrogens (poorly effective)
- Hair reduction with eflornithine cream.

## Long-term outcomes

As yet there is little evidence of the longitudinal outcomes. Psychological support and puberty suppression may be associated with an improved global psychosocial functioning. Frequent change in nominal and legal identity can hinder follow-up. The few longitudinal follow-up studies that have been published have generally shown a high satisfaction outcome (Box 12.3).

## Box 12.3  A glossary of useful terminology

*Gender identity*: the individual's deeply held personal sense of their own gender as male or female, neither, or both.

*Gender incongruence or dysphoria*: refers to an individual's discontent with their birth gender and their identification with a gender other than that associated with their birth sex based on physical sex characteristics. 'Dysphoria' relates to the distress and unease experienced.

*Transgender*: individuals who identify with a gender other than that associated with their birth sex.

*Gender variance and gender diversity*: the wide range of gender identifications outside conventional gender categories.

*Non-binary*: a lack of identification with conventional maleness or femaleness. Non-binary people may express features of both genders or neither.

*Transman/transboy*: a person born phenotypically female (natal female), registered (assigned) female at birth, who identifies as male. Also known as female-to-male (FtM).

*Transwoman/transgirl*: a person born phenotypically male (natal male), registered (assigned) male at birth, who identifies as female. Also known as male-to-female (MtF).

*GnRH analogue*: known colloquially as 'the blocker', used to prevent FSH and LH secretion by competitive inhibition of the GnRH receptor.

*Cross-sex hormones (also known as gender-affirming hormones)*: physiological doses of testosterone in transboys and oestradiol in transgirls used to induce $2°$ sex changes associated with the gender of identification.

# Further reading

American Psychiatric Association. *Diagnostic and Statistical Manual of Mental Disorders* (5th ed). Arlington, VA: American Psychiatric Association, 2013.

Butler G, De Graaf N, Wren B, et al. The assessment and support of children and adolescents with gender dysphoria. *Arch Dis Child* 2018;103:631–636.

Coleman E, Bockting W, Botzer M, et al. Standards of care for the health of transsexual, transgender, and gender-nonconforming people, version 7. *Int J Transgenderism* 2012;13:165–232.

De Vries AL, McGuire JK, Steensma TD, et al. Young adult psychological outcome after puberty suppression and gender reassignment. *Pediatrics* 2014;134:696–704.

Hembree WC, Cohen-Kettenis PT, Gooren L, et al. Endocrine treatment of gender-dysphoric/gender-incongruent persons: an Endocrine Society clinical practice guideline. *J Clin Endocrinol Metab* 2017;102:1–35. ℰ https://www.england.nhs.uk/wp-content/uploads/2017/04/gender-development-service-children-adolescents.pdf

Richards C, Bouman WP, Seal L, et al. Non-binary or genderqueer genders. *Int Rev Psych* 2016;28:95–102.

# Chapter 13

# Endocrine emergencies

# Introduction

This chapter is intended to be brief with readily accessible information that is needed in an endocrine emergency in an infant, child, or adolescent. Endocrine emergencies are rare but because of this they are usually unexpected. Always take a few moments to assess the situation. Getting the clinical signs and obtaining the right biochemical samples at the time is often the key to getting the correct diagnosis and management. The theory and background about each problem are dealt with in the relevant chapter.

The key endocrine emergencies are:
- diabetic ketoacidosis (DKA)
- hypoglycaemia
- adrenal insufficiency
- hypocalcaemia
- hypercalcaemia
- acute diabetes insipidus
- syndrome of inappropriate antidiuretic hormone secretion
- hyperthyroid crisis
- hypothyroid coma
- unclear sex (ambiguous genitalia—disorders or differences of sex development).

# Diabetic ketoacidosis

(⮌ See also Chapter 5.)

DKA is probably the commonest endocrine emergency. The management is complex and it is very important to proceed cautiously.

This section is based on the BSPED national guidelines (⅏ https://www.bsped.org.uk/clinical-resources/guidelines/) (Figs. 13.1–13.3).

## Diagnosis of DKA

Children with:
- hyperglycaemia (blood glucose >11 mmol/L)
- pH <7.3
- bicarbonate <15 mmol/L

and who are:
- >5% dehydrated
- and/or vomiting
- and/or drowsy
- and/or clinically acidotic.

In A&E, check ABC: Airway, Breathing, Circulation.

If shocked, give 0.9% saline 10 mL/kg as a bolus, and repeat only after consultation with a senior paediatrician.

## Confirm diagnosis

- History: polyuria, polydipsia
- Clinical: acidotic respiration, dehydration drowsiness, abdominal pain, vomiting
- Biochemical: hyperglycaemia, acidosis, ketonaemia/ketonuria.

## Investigations

- Blood glucose
- U&E
- Blood gases (venous is fine)
- Blood ketones (superior to urine)
- Other investigations: FBC, chest X-ray, cerebrospinal fluid, throat swab, blood cultures, urine microscopy, culture, and sensitivity only if indicated.

## Clinical assessment and observations

- Level of dehydration: assume 5% if moderate, 10% if severe
- Conscious level: using Glasgow Coma Scale (GCS) score.

Examination, looking for evidence of:
- cerebral oedema: headache, irritability, slow pulse, raised blood pressure, reduced consciousness; NB: papilloedema is a late sign
- infection
- ileus.

## Consider transfer to paediatric intensive care unit if

- severe acidosis pH <7.1
- severe dehydration and shock
- decreased GCS score
- very young child, <2 years
- inadequate ward staffing.

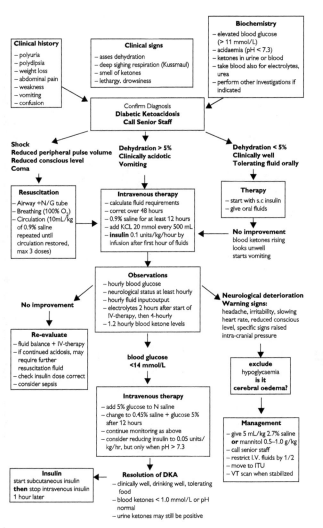

**Clinical history**
– polyuria
– polydipsia
– weight loss
– abdominal pain
– weakness
– vomiting
– confusion

**Clinical signs**
– asses dehydration
– deep sighing respiration (Kussmaul)
– smell of ketones
– lethargy. drowsiness

**Biochemistry**
– elevated blood glucose (> 11 mmol/L)
– acidaemia (pH < 7.3)
– ketones in urine or blood
– take blood also for electrolytes, urea
– perform other investigations if indicated

Confirm Diagnosis
**Diabetic Ketoacidosis**
**Call Senior Staff**

**Shock**
**Reduced peripheral pulse volume**
**Reduced conscious level**
**Coma**

**Dehydration > 5%**
**Clinically acidotic**
**Vomiting**

**Dehydration < 5%**
**Clinically well**
**Tolerating fluid orally**

**Resuscitation**
– Airway +N/G tube
– Breathing (100% O₂)
– Circulation (10mL/kg of 0.9% saline repeated until circulation restored, max 3 doses)

**Intravenous therapy**
– calculate fluid requirements
– corret over 48 hours
– 0.9% saline for at least 12 hours
– add KCL 20 mmol every 500 mL
– **insulin** 0.1 units/kg/hour by infusion after first hour of fluids

**Therapy**
– start with s.c insulin
– give oral fluids

**No improvement**
blood ketones rising
looks unwell
starts vomiting

**Observations**
– hourly blood glucose
– neurological status at least hourly
– hourly fluid input:output
– electrolytes 2 hours after start of IV-therapy, then 4-hourly
– 1.2 hourly blood ketone levels

**No improvement**

**Neurological deterioration**
**Warning signs:**
headache, irritability, slowing heart rate, reduced conscious level, specific signs raised intra-cranial pressure

**Re-evaluate**
– fluid balance + IV-therapy
– if continued acidosis, may require further resuscitation fluid
– check insulin dose correct
– consider sepsis

**blood glucose**
**<14 mmol/L**

**exclude**
hypoglycaemia
**is it**
**cerebral oedema?**

**Intravenous therapy**
– add 5% glucose to N saline
– change to 0.45% saline + glucose 5% after 12 hours
– continue monitoring as above
– consider reducing insulin to 0.05 units/ kg/hr, but only when pH > 7.3

**Management**
– give 5 mL/kg 2.7% saline **or** mannitol 0.5–1.0 g/kg
– call senior staff
– restrict I.V. fluids by 1/2
– move to ITU
– VT scan when stabilized

**Insulin**
start subcutaneous insulin **then** stop intravenous insulin 1 hour later

**Resolution of DKA**
– clinically well, drinking well, tolerating food
– blood ketones < 1.0 mmol/L or pH normal
– urine ketones may still be positive

**Fig. 13.1** Algorithm for the management of diabetic ketoacidosis.

Reproduced with permission from BSPED, http://www.bsped.org.uk. Copyright © 2019 British Society for Paediatric Endocrinology and Diabetes (BSPED).

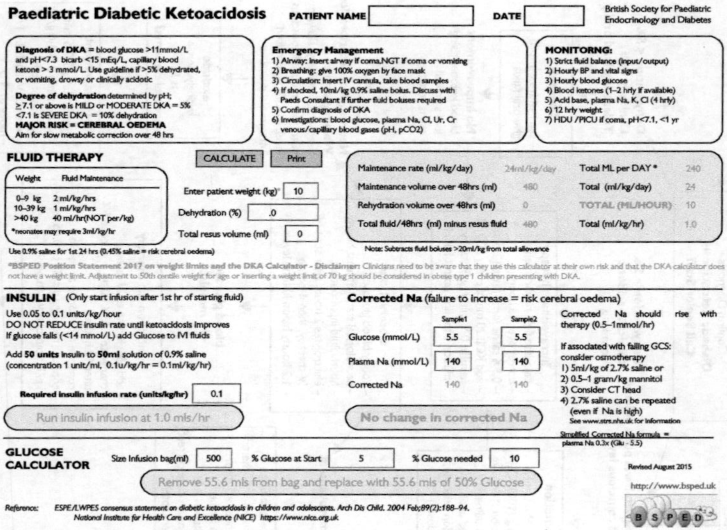

**Fig. 13.2** DKA calculator.

Reproduced with permission from BSPED guidelines on Clinical Standards for Management of an Infant or Adolescent presenting with a suspected disorder of sex development (DSD), https://www.bsped.org.uk/media/1371/dsd-standards-november-2017.pdf. Copyright © 2019 British Society for Paediatric Endocrinology and Diabetes (BSPED).

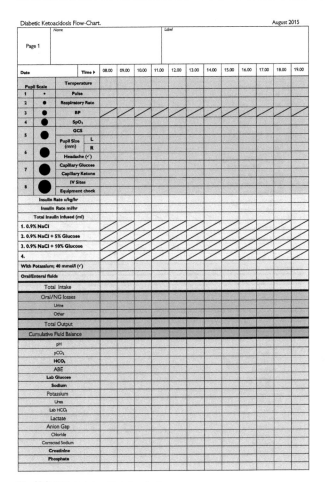

**Fig. 13.3** Diabetic ketoacidosis flowchart.

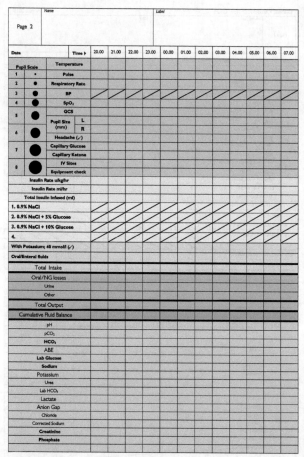

| | | Time ▶ | 20.00 | 21.00 | 22.00 | 23.00 | 00.00 | 01.00 | 02.00 | 03.00 | 04.00 | 05.00 | 06.00 | 07.00 |
|---|---|---|---|---|---|---|---|---|---|---|---|---|---|---|
| **Pupil Scale** | | **Temperature** | | | | | | | | | | | | |
| 1 | | Pulse | | | | | | | | | | | | |
| 2 | | Respiratory Rate | | | | | | | | | | | | |
| 3 | | BP | | | | | | | | | | | | |
| 4 | | SpO₂ | | | | | | | | | | | | |
| 5 | | GCS | | | | | | | | | | | | |
| 6 | | Pupil Size (mm) L | | | | | | | | | | | | |
| | | R | | | | | | | | | | | | |
| | | Headache (✓) | | | | | | | | | | | | |
| 7 | | Capillary Glucose | | | | | | | | | | | | |
| | | Capillary Ketone | | | | | | | | | | | | |
| 8 | | IV Sites | | | | | | | | | | | | |
| | | Equipment check | | | | | | | | | | | | |
| **Insulin Rate u/kg/hr** | | | | | | | | | | | | | | |
| **Insulin Rate ml/hr** | | | | | | | | | | | | | | |
| **Total Insulin Infused (ml)** | | | | | | | | | | | | | | |
| 1. 0.9% NaCl | | | | | | | | | | | | | | |
| 2. 0.9% NaCl + 5% Glucose | | | | | | | | | | | | | | |
| 3. 0.9% NaCl + 10% Glucose | | | | | | | | | | | | | | |
| 4. | | | | | | | | | | | | | | |
| With Potassium; 40 mmol/l (✓) | | | | | | | | | | | | | | |
| Oral/Enteral fluids | | | | | | | | | | | | | | |
| Total Intake | | | | | | | | | | | | | | |
| Oral/NG losses | | | | | | | | | | | | | | |
| Urine | | | | | | | | | | | | | | |
| Other | | | | | | | | | | | | | | |
| Total Output | | | | | | | | | | | | | | |
| Cumulative Fluid Balance | | | | | | | | | | | | | | |
| pH | | | | | | | | | | | | | | |
| pCO₂ | | | | | | | | | | | | | | |
| HCO₃ | | | | | | | | | | | | | | |
| ABE | | | | | | | | | | | | | | |
| Lab Glucose | | | | | | | | | | | | | | |
| Sodium | | | | | | | | | | | | | | |
| Potassium | | | | | | | | | | | | | | |
| Urea | | | | | | | | | | | | | | |
| Lab HCO₃ | | | | | | | | | | | | | | |
| Lactate | | | | | | | | | | | | | | |
| Anion Gap | | | | | | | | | | | | | | |
| Chloride | | | | | | | | | | | | | | |
| Corrected Sodium | | | | | | | | | | | | | | |
| Creatinine | | | | | | | | | | | | | | |
| Phosphate | | | | | | | | | | | | | | |

**Fig. 13.3** Contd

Emphasize need for
- strict fluid balance
- measurement of urine output (urinary catheterization may be required but only in young/sick children)
- hourly capillary blood glucose measurements (may be inaccurate with severe dehydration/acidosis but useful in documenting trends); check with a venous laboratory glucose measurement

- capillary blood ketone levels every 1–2 hours (if available, alternatively urine ketone testing)
- half-hourly blood pressure and basic observations
- twice-daily weight; helpful in assessing fluid balance
- hourly or more frequent neurological observations initially (half-hourly <2 years)
- reporting immediately to the medical staff, even at night, symptoms of headache, slowing of pulse rate, or any change in either conscious level or behaviour
- reporting any electrocardiogram changes, especially T-wave changes suggesting hyper/hypokalaemia.

## Fluids

(See 🔗 https://www.bsped.org.uk/media/1629/bsped-dka-aug15_.pdf.)

Requirement = maintenance + deficit − fluid already given

- For most children, use 5% dehydration to calculate fluids:
  - if they weigh <10 kg, give 2 mL/kg/hour
  - if they weigh between 10 and 40 kg, give 1 mL/kg/hour
  - if they weigh >40 kg, give a fixed volume of 40 mL/hour.
- Hourly rate = 48-hour maintenance + deficit − resuscitation fluid already given/48.
- Initially 0.9% saline and continue for at least 12 hours.
- Once blood sugar has fallen to 14 mmol/L add glucose (usually 5%) to the fluid.
- After 12 hours, if plasma sodium level stable or increasing, change to 0.45% saline/5% glucose/20 mmol KCl.
- Oral fluids should only be offered only after clinical improvement and no vomiting.
- If good clinical improvement occurs before end of rehydration period, IV fluids can be reduced to take into account oral intake.

## Potassium

- Blood levels will fall once insulin is started.
- Should be commenced immediately after resuscitation with rehydration fluid unless anuria suspected.
- ▶ *Use potassium 40 mmol/L even if plasma level normal (cellular depletion).*
- Check U&E 2 hours after resuscitation begun and then at least 4-hourly; alter potassium replacement accordingly. May require >40 mmol/L electrolytes. A blood gas machine can be helpful for trends.
- Use a cardiac monitor; observe frequently for T-wave changes.

## Insulin

- Should be omitted for first hour.
- Continuous low-dose insulin is preferred method (0.1 U/kg/hour).
- Once pH is >7.3, blood sugar down to 14 mmol/L, and glucose-containing fluid started, consider reducing insulin infusion rate, but not <0.05 U/kg/hour and not if ketones >3 mmol/L.
- Don't stop insulin if blood sugar <4 mmol/L; if necessary, give bolus of 2 mL/kg of 10% dextrose and increase glucose concentration to 10%.

### Others

- *Bicarbonate* is rarely used. Ongoing acidosis indicates insufficient resuscitation or insulin.
- *Phosphate* is often low, but little published benefit of replacement.
- *Anticoagulation* should be considered in:
  - young
  - very sick
  - significant hyperosmolarity.

### Cerebral oedema

(⮕ See also Chapter 5.)

#### Signs and symptoms

- Headache
- Bradycardia, raised blood pressure
- Altered neurological state
- Abnormal posturing.

Late signs include convulsions, papilloedema, and respiratory arrest.

#### Treatment

- Hypertonic saline (2.7%) 5 mL/kg, or mannitol 0.5–1.0 g/kg over 10–15 minutes. The latter may be repeated after 2 hours if no response.
- Restrict fluids to 1/2 maintenance and rehydrate over 72 hours.
- Move child to intensive therapy unit if not already there.

# Hypoglycaemia

(For a detailed account, see Chapter 7.)

## When to suspect it

- In a child/adolescent with established diabetes
- Unexpected drowsiness or loss of consciousness
- Seizure with no neurological disease
- In a severely unwell child with a trivial illness.

## Other relevant drug treatments/inter-reactions

- Insulin
- (Accidental) ingestion of oral hypoglycaemic agents
- Under-replacement or missed dose of glucocorticoids.

## Age group

### Neonatal

- Premature infants
- SGA/light for gestational age
- Infant of a diabetic mother.

### Toddler and child

- Metabolic causes if inappropriately ill for underlying cause
- Accidental/non-accidental poisoning.

### Adolescent

- Severe illness
- Alcohol or other substance abuse.

## Presenting symptoms

- Drowsiness, slow mentation
- Unconsciousness
- Fitting
- Headache.

## Presenting signs

- Pallor
- Sweating
- Tachycardia
- Tachypnoea.

## Samples to take

- Plasma/blood glucose: do not rely on bedside blood glucose testing
- Ketone bodies
- Free fatty acids
- Acyl carnitine
- Insulin and C-peptide
- Growth hormone
- Cortisol
- ACTH
- *First urine passed* for organic acids, ketone bodies.

Immediate management
- If awake and orientated, give a glucose drink or three glucose tablets
- If *drowsy* or unconscious, 10% glucose IV 2 mL/kg bolus dose
- ▶ *Never* use 50% glucose IV.

Next steps
- Repeat 2 mL/kg bolus of 10% glucose. Recheck bedside/laboratory blood glucose. The aim should be to raise blood glucose to 5–9 mmol/L and *no higher*.
- If glucose becomes normal and symptoms do not improve, look for another cause
- IV 10% glucose infusion (0.1 mL/kg/min) for repeated hypoglycaemia.

Stabilization
- In most cases when there is a failure of the hypoglycaemic response, this is usually satisfactory.
- Persistent hypoglycaemia requiring high glucose infusion rates (>8 mg/kg/minute) suggests hyperinsulinism:
  - hyperinsulinism of infancy in a neonate
  - insulin excess in a diabetic patient
  - insulin/oral hypoglycaemic agent poisoning in a non-diabetic patient.

# Adrenal insufficiency/adrenal crisis

When to suspect it

- Shocked child
- Unexplained hypoglycaemia
- Non-surgical acute abdomen
- Inappropriately ill for underlying cause
- In acute meningococcal septicaemia
- Developing hyperpigmentation.

Other relevant drug treatments/inter-reactions

- Current or recent glucocorticoid therapy (any type including inhaled steroids and any dose)
- Antifungal therapy (ketoconazole)
- Antiandrogen (cyproterone acetate).

Age group

- Any age.

Presenting symptoms

- Drowsiness may be with history of lethargy
- Dizziness
- Unconsciousness
- Vomiting (often profuse).

Presenting signs

- Pallor of shock, but
- Hyperpigmentation (check skin creases, scars, buccal cavity, and areas not usually sun-exposed such as buttocks)
- Dehydration
- Acute abdomen
- Tachypnoea
- Tachycardia.

Samples to take

- Glucose
- Electrolytes
- Cortisol
- Adrenal steroids
- ACTH (need urgent transport to laboratory on ice).

Immediate management

- Treat shock with IV 0.9% saline boluses 10 mL/kg.
- Treat hypoglycaemia with IV 10% glucose boluses 2 mL/kg.
- Continue infusion (0.9% saline with 5% glucose) at maintenance plus calculated deficit.
- Treat hyperkalaemia if present.
- IV bolus hydrocortisone 4 mg/kg or if weight not known:
  - Infant: 25 mg
  - 2–5 years: 50 mg
  - >5 years: 100 mg

### Next steps

- Treat other underlying condition, e.g. infection even if only suspected.
- Establish hydrocortisone infusion (2.0 mg/kg/day).
- Monitor and correct sodium and potassium disturbances.

### Stabilization

- Fully rehydrate and normalize blood glucose.
- Start physiological replacement steroids:
  - Hydrocortisone 10–12 mg/m$^2$/day in three divided doses, usually 50% on waking, 25% at lunchtime, and 25% in the evening.
  - Fludrocortisone 150 mcg/m$^2$/day once daily.
  - Oral saline 30% (5 mmol/mL) 1–3 mmol/kg/day in three divided doses in infants <1–2 years.

# Hypocalcaemia

**When to suspect it**

- Unexplained movements or seizures.

**Other relevant drug treatments/inter-reactions**

- May be caused by maternal rickets or clinical rickets in the child.

**Age group**

- Neonate: anytime from birth, usually within the first week
- Child/adolescent: any age.

**Presenting symptoms**

- Twitching
- Irritability
- Tingling fingers, toes, or lips
- Numbness of fingers, toes, or lips
- Stridor
- Seizures.

**Presenting signs**

- Carpopedal spasm
- Seizures
- Chvostek's sign
- Trousseau's sign.

**Samples to take**

- Calcium
- Phosphate
- Magnesium
- Alkaline phosphatase
- 25-hydroxyvitamin $D_3$
- PTH.

**Immediate management**

- IV bolus of 10% calcium gluconate (226 µmol Ca/mL) 0.1 mL/kg.
- Dilute with 0.9% saline or 5% glucose and infuse over 10 minutes into central line or large cannula in *large* vein as severe risk of calcium burns with tissue leak from peripheral site.
- Do not co-administer with sodium bicarbonate as this causes calcium carbonate precipitation.

**Next steps**

- Calcium infusion 1–2 mmol/kg/day via a central line
- Magnesium infusion if low.

**Stabilization**

- Oral calcium supplements
- Vitamin D analogue (alfacalcidol if hypoparathyroidism)
- Oral magnesium supplements.

# Hypercalcaemia

## When to suspect it

- Excessive vitamin D treatment
- Pre-existing bone disorder
- Prolonged immobilization
- During chemotherapy.

## Other relevant drug treatments/inter-reactions

- Vitamin D (cholecalciferol, ergocalciferol) and analogues (alfacalcidol, calcitriol)
- Rarely a presenting feature of leukaemia, lymphomas, or solid tumours.

## Age group

- Any.

## Presenting symptoms

### Gastrointestinal

- Anorexia
- Vomiting
- Abdominal pain
- Constipation.

### Renal

- Polyuria
- Polydipsia.

### Central nervous system

- Confusion
- Lethargy
- Mood changes.

### Other

- Muscular hypotonia
- Pruritus
- Sore eyes.

## Presenting signs

- Usually none.

## Samples to take

- Calcium
- Magnesium
- Phosphate
- Alkaline phosphatase
- PTH
- U&E, creatinine
- LFTs
- TFTs
- Urine calcium, phosphate, creatinine, albumin.

Immediate management
- 0.9% saline infusion at maintenance plus deficit (if present)
- IV furosemide infusion 0.5–1.5 mg/kg daily, maximum 20 mg daily
- IV pamidronate infusion 0.5 mg/kg daily for 2–3 days if persistent.

Next steps
- Pamidronate may be repeated if required.

Stabilization
- 1° management dependent upon cause of hypercalcaemia (rare).

## Acute diabetes insipidus

### When to suspect it

- Polyuria (and polydipsia if conscious) following physical disturbance of the HP axis:
  - midline cranial surgery, e.g. craniopharyngioma
  - traumatic brain injury, e.g. road traffic accident.

### Other relevant drug treatments/inter-reactions

- None.

### Age group

- Any.

### Presenting symptoms

- Dehydration in patient possibly unconscious or sedated, intubated, and ventilated.

### Presenting signs

- Polyuria >120 mL/m$^2$/hour (~2.5 mL/kg/hour).

### Samples to take

- Plasma: electrolytes, glucose, osmolality, cortisol, free T$_3$, and free T$_4$.
- Urine: electrolytes and osmolality.

### Immediate management

- Hourly fluid balance with replacement of losses usually starting with 0.45% saline/5% glucose and adjusting according to osmolality, glucose, and electrolytes.

### Next steps

- Persistent or increasing polyuria and dehydration may require AVP infusion (▶ arginine vasopressin—aqueous pitressin which is *not* the same as DDAVP).
- Ensure normal adrenal and thyroid function first, as cortisol and thyroxine are necessary for normal renal tubular function and hence water excretion.
- Vasopressin infusion rate starts at 1.5–2.5 mU/kg/hour and titrate according to urine flow.
- Fluid infusion rates should be reduced accordingly, usually to around 1.0 L/m$^2$/day

### Stabilization

- If diabetes insipidus is likely to be permanent, switch treatment to desmopressin (DDAVP).
- Use lowest possible dose and titrate dose and frequency to the antidiuretic effect.
- Suggested starting doses: nasal 2.5 mcg; oral 50 mcg (caution in infants—need lower doses, e.g. 10 mcg—need to be prepared by pharmacy).
- NB: overdosing causes fluid retention, anuria, and hyponatraemia. This is very dangerous and difficult to treat.

# Syndrome of inappropriate antidiuretic hormone secretion

When to suspect it
- Unexplained hyponatraemia with normovolaemia, i.e. absence of shock
- Low plasma osmolality <270 mOsmol/kg
- Inappropriate urine osmolality >300 mOsmol/kg
- Renal sodium loss—urine Na >30 mmol/L.

Other relevant drug treatments/inter-reactions
### CNS disorders
- Infections, e.g. meningitis
- Head injury
- Cranial surgery
- Intracranial bleed
- Guillain–Barré syndrome.

### Chest diseases
- Infection, e.g. pneumonia
- Asthma
- Pneumothorax
- Positive pressure ventilation.

### Malignancy metabolic disorders
- Cortisol deficiency
- Thyroxine deficiency.

### Drugs
- Chemotherapy agents
- Antiepileptics, e.g. carbamazepine, valproate
- Antipsychotics.

### Idiopathic

Age group
- Any.

Presenting symptoms
- Mild—none
- Severe—symptoms of cerebral oedema.

Presenting signs
- Severe—signs of raised intracranial pressure.

Samples to take
### Plasma
- Osmolality
- Electrolytes
- Glucose
- Cortisol
- TFTs.

*Urine*
- Osmolality
- Electrolytes
- Glucose.

## Immediate management
- Mild—plasma sodium >120 mmol/L:
  - fluid restriction to 600–800 mL/m²/day
  - aim to raise plasma Na maximum rate 0.5 mmol/L/hour
- Severe—plasma sodium <120 mmol/L:
  - fluid restriction as for mild cases
  - hypertonic saline infusion: 3% saline 1–2 mL/kg/hour
  - aim to raise plasma sodium 1–2 mmol/L/hour (0.5–1.0 mmol/L/hour in longstanding SIADH).

## Next steps
- Consider loop diuretics (furosemide).

## Stabilization
- Beware over-rapid increase in plasma sodium concentrations >15 mmol/kg/24 hours
- Associated with changes in mental state and brain injury.

## Differential diagnosis
- *Cerebral salt* wasting is usually associated with dehydration, hypovolaemia, and greater renal sodium losses than in SIADH. The management differs, consequently requiring rehydration therapy often with hypertonic saline fluids as opposed to fluid restriction.

# Hyperthyroid crisis

**When to suspect it**
- Infant of mother with active or previously thyroidectomized for Graves' disease
- Neonatal persistent tachycardia and cardiac compromise.

**Other relevant drug treatments/inter-reactions**
- None.

**Age group**
- Neonatal mostly, but rare
- Severe thyrotoxicosis in an older child or adolescent extremely rare.

**Presenting symptoms**
- Irritability
- Restlessness
- Voracious feeding
- Weight loss or failure to gain weight.

**Presenting signs**
- Tachycardia
- Tachypnoea
- Signs of cardiac failure
- Goitre.

**Samples to take—from infant *and* mother**
- Free T$_3$
- Free T$_4$
- TSH
- Thyroid receptor antibody titre (TRAb/TSI).

**Immediate management**
- Antithyroid drugs:
  - carbimazole 0.25 mg/kg 8-hourly
  - propylthiouracil 0.5–1.5 mg/kg/day once daily (only if failure of control with carbimazole—risk of idiosyncratic liver failure)
- β-blockade: propranolol 0.25–0.75 mg/kg 8-hourly.

**Next steps**
- Dosage titration to control cardiac hyperfunction and high-output cardiac failure.
- Aqueous iodine oral solution (Lugol's solution 1–2 drops) only considered in uncontrollable thyrotoxicosis.

**Stabilization**
- β-blockade can be withdrawn once cardiac compromise resolves.
- Antithyroid drug treatment may be needed for up to 9 months until maternally transmitted antibody levels spontaneously fall.

# Hypothyroid coma

**When to suspect it**

- Failure to respond or awaken following CNS insult, e.g. surgery in patient who may have had pre-existing HP disease.
- Coma in child/adolescent who has received high-dose cranial irradiation previously for a central brain tumour.

**Other relevant drug treatments/inter-reactions**

- None.

**Age group**

- Usually older children/adolescents.

**Presenting symptoms**

- Failure to awaken in the absence of metabolic disturbance and with normal blood glucose and cortisol levels.

**Presenting signs**

- Reduced GCS score (<8)
- Hypothermia.

**Samples to take**

- Free $T_3$—low
- Free $T_4$—low
- TSH—inappropriately low if a central cause.

**Immediate management**

- Tri-iodothyronine (liothyronine, $T_3$) by slow IV injection, 5–20 mcg repeated every 12 hours or as often as every 4 hours if necessary.

**Next steps**

- Start L-thyroxine ($T_4$) 2–5 mcg/kg/day once daily orally or via nasogastric tube at the same time as $T_3$.
- Titrate $T_3$ doses to plasma free $T_3$ levels to achieve a biochemical euthyroid state.

**Stabilization**

- Once patient has awoken from coma and is neurologically normal, gradually withdraw $T_3$ therapy, continuing with $T_4$.
- Manage $T_4$ replacement conventionally, keeping free $T_4$ levels in upper normal range. Free $T_4$ levels may take 1–2 weeks to stabilize.
- NB: TSH measurements may be unhelpful.

# Unclear sex (ambiguous genitalia—differences of sex development)

(➲ See also Chapter 11.)

### When to suspect it

- Sex not immediately clear at birth.

### Other relevant drug treatments/inter-reactions

- Family history
- Closely inter-related parents and family
- Occupational or environmental exposure to organic chemicals
- Maternal virilizing adrenal or ovarian tumour.

### Age group

- At birth.

### Presenting symptoms

- Associated with any other congenital anomaly
- Infant usually otherwise well.

### Presenting signs

- Varying degrees of virilization of a female infant or undermasculinization of a male infant. Stage according to Prader (➲ see Table 11.3, p. 347).
- Signs of other recognizable dysmorphic syndrome.

### Samples to take

- Cord blood or venous blood: karyotype and DNA for FISH analysis.
- Testosterone, FSH, LH, and 17OHP.
- *No* samples for electrolytes until day 3.

### Immediate management

- Manage any 1° clinical condition.
- Examine the infant fully and document genital findings.
- Frank open explanation to the parents.
- Provide support and do not leave them alone initially.
- Discuss management plan with medical, midwifery, and nursing teams.

### Next steps

- Call for expert help—neonatal, endocrine, and surgical teams.
- Pelvic ultrasound by experienced radiologist.
- Blood/urine samples for electrolytes, 17OHP.

### Stabilization

- Depends on 1° cause.
- Salt-wasting in virilized female with CAH may take up to 2–3 weeks to present clinically, so monitor plasma and urine electrolytes daily.
- Long-term management is best performed with a specialist multidisciplinary team (➲ see Chapter 11).

# Endocrine investigations and laboratory reference ranges

# General guidelines

Some endocrine investigations are complex and may involve the collection of several types of samples for different types of tests. When performing complex investigations please take into consideration the following guidelines:

• If clinically possible, collect blood samples during the morning or early afternoon of a working day.
• Very sick neonates/infants can present at any time and samples for metabolic investigations are best taken during the acute episode.
• Samples may need to be transported to the referral laboratory during normal working hours.
• Investigation of endocrine disorders should be done in stages.
• Blanket requesting of tests without taking into consideration the results of first-line routine tests is unhelpful to the patient and wasteful of resources.

2 It is important that the laboratory is given full clinical details so that investigations are narrowed down to the specific enzyme panel.

### Filling in request cards

If you are collecting serial specimens it is very important to label both request cards and specimens with the *date* and *time*. This is necessary whether you are using a single request card with several specimens or one card with each specimen.

Please put a *hospital number* and/or patient identification details on every request card. Electronic processes are generally superior but please check specimen labels match the patient.

### Liaison with clinical biochemistry

It is usually helpful to contact the duty biochemistry team for advice on carrying out dynamic tests and they will organize rapid analyses and special sampling transport and preparation where necessary if requested.

### A note on the suggested protocols

This chapter contains information on reference laboratory ranges and suggested investigation protocols derived from several major units. It is advisable to have a discussion with your biochemistry team prior to undertaking any of the protocols so any local issues can be clarified.

# Growth hormone provocation tests

## Choice of test

The *insulin stress (tolerance) test* is the gold standard for assessment of GH production. However, the BSPED recommends that its use is limited to centres with experience of its use and full back-up emergency paediatric teams and intensive care facilities should (rare) complications arise. This test is not suitable for use in babies and young children and those with bodyweight <15 kg. This test measures the GH response to induced hypoglycaemia.

The *glucagon test* is used in babies and young children but is commonly used as a first-line test in children and adolescents of any age. It has a central effect on the hypothalamus stimulating GH release. It is *not necessary* or indeed desirable to induce hypoglycaemia during this test.

*Arginine* infusion stimulates GH release by reducing somatostatin tone. It also may stimulate GHRH release via α-adrenergic receptors. It is generally free from side effects. GH release may be impaired with coexisting hypothyroidism.

*Clonidine* also acts as a central releasing agent via the stimulation of GHRH. It can cause prolonged hypotension which is unpleasant for the child, and is probably the least effective stimulus to GH release.

## Priming

Children with bone age >10 years who are not yet in puberty may not show an optimal GH response to insulin (or any other provocation tests) unless the patient is primed with testosterone or oestrogen. This produces an improved releasability of GH, mimicking the normal pubertal increase in physiological GH secretion. Girls require ethinyloestradiol 10 mcg orally or oestradiol valerate 1 mg once a day for 5 days immediately beforehand. Boys require injectable testosterone esters 100 mg IM, given 1 week before the investigation.

It is also possible to prescribe oral testosterone undecanoate 40 mg for 5 days prior to the investigation. This may be helpful if the child is needle phobic.

Alternatively, both sexes can be given stilboestrol 1 mg twice a day orally for 2 days before the test.

# Stimulation tests for growth hormone secretion

## Glucagon stimulation test

### Indication

Standard investigation of GH deficiency in children. The triple test (⊙ see p. 394) is rarely necessary.

▶ NB: ensure that this is the test you really want, and that you are not investigating hypoglycaemia.

### Interpretation

Induces a peak of GH secretion due to central action. A peak response of >6.5 mcg/L is considered normal, 3–6.5 mcg/L as partial GH deficiency, and <3.0 mcg/L as severe GH deficiency. May also act as stimulant for ACTH/cortisol release but less reliable if >10 years of age.

### Preparation for the test

- *Fasting*: yes, nil by mouth except water from midnight.
  - If the child weighs <10 kg, they can have a milk feed 4 hours beforehand.
- *Calculate drug dosage*: 100 mcg/kg bodyweight of insulin-free glucagon given as a single IM dose.
- (▶ Maximum dose = 1 mg.)

It is possible to give IV glucagon in exceptional circumstances, please discuss with local endocrinology team for further advice.

### Procedure

1. Test to be commenced 09:00–10:00.
2. Prepare rescue drugs including 10% glucose solution (2 mL/kg equivalent to 0.2 g/kg) and hydrocortisone 100 mg.
3. Site IV cannula at time −15 minutes.
4. Draw baseline bloods (at −15 and 0 minutes).
5. Give IM glucagon.
6. Take blood specimens as charted, checking fingerprick glucose with each specimen.
7. Doctor must attend the patient if hypoglycaemia occurs, If symptomatic hypoglycaemia occurs, oral glucose drink (Lucozade® or Polycal®) can be given, but continue with sampling schedule. If this does not help the patient or they are vomiting, give 2 mL/kg 10% glucose IV slowly, *but continue with sampling*. If severe hypoglycaemia develops or recovery after IV glucose is slow, give IV hydrocortisone (100 mg) in addition to a second glucose bolus. Call for additional emergency help as well. Maintain normal blood glucose (4–8 mmol/L) and no higher. Dangers arise, not only from hypoglycaemia, but from overenthusiastic administration of *hypertonic* glucose solutions. Always check fingerprick blood glucose sample before repeating a dose of IV glucose. Do not repeat IV glucose if blood glucose sample is >10 mmol/L.

### Samples

See Table 14.1.

**Table 14.1** Samples

| Time (minutes) | IGF-1 | Glucose | GH | Cortisol |
|---|---|---|---|---|
| −15 | + | + | + | + |
| 0 | | + | + | + |
| 30 | | + | + | |
| 60 | | + | + | + |
| 90 | | | + | + |
| 120 | | + | + | + |
| 150 | | + | | |
| 180 | | + | + | + |

*Side effects*
*Vomiting is relatively common.* Severe reactive hypoglycaemia at around 2 hours into the test is unusual. If this occurs, give 2 mL/kg (0.2 g/kg) 10% glucose IV slowly, *but continue with sampling*. If severe hypoglycaemia develops or recovery after treatment with IV dextrose is slow, give 100 mg IV hydrocortisone in addition. Maintain normal blood glucose. Dangers arise, not only from hypoglycaemia, but from overenthusiastic administration of *hypertonic* glucose solutions. Always check fingerprick blood glucose sample before repeating a dose of intravenous glucose. Do not repeat IV glucose if blood glucose sample is >10 mmol/L. Continue with test sampling protocol if possible

### Insulin tolerance test
The dose of soluble insulin is 0.15 IU/kg IV. This should be reduced to 0.1 IU/kg if hypopituitarism is strongly suspected and if the cortisol response is likely to be impaired. Ensure the dose of insulin is double checked by at least two doctors. The test sampling protocol is as given for the glucagon stimulation test (◉ see above) up to 120 minutes. Hypoglycaemia awareness is vital. Comments as given for the glucagon stimulation test are very pertinent.

### Arginine
The dose is 0.5 g/kg to a maximum of 30 g. This should be administered as a 10% solution of arginine monochloride dissolved in 0.9% saline and infused at a constant rate over 30 minutes. The protocol is as given for the glucagon stimulation test (◉ see above).
   Arginine does not promote ACTH/cortisol release so do not measure cortisol.

### Clonidine
The dose is 0.15 mg/m² orally. Monitor blood pressure beforehand and every 30 minutes during the test as it can dip markedly.
   The protocol is as given for the glucagon stimulation test (◉ see above).
   Clonidine does not promote ACTH/cortisol release so do not measure cortisol.

# IGF-1 generation test

Indication

The investigation of possible GH insensitivity, with high baseline or stimulated GH levels. Does *not* need to be performed if baseline IGF-1 levels are normal.

Can be performed immediately after an unprimed GH provocation test. If priming is needed for the provocation test, the generation test should be delayed for at least 2 weeks.

*Interpretation*

In severe 1° IGF-1 deficiency, IGF-1 levels are extremely low and show no response to GH stimulation. Partial IGF-1 deficiency may show a slight response to GH but levels do not rise into the age-related predicted normal range.

Procedure

- Day 1:
  - Patient has nothing by mouth from midnight. Basal blood samples are preferably taken in the morning. Then give GH injection 0.03 mg/kg SC (the technique for GH injections can normally be taught to the parents on the first day).
  - Therefore injections on days 2–4 can be administered by the family at home, before bedtime. If this is not possible, then the timing of the GH injections on these days may need to be brought forward.
- Day 2: GH (0.03 mg/kg) SC before bedtime.
- Day 3: GH (0.03 mg/kg) SC before bedtime.
- Day 4: GH (0.03 mg/kg) SC before bedtime.
- Day 5: blood specimens taken in the morning.

Blood samples

- Day 1:
  - IGF-1
  - IGFBP3
- Day 5:
  - IGF-1
  - IGFBP3.

# Glucose tolerance test for investigating excess GH

## Indication

To ensure that GH can be suppressed in tall children suspected of autonomous GH release. ► Check that you do not want to use the glucose tolerance test for the investigation of impaired glucose tolerance (see p. 418).

## Interpretation

Baseline GH levels are usually low (<2 mcg/L) but as GH is released in a pulsatile manner and in response to stress, higher levels may reflect sampling during a GH pulse. GH levels should not increase during the test, and if a GH peak has occurred during initial sampling, GH levels should subsequently decrease. An abnormal result follows if GH levels do not decrease from baseline values and indeed show an increase. A raised baseline IGF-1 together with abnormal glucose tolerance may suggest the diagnosis of GH excess.

## Fasting

Not required.

## Order drugs from pharmacy

Oral glucose solution 1.75 g/kg up to maximum of 75 g.
   *Alternatively*, Polycal® can be used.

## Procedure

1. Take basal blood samples.
2. Give oral glucose drink. Drink should be consumed in 5–10 minutes.
3. Take blood samples as charted (Table 14.2).

**Table 14.2** Samples

| Time (minutes) | Glucose | GH | IGF-1 | IGFBP3 |
|---|---|---|---|---|
| Baseline | + | + | + | + |
| 30 | + | + | | |
| 60 | + | + | | |
| 90 | + | + | | |
| 120 | + | + | | |
| 180 | + | + | | |

# Thyrotropin-releasing hormone test

## Indication

This investigation is rarely needed and is used only for the investigation of the integrity of the HP–thyroid axis, the suspicion of a TSH-secreting tumour, or in TSH resistance.

## Interpretation

This is subject to much controversy. A rise in TSH indicates that the HP axis is intact. The timing of the peak TSH response *does not*, as formerly thought, point to the site of the abnormality in this axis. An exaggerated peak (>50 mU/L) may suggest a hyper-responsive state, either due to a TSH resistance state (abnormality of TSH receptor, or a pituitary adenoma). Both of these are extremely rare. Diurnal TSH sampling and pituitary imaging may be needed (Table 14.3).

## Fasting

Not required.

## Order drugs from pharmacy

TRH 7 mcg/kg IV (maximum dose 200 mcg).

## Procedure

1. Draw baseline blood specimen. Occasionally TBG also required.
2. Give TRH IV.

## Side effects

Include bitter taste in mouth, flushing, nausea, and occasional vomiting, especially if TRH injected rapidly.

NB: can be done concurrently with other investigations.

**Table 14.3** Samples

| Time (minutes) | TSH and prolactin | Free $T_3$, free $T_4$ |
|---|---|---|
| Baseline | + | + |
| 20 | + | |
| 60 | + | |

# Luteinizing hormone-releasing hormone/ gonadotropin-releasing hormone stimulation test

## Indication

For investigation of the HP–gonadal axis. It is useful in paediatric endocrinology to assist in the differential diagnosis of central gonadotropin-dependent precocious puberty and the monitoring of treatment in this condition, and in the investigation of extremes of delayed puberty and hypogonadotropic hypogonadism (Table 14.4).

## Interpretation

- *Normal prepubertal state*: LH and FSH levels usually <1.0 mU/L; peak LH and FSH responses usually <5 mU/L. FSH peak usually slightly greater than LH.
- *Central precocious puberty*: baseline LH and FSH levels may be diagnostic both >3.0 mU/L. In early normal and precocious puberty, the LH peak is usually greater than that of FSH (LH:FSH ratio >1.0) and the peak LH response is >5.0 mu/L over the baseline value.
- *Monitoring of GnRH analogue treatment in central precocious puberty*: a prepubertal or absent LH and FSH response should be seen.

NB: this test cannot be performed after an hCG test, or if the child has been primed with sex steroids for a GH provocation test. At least 2 weeks should be left between these investigations. An hCG test *can* follow immediately after completing the LHRH stimulation test.

## Fasting

Not required.

## Order drugs from pharmacy

LHRH 25 mcg/m$^2$ or 2.5 mcg/kg, maximum dose 100 mcg.

## Procedure

1. Collect baseline blood samples.
2. Give LHRH IV.

## Side effect

Rare. May in exceptional circumstances cause allergic reactions.

**Table 14.4** Samples

| Time (minutes) | LH | FSH | Testosterone (boys)/oestradiol (girls) |
|---|---|---|---|
| Baseline | + | + | + |
| 20 | + | + | |
| 60 | + | + | |

# Triple pituitary stimulation test

## Indication

This is an exceptional investigation in children >10 years old where panhypopituitarism is suspected.

2 NB: the gonadotrophin stimulation part of this test cannot be performed after an hCG test.

## Fasting

Yes, nil by mouth except water from midnight.

## Order drugs from pharmacy

Before test note height and weight, calculate surface area, and order:
- GH stimulant—glucagon or insulin as for the glucagon stimulation test (⊃ see p. 388)
- TRH 7 mcg/kg (maximum = 200 mcg)
- LHRH 2.5 mcg/kg (25 mcg/m$^2$).

## Procedure

1. Test to be commenced at 09:00–10:00
2. Prepare drugs including 10% glucose solution, 0.2 g/kg (2 mL/kg) and hydrocortisone 100 mg.
3. Site IV cannula at −15 minutes.
4. Draw baseline bloods (at −15 and 0 minutes).
5. Give IV drugs.
6. Take blood specimens as charted, checking bedside glucose analysis with each specimen.
7. Doctor must attend the patient if hypoglycaemia occurs. If symptomatic hypoglycaemia occurs, an oral glucose drink (Lucozade® or Polycal®) can be given, but continue with sampling schedule. If this does not help the patient or they are vomiting, give 2 mL/kg 10% glucose IV slowly, *but continue with sampling*. If severe hypoglycaemia develops or recovery after IV glucose is slow, give IV hydrocortisone (100 mg) in addition to a second glucose bolus. Maintain normal blood glucose (4–8 mmol/L) and no higher. Dangers arise, not only from hypoglycaemia, but from overenthusiastic administration of *hypertonic* glucose solutions. Always check fingerprick blood glucose sample before repeating a dose of IV glucose. Do not repeat IV glucose if fingerprick glucose is >10 mmol/L.

## Samples

### Baseline samples

IGF-1, IGFBP3, testosterone/oestradiol, and prolactin (Table 14.5).

**Table 14.5** Samples

| Time (minutes) | Glucose | GH | Cortisol | TSH | FSH/LH |
|---|---|---|---|---|---|
| −15 | + | + | + | + | + |
| 0 | + | + | + | + | + |
| 20 | + | + | + | + | + |
| 60 | + | + | + | + | + |
| 90 | + | + | + | | |
| 120 | + | + | + | | |
| 150 | + | + | + | | |
| 180 | + | + | + | | |

# Water deprivation test

## Indication

For the investigation of pituitary and nephrogenic diabetes insipidus. If diabetes insipidus is not likely then arrange a paired early-morning plasma and urine osmolality from clinic. If the urine osmolality is >750 mOsmol/kg, the child does not have diabetes insipidus. If this is a 're-test', DDAVP must be stopped 24 hours prior to the test.

## Interpretation

Loss of 5% body weight, rise of plasma Na to >145 mmol/L, and/or no urinary concentration confirms cranial diabetes insipidus. For discussion of interpretation in partial forms and in chronic polydipsia, ➔ see Chapter 5.

## Fasting

Not required. Allow to eat and drink freely until start of test especially in an infant or young child. No food or fluids allowed during the test.

## Preparation

This test needs to be discussed with the clinical biochemistry department beforehand, discuss with them the necessity for *rapid* measurements of plasma and urine osmolalities phoned back to you urgently in order to complete the test *safely*.

## Procedure

- Test starts at 08:30.
- Use a flow sheet (Fig. 14.1) to record the timing of specimens, results, and the patient's weight, blood pressure, and thirst.
- Insert sampling cannula. Baseline blood sample for osmolality, plasma Na.
- Weigh child.
- Child to empty bladder—send urine for osmolality, Na. Make sure urine is not already concentrated. If osmolality >750 mOsmol/kg, no need to perform test.
- Start fluid fast. It is seldom necessary to fast for >12 hours (in infants 6–8 hours).
- Collect each urine sample passed:
  • record volume and time
  • send aliquot to laboratory for Na, osmolality.
- Take blood specimens for Na and osmolality at the same time as each urine sample, or hourly, if none passed.
- Record weight, estimate of thirst, and urine samples on forms provided and file in notes.
- Weigh child and record blood pressure hourly.
- Test is terminated when:
    a. urine osmolality concentrates to >750 mOsmol/kg,
  *or*
    b. plasma Na >145 mmol/L
  *or*
    c. plasma osmolality >305 mOsmol/kg

**Flow chart for water deprivation test (please file in patient's notes)**

Patient addressograph:

Date (start/finish time):

Reason for test:

Symptoms during test:

DDAVP (time and dosage):

| Time | Weight | Thirst* | BP | Urine volume passed | Urinary Na | Urine osmolality | Plasma osmolality | Plasma Na | AVP |
|------|--------|---------|----|--------------------|-----------|------------------|-------------------|-----------|-----|
|      |        |         |    |                    |           |                  |                   |           |     |
|      |        |         |    |                    |           |                  |                   |           |     |
|      |        |         |    |                    |           |                  |                   |           |     |
|      |        |         |    |                    |           |                  |                   |           |     |
|      |        |         |    |                    |           |                  |                   |           |     |
|      |        |         |    |                    |           |                  |                   |           |     |
|      |        |         |    |                    |           |                  |                   |           |     |
|      |        |         |    |                    |           |                  |                   |           |     |
|      |        |         |    |                    |           |                  |                   |           |     |
|      |        |         |    |                    |           |                  |                   |           |     |
|      |        |         |    |                    |           |                  |                   |           |     |
|      |        |         |    |                    |           |                  |                   |           |     |
|      |        |         |    |                    |           |                  |                   |           |     |
|      |        |         |    |                    |           |                  |                   |           |     |
|      |        |         |    |                    |           |                  |                   |           |     |
|      |        |         |    |                    |           |                  |                   |           |     |

* Thirst - score 1-10 each hour, 1= no thirst, 10- severe thirst

**Fig. 14.1** Example of flowchart for water deprivation test.

*or*
    d. child loses >5% body weight from baseline weight.
*Always* collect blood for Na, osmolality, and urine for Na and osmolality at the end of the test.

Allow the child to drink *after* you have obtained the most recent re-sults when the decision has been made to terminate the test. If the child has become hyperosmolar (i.e. plasma osmolality >305 mOsmol/kg, or plasma Na >148 mmol/L), drinking should be limited to the volume of urine passed out during the test (or to maintenance fluid volumes for age) during the first 4 hours following the test. Allow free fluids once the child is passing urine freely again.

### Samples

• Blood: Na, osmolality
• Urine: plain universal container to laboratory.

### Prolonged water deprivation test

Where severe diabetes insipidus has been excluded as previously described, prolonged water deprivation from 24:00 may be considered.

# Standard-dose short Synacthen test

(For 1° adrenal insufficiency, see separate protocol for investigation of possible CAH, p. 404.)

### Indication

Investigation of 1° adrenal insufficiency, including Addison's disease.

All steroid therapy other than dexamethasone or betamethasone interferes with the assay of cortisol. Hydrocortisone should have been stopped for at least 12 hours, ideally 48 hours if hypoadrenalism is *not* strongly suspected (may need to be admitted for monitoring). Prednisone, prednisolone, or other interfering therapy should have been stopped for at least 3 days. Cover may be provided by a physiological dose of dexamethasone if strictly necessary.

### Interpretation

Peak cortisol should be >415 nmol/L (assay dependent). This is usually combined with a rise of >200 nmol/L over baseline values.

### Fasting

Not required.

### Side effects

Synacthen very rarely may cause a hypersensitivity reaction (usually within 30 minutes) particularly in children with atopic tendency. Have hydrocortisone and antihistamine chlorphenamine available in such cases.

### Order Synacthen from pharmacy

Dose:
- 0–6 months: 62.5 mcg
- 6 months–2 years: 125 mcg
- Over 2 years: 250 mcg.

### Procedure

1. Collect baseline bloods
2. Give IV Synacthen.

### Samples

See Table 14.6.

**Table 14.6** Samples

| Time (minutes) | Cortisol | ACTH |
|---|---|---|
| Baseline | + | + |
| 30 | + | |
| 60 | + | |

ACTH: send immediately to laboratory in iced water. Must be marked urgent. Contact laboratory before sending the sample.

# Prolonged adrenocorticotropic hormone test (long Synacthen test)

## Indication

Diagnostic uncertainty following short and low-dose Synacthen tests, particularly concerning whether adrenals are completely suppressed.

All steroid therapy other than dexamethasone or betamethasone interferes with the assay of cortisol. Hydrocortisone should have been stopped for at least 12 hours, ideally 48 hours if hypoadrenalism is *not* strongly suspected (may need to be admitted for monitoring). Prednisone, prednisolone, or other interfering therapy should have been stopped for at least 3 days. Cover may be provided by a physiological dose of dexamethasone.

## Interpretation

As per the SST, but as this test is, by definition, used in cases of diagnostic uncertainty, discussion with the endocrine team is suggested.

## Order drugs from pharmacy

Depot Synacthen (dose 1 mg for injection). Three doses are required.

## Procedure

- Day 1:
  - take blood for cortisol and ACTH (09:00)
  - inject depot Synacthen (dose 1 mg) IM at 09:00.
- Day 2: inject depot Synacthen (dose 1 mg) IM at 09:00.
- Day 3: inject depot Synacthen (dose 1 mg) IM at 09:00.
- Day 4: repeat the blood collection for cortisol at 09:00.

Send each of the blood samples to the laboratory as it is collected. ▶ State the day and timing clearly on each request.

## Samples

ACTH: transport immediately to the laboratory, on ice. Contact laboratory before sending.

## Side effects

The test is liable to cause fluid retention which may be dangerous in some patients.

# Short Synacthen test for investigation of possible congenital adrenal hyperplasia

## Indications
Investigation of possible CAH.

## Interpretation
Elevated basal 17OHP or a rise to >30 nmol/L is associated with CAH. Higher rises are seen in more severe (classical) forms. Lesser rises may be seen in heterozygotes (carriers), but genotype analysis gives a more reliable and absolute result as to status.

## Fasting
Not required.

## Order drugs from pharmacy
Dose:
- 0–6 months: 62.5 mcg
- 6 months–2 years: 125 mcg
- >2 years: 250 mcg.

## Procedure
1. If a basal 24-hour urinary steroid profile is required, this should be collected in the previous 24 hours.
2. Collect baseline bloods.
3. Give IV Synacthen at time 0 minutes.
4. Collect two urine samples if possible. Collect all urine passed 0–2 hours and 2–4 hours post Synacthen in separate containers. Record volume and exact times and save for stimulated steroid profile if required. Send a 20 mL aliquot from each sample for urinary steroid profiling, along with serum steroid results and details of dose of Synacthen.

## Samples
See Table 14.7.

## Side effects
Synacthen very rarely may cause a hypersensitivity reaction (usually within 30 minutes) particularly in children with atopic tendency. Have IV hydrocortisone and chlorphenamine available in such cases

**Table 14.7** Samples

| Time (minutes) | Cortisol | 17OHP | 11-deoxycortisol | A4 | ACTH | Renin |
|---|---|---|---|---|---|---|
| 0 | + | + | + | + | + | + |
| 30 | + | + | + | + | | |
| 60 | + | + | + | + | | |

# Low-dose short Synacthen test

For 2° adrenal insufficiency when central CRH/ACTH deficiency is suspected as the cause for adrenal failure *or* to investigate the subtle inhibition of the HPA axis, e.g. in high-dose inhaled corticosteroids in asthma treatment.

## Indication

Investigation of 2° adrenal insufficiency, where a HP cause may be implicated such as after cranial surgery andor radiotherapy, or to document the recovery of the HPA axis to (especially prolonged) exogenous steroid treatment. This positive predictive value may be improved by combining this test with a measure of spontaneous adrenocortical activity—morning peak 08:00 cortisol and ACTH levels.

## Interpretation

A morning peak cortisol >415 nmol/L is normal, but values >250 nmol/L can be seen in healthy subjects.

The peak stimulated cortisol level should rise to >415 nmol/L. This is usually combined with an increase of >200 nmol/L over baseline values.

## Fasting

Not required. Possibly best done in the afternoon to avoid the morning cortisol peak.

## Side effects

Synacthen in this extremely low dose is unlikely to cause a hypersensitivity reaction (usually within 30 minutes) even in children with atopic tendency. Have hydrocortisone and antihistamine chlorphenamine available in such cases.

## Order Synacthen from pharmacy

Dose: 500 ng/1.73 m² body surface area.

Body surface area = $\sqrt{[\text{height (cm)} \times \text{weight (kg)}/3600]}$ m²

Dilute standard 250 mg vial in 1000 mL 0.9% saline. Shake the bag vigorously. 2 mL of the mixture contains 500 ng of Synacthen.

Calculate dose required as: dose (mL) = 2 × body surface area/1.73.

## Samples

See Table 14.8.

**Table 14.8** Samples

| Time (minutes) | Cortisol | ACTH |
|---|---|---|
| Baseline 1 = 08:00 | + | + |
| Baseline 2 = 0 min | + | |
| *Administer Synacthen* | | |
| 5 | + | |
| 10 | + | |
| 15 | + | |
| 20 | + | |
| 25 | + | |
| 30 | + | |
| 35 | + | |
| 40 | + | |
| 45 | + | |

ACTH: send immediately to laboratory. Must be marked urgent. Contact laboratory before sending the sample.

# Day curve and baseline investigations for patients with congenital adrenal hyperplasia

### Indication

To establish treatment and measure control in poorly controlled patients by showing if current doses are suppressing adrenal androgen production.

### Interpretation

Individual interpretation required, but in general cortisol levels should mimic the diurnal pattern where possible with morning peaks of >415 nmol/L and appropriate troughs to prevent over-replacement. 17OHP levels should also show a diurnal rhythm. Levels >30 nmol/L suggest under-replacement with glucocorticoid. Completely suppressed levels suggest over-replacement.

### Patient preparation

Patients should stay on their normal doses of hydrocortisone and fludrocortisone ± salt supplements. Give hydrocortisone at usual times, but ensure the first set of bloods are taken before the morning dose.

Patients ideally should lie supine for 20 minutes before the renin sample (but in practice this makes little difference when already on treatment).

### Specimens

See Table 14.9.

Label request cards and specimens with:
- test required and
- time and number of specimen.
▶ ACTH: send to laboratory within *30 minutes*, contact before sending.
▶ Renin: send to laboratory within *30 minutes*.

**Table 14.9** Specimens

|  | Cortisol | ACTH | 17OHP | Testosterone | Renin |
|---|---|---|---|---|---|
| 08:00 (pre morning dose) | + | + | + | + | + |
| 10.00 | + | + | + | + | + |
| 12:00 (pre lunch dose) | + |  | + |  |  |
| 14:00 (pre afternoon dose) | + |  | + |  |  |
| 16:00 | + |  | + |  |  |
| 18:00 (pre bed dose) | + |  | + |  |  |
| 20:00 (pre bed dose) | + |  | + |  |  |
| 24:00 | + |  | + |  |  |

# Overnight dexamethasone suppression

Indication

Screening test to exclude Cushing's syndrome.

Interpretation

Cortisol levels should fully suppress if the adrenals are functioning normally.

Seek advice about possible interference in the test from any currently prescribed steroids in individual patients.

Let the laboratory know in advance that you are taking a midnight ACTH sample.

Fasting

Not required.

Procedure

1. Admit child for overnight stay.
2. Insert indwelling IV catheter.
3. Collect blood sample at 23:00–24:00 for cortisol and ACTH from IV line, *ensuring patient is asleep* (▶ the midnight sample must be taken with the child asleep, if not, wait until asleep and write the time on the request form).
4. Give dexamethasone 1 mg orally immediately.
5. Repeat blood sample at 08:00 for cortisol and ACTH.

Specimens

- ACTH—take immediately to the laboratory (if out of hours, ask duty biochemist to separate and freeze serum immediately).
- Cortisol.

# Low-dose dexamethasone suppression test

## Indications

Diagnosis of Cushing syndrome.

## Interpretation

Plasma cortisol <50 nmol/L on day 4 excludes Cushing syndrome. Failure to suppress confirms hypercortisolism, but does not necessarily provide information about the cause.

## Precautions

Diabetes mellitus: this investigation may cause worsening of glycaemic control.

## Procedure

1. Admit patient: day 1.
2. Insert IV cannula for sampling.
3. Collect samples for ACTH and cortisol at 24:00 and the following morning at 09:00 (▶ the midnight sample must be taken with the child asleep, if not, wait until asleep and write the time on the request form).
4. Day 2: start dexamethasone 0.5 mg 6-hourly for eight doses, i.e.:
   • Day 2: 12:00 18:00 24:00
   • Day 3: 06:00 12:00 18:00 24:00
   • Day 4: 06:00
5. Day 4: repeat samples for ACTH and cortisol at 09:00.

## Samples required

- ACTH—take immediately to laboratory: phone and inform laboratory before sending the sample.
- Cortisol.

# High-dose dexamethasone suppression test

### Indications
Differential diagnosis of Cushing syndrome.

### Interpretation
Pituitary-dependant hypercortisolaemia (Cushing disease): plasma cortisol usually (but not invariably) suppresses to at least 50% of basal levels.
  Adrenal tumours and ectopic ACTH: failure to suppress.

### Precautions
Diabetes mellitus; worsening of glycaemic control.

### Procedure
Identical to low-dose dexamethasone suppression test except 2 mg dexamethasone is used per dose. Often the high-dose dexamethasone suppression test will follow directly on from the low-dose test.
1. Admit patient: day 1.
2. Insert IV cannula for sampling.
3. Collect samples for ACTH and cortisol at 24:00 and the following morning at 09:00 (▶ the midnight sample must be taken with the child asleep, if not, wait until asleep and write the time on the request form).
4. Day 2: start dexamethasone 2.0 mg 6-hourly for eight doses, i.e.:
   • Day 2: 12:00  18:00  24:00
   • Day 3: 06:00  12:00  18:00  24:00
   • Day 4: 06:00
5. Day 4: repeat samples for ACTH and cortisol at 09:00.

### Samples required
• ACTH—take immediately to laboratory. Phone and inform laboratory before sending.
• Cortisol.

# Corticotrophin-releasing hormone test

### Indication

Differential diagnosis of Cushing syndrome. May be helpful in determining the source of ACTH in ACTH-dependent Cushing syndrome, after adrenal adenoma has been ruled out by baseline plasma ACTH level and high-dose dexamethasone suppression test.

### Interpretation

ACTH and cortisol are secreted in response to CRH in normal subjects. An exaggerated response is seen in Cushing disease (pituitary ACTH overproduction). In ectopic ACTH syndrome, ACTH and cortisol fail to respond to CRH.

### Precautions

- Patient should be warned that facial flushing is likely.
- Transient hypotension may occur.

### Procedure

1. Fast from midnight.
2. 08:30: site IV cannula.
3. 08:45: take −15-minute blood specimen.
4. 09:00: take 0-minute blood sample, give CRH 1 mcg/kg body weight over 1 minute. This is time = 0.

### Blood samples

See Table 14.10.

### Collecting specimens

The specimen volume requirements given are the *minimum* amounts required to perform each analysis once. It is essential to collect at least the amounts stated.

▶ If smaller specimens are sent, some tests will have to be *omitted*.

### Specimen requirements

- Cortisol
- ACTH sample *taken immediately to laboratory*. Phone and inform laboratory before sending.

**Table 14.10** Samples

| Time (minutes) | Cortisol | ACTH |
| --- | --- | --- |
| −15 | + | + |
| 0 | + | + |
| 5 | + | + |
| 15 | + | + |
| 30 | + | + |
| 45 | + | + |
| 60 | + | + |
| 90 | + | + |
| 120 | + | + |

# Human chorionic gonadotropin stimulation test (3 days)

## Indication

To investigate testicular response to gonadotrophin in the diagnosis of hypo- and hypergonadotropic hypogonadism, and investigation of disorders of sex development (see later in this topic).

## Interpretation

A rise of testosterone to >5 nmol/L indicates good testicular (Leydig cell) function.

▶ hCG interferes with LH and FSH estimations and these measurements should be complete before carrying out the hCG test.

## Dose

- 1000 IU hCG IM daily for 3 days (in infants)
- 1500 IU or 2000 IU hCG IM daily for 3 days (older children). When it is not possible to give three injections on consecutive days, an alternative is to give a single dose of 1500 IU (infants) 5000 IU (older children) of hCG IM.

## Procedure

- Day 1:
  - specimen for testosterone and DHT
  - give hCG.
- Day 2: give hCG.
- Day 3: give hCG.
- Day 4: specimen for testosterone and DHT.

### ▶ Ambiguous genitalia/DSD

If you are investigating a DSD, measurement of testosterone precursors (androstenedione, dehydroepiandrosterone, 11-deoxycortisol) will be required before and after hCG. Check with a member of the endocrine team *before* doing the test. An additional blood sample will then be needed with the samples on days 1 and 4 and requested on the cards. Please take separate samples for these.

# Prolonged human chorionic gonadotropin stimulation test

## Indication

This may be indicated instead of the short hCG stimulation test if 1° hypo-gonadism (i.e. absent or hypoplastic testes) is strongly suspected. The test will normally follow a standard LHRH stimulation rest.

## Interpretation

Requires individual interpretation. A rise of testosterone to >5 nmol/L indicates good testicular (Leydig cell) function.

## Procedure

- Week 1:
  - *Monday*: collect baseline plasma testosterone/FSH/LH. Give hCG 2000 U IM
  - *Thursday*: hCG 2000 U
- Week 2:
  - *Monday*: hCG 2000 U
  - *Thursday*: hCG 2000 U
- Week 3:
  - *Monday*: hCG 2000 U
  - *Thursday*: hCG 2000 U
  - *Friday*: collect blood for post-hCG plasma testosterone.

# Oral glucose tolerance test

## Indication

For investigation of impaired glucose tolerance, T1DM or T2DM, or MODY. Occasionally an OGTT is used to check that GH can be suppressed in tall children suspected of autonomous GH release, please consult the protocol entitled 'Glucose tolerance test for GH hypersecretion' (see p. 391).

## Interpretation: criteria for diagnosis of diabetes mellitus

1. Symptoms of diabetes plus random plasma glucose concentration ≥ 11.1 mmol/L, or
2. Fasting plasma glucose ≥7.0 mmol/L, or
3. Plasma glucose ≥11.1 mmol/L 2 hours after an oral 75 g anhydrous glucose load.
4. Impaired glucose tolerance—plasma glucose >7.8 but <11.1, 2 hours after an oral 75 g anhydrous glucose load.

## Fasting

Yes, nil by mouth except water from midnight.

## Order drugs from pharmacy

Oral glucose solution 1.75 g/kg up to maximum of 75 g
   Alternatively, Polycal® can be used.

## Procedure

1. Baseline fasting bloods for glucose, insulin, islet cell antibodies, HbA1c, and C-peptide.
2. Give oral glucose solution. Drink should be consumed in 5–10 minutes.
3. Take blood samples as charted, checking fingerprick blood glucose at each time point.

## Samples

See Table 14.11.

**Table 14.11** Samples

| Time (minutes) | Glucose | Insulin/C-peptide | HbA1C | Islet cell/GAD antibodies |
|---|---|---|---|---|
| Baseline | + | + | + | + |
| 30 | + | | | |
| 60 | + | | | |
| 90 | + | | | |
| 120 | + | | | |

Continue sampling until blood glucose returns to normal.

# Intravenous glucose tolerance test

## Indication

For investigation of first- and second-phase insulin response in suspected glucose intolerance (e.g. 2° to cystic fibrosis, thalassaemia).

By giving glucose intravenously, variations of the rate of absorption from the GI tract are avoided but the test is complex and only rarely needed.

## Interpretation

The results are interpreted by plotting log glucose against time and calculating the rate of disappearance (Kt).

Normal values:

- Zuppinger: Kt = 2.10%/min (1 SD = 0.47)
- Loeb: Kt = 2.8%/min (1 SD = 0.55).

## Fasting

Fast overnight (12–15 hours) but only 6 hours for babies <6 months. (If the child is liable to develop hypoglycaemia, the fast should be as long as he/she can tolerate.)

## Procedure

1. Insert indwelling cannula and take fasting bloods for glucose and insulin.
2. Give glucose IV at 2–4 minutes, preferably via a different vein from that which the specimens are to be collected.
   - Dose of glucose: (25% solution) 0.33 g/kg up to a maximum of 25 g. Note *exact* time when injection finished.
3. Blood samples are collected at precise times. If specimens are collected late, please note *exact* time.

## Samples

See Table 14.12.

**Table 14.12** Samples

| Time (minutes) | Glucose | Insulin |
|---|---|---|
| −10 | + | + |
| −5 | + | + |
| 0 | + | + |
| 1 | + | + |
| 3 | + | + |
| 5 | + | + |
| 10 | + | + |
| 15 | + | + |
| 20 | + | + |
| 30 | + | + |
| 45 | + | + |
| 60 | + | + |
| 75 | + | + |
| 90 | + | + |
| 120 | + | + |
| 180 | + | + |

# Prolonged fast (hypoglycaemia screen)

## Indication

For investigation of unexplained hypoglycaemia (non-neonatal).
   Warn the duty biochemist the day *before*.

## Precautions

The test must be performed as an inpatient under close supervision.
   Every child undergoing a starvation test *must* have IV access.

## Length of the test

This will depend on the age of the child, see Table 14.13.

## Procedure

1. During the fast children require close monitoring and supervision.
   Check blood glucose using a bedside test starting from halfway through
   the test (after 6 hours for the longer fasts) and then continue hourly.
   Earlier testing is required if the child is symptomatic.
   ▶ NB: very rapid laboratory blood glucose estimations are available for
   prolonged fasts and it is advisable to use them in addition to bedside
   monitoring. For this service, contact the duty biochemist early in the
   fasting period.
2. Collect blood specimens (Table 14.14) for laboratory analysis:
   • when bedside fingerprick blood glucose is ≤3.0 mmol/L, and
   • at the end of test.
   If there is concern over compliance it may be helpful to collect specimens
   at more frequent intervals for β-hydroxybutyrate, free fatty acids, and
   insulin.
3. Test is ended when:
   • there are clinical signs of hypoglycaemia
   • or blood glucose ≤2.6 mmol/L by rapid laboratory measurement or
   after the pre-arranged duration of fast.
   Once the blood samples are taken, terminate the test and treat any
   hypoglycaemia.
4. ▶ *Very important*—collect *urine* during last few hours of fast and/
   or immediately afterwards for organic acid and amino acid analysis.
   NB: do not wait for urine sample before treating the hypoglycaemia.
5. Ensure that the child has eaten a good meal before discharge.

## Blood samples

See Table 14.14.

## Urine sample

Send the specimen of urine collected closest to the time of maximum fast
or hypoglycaemia for:
• amino acids: at least 2 mL urine—send to laboratory same day
• organic acids: at least 5 mL urine—send to laboratory within 3 hours of
   collection.

**Table 14.13** Length of test

| Age | <6 months | 6–8 months | 8–12 months | 1–2 years | 2–4 years | 4–7 years | >7 years |
|-----|-----------|------------|-------------|-----------|-----------|-----------|----------|
| Duration (hours) | 8 | 12 | 16 | 18 | 20 | 20 | 24 |

NB: for the longer fasts it will be necessary to start overnight in order to ensure that the end of the fast coincides with normal working hours for both clinical and laboratory staff (do not start fasts at home).

**Table 14.14** Samples (laboratory will run full screen only if laboratory glucose ≤3.0 mmol/L)

| | |
|---|---|
| Glucose | |
| Lactate | On ice to laboratory immediately |
| β-hydroxybutyrate and free fatty acids | On ice immediately to the laboratory |
| Insulin and C-peptide | Immediately to the laboratory |
| Cortisol | |
| GH | |
| Amino acids | To laboratory immediately, or four blood spots on neonatal screening card (qualitative) |
| Ammonia | To laboratory immediately on ice |
| Venous gases | Capillary tube/blood gas syringe |
| Acylcarnitine profile (if not already done) | 4 drops blood on Guthrie card, need separate Guthrie card from amino acids |
| Free carnitine (already included in acylcarnitine profile) | |
| Glucagon | On ice to laboratory immediately |
| Adrenaline | Not always available. Refer to local protocols. Alternative is plasma/urine metanephrine |

# Investigation of a child with osteopenia

## Indication

Outlined here are the investigations for a child who presents with recurrent fractures and/or radiological evidence of osteopenia.

Interpretation: this depends on the pattern of any abnormalities detected (→ see Chapter 7 on hypocalcaemia). Advice should be sought.

## History and examination

A full clinical history and physical examination should always be performed. Particular attention to the following should be taken:
- nature of any fractures (i.e. cause and severity of any associated trauma)
- bone pain
- drug history
- family history of fracture and/or osteoporosis
- height, weight, and pubertal assessment
- extensibility of joints (Beighton scoring)
- colour of sclera
- dentition
- striae
- hearing

## Biochemical investigations

### Blood
- FBC and film
- ESR
- Calcium
- Phosphate
- Magnesium
- U&E and creatinine
- LFTs including alkaline phosphatase
- TFT
- PTH
- IGF-1
- 1,25 dihydroxy- and 25-hydroxyvitamin D
- Alkaline phosphatase
- P1NP
- tissue transglutaminase (for coeliac screening).

### Urine
- 24-hour urine for urinary free cortisol
- Random urine for calcium, phosphate, and creatinine ratio (request calcium/creatinine ratio and tubular reabsorption of phosphate calculation).

## Radiological investigations

DXA scan for bone density of the left hip and lumbar spine.

## Other investigations

Consider bone biopsy.

# Investigation of severe obesity

Admit patient following an overnight fast (nil by mouth except water from midnight). Record current height and weight.

## Baseline samples

- Fasting leptin (must be requested by consultant paediatrician usually as part of a research study (Genetics of Obesity Study, University of Cambridge)
- Free $T_4$, TSH, cortisol, Ca, $PO_4$, PTH, alkaline phosphatase
- Fasting lipids (cholesterol and triglyceride)
- DNA from patient and *both parents* if possible (for PWS)
- Fasting glucose and insulin (if not proceeding to OGTT).

## Oral glucose tolerance test

### Dose

Oral glucose solution 1.75 g/kg up to a maximum of 75 g.
  *Alternatively*, Polycal®.

### Interpretation

➔ See 'Oral glucose tolerance test', p. 418.

### Procedure

1. Baseline fasting bloods.
2. Give oral glucose solution (or Lucozade®). This should be consumed in 5–10 minutes.
3. Take blood samples as shown in Table 14.15, checking blood glucose at the bedside at each time point.

### Samples

See Table 14.15.

## Specimens

- $T_4$, TSH, Ca, $PO_4$, alkaline phosphatase
- Glucose, cortisol
- AFP, HCG
- Leptin
- Insulin and C-peptide *to laboratory immediately*
- PTH to laboratory within 60 minutes.

**Table 14.15** Samples

| Time (minutes) | Glucose | Insulin | C-peptide |
|---|---|---|---|
| Baseline | + | + | + |
| 30 | + | | |
| 60 | + | | |
| 90 | + | | |
| 120 | + | | |

Continue sampling until the bedside blood glucose returns to normal.

# Laboratory reference ranges

Each laboratory will have their own assay systems and links with regional laboratories for specialist analyses. The values given here are as a guide only.

## Samples

It is essential that samples are taken into the right container to prepare the blood or urine for analysis. The additive will either promote clotting (as in SST gel or a plain tube) to obtain serum for analysis, prevent clotting (as in lithium–heparin tubes) to obtain plasma, or stabilize the sample to prevent breakdown of the analyte (as with EDTA or fluoride preservative for glucose).

Urine is either collected as a single spot sample into a plain universal container (usually for acute samples) or if a 24-hour collection is required, a plain container or one containing acid as a preservative. Always check with the biochemistry laboratory.

## Tube types

This will vary by hospital and laboratory and whether specialized tubes are available for neonatal use. Table 14.16 is a guide to what is commonly available in UK hospitals for biochemistry investigations.

## Sample requirements and reference ranges of common endocrine tests

See Table 14.17.

**Table 14.16** Biochemistry investigations

| Tube type | General use | Neonatal use |
| --- | --- | --- |
| EDTA anticoagulant | Purple top | Pink or red top |
| Lithium–heparin | Green top | Orange top |
| Plain | Red top | White top |
| SST gel separator | Gold top | – |
| Fluoride preservative | Grey top | Yellow top |

**Table 14.17** Sample requirements

| Adreno-corticotropic hormone (ACTH) | 4 mL blood EDTA purple top tube—kept cold, centrifuged immediately | <46 ng/L (09:00) |
|---|---|---|
| Aldosterone, blood | 4 mL EDTA purple top tube or SST gel gold top tube | 1–3 months: 1000–3500 pmol/L<br>3–12 months: 400–1500 pmol/L<br>1–4 years: 300–1000 pmol/L<br>Adult, ambulant: 90–700 pmol/L |
| Aldosterone, urine | 24-hour urine collected in plain bottle | 10–50 nmol/24 hours |
| Alkaline phosphatase, total | 5 mL blood gold top SST gel tube | 0–5 days: 0–250 IU/L<br>5–180 days: 0–449 IU/L<br>180–365 days: 0–462 IU/L<br>1–3 years: 0–281 IU/L<br>3–6 years: 0–269 IU/L<br>6–12 years: 0–300 IU/L<br>Male 12–17 years: 0–390 IU/L<br>Female 12–17 years: 0–187 IU/L<br>Male >17 years: 40–129 IU/L<br>Female >17 years: 35–104 IU/L |
| Ammonia | 4 mL blood EDTA purple top tube | Preterm neonate: <150 µmol/L<br>Term neonate: <100 µmol/L<br>1 month–14 years: <40 µmol/L<br>>14 years: 11–32 µmol/L |
| Androstenedione | 5 mL blood gold top SST gel tube | Prepubertal: <1.1 nmol/L<br>Male: 2.0–10.0 nmol/L<br>Female: 1.4–11.5 nmol/L |
| Calcitonin | 5 mL blood plain red top tube or SST gel gold top tube *on ice* | Male: <8.4 ng/L<br>Female: <5.0 ng/L |
| Calcium | 5 mL blood gold top SST gel tube | 2.20–2.60 mmol/L |
| Calcium, urine | 24-hour urine collected in bottle with acid | 0.08–0.79 mmol/mmol creatinine<br>2.5–8.0 mmol/24 hours |

*(Continued)*

Table 14.17 (Contd.)

| | | |
|---|---|---|
| Catecholamines (plasma/urine metanephrines recommended) | 2 × 4 mL blood purple top EDTA *on ice* 24-hour urine collected in bottle with acid | Normetanephrine 120–1180 pmol/L Metanephrine 80–510 pmol/L Refer to laboratory report |
| Cortisol | 5 mL blood gold top SST gel tube 24-hour urine collected in plain bottle | Midnight <100 nmol/L 09:00 142–497 nmol/L 0–250 nmol/24 hours |
| C-peptide | 5 mL blood gold top SST gel tube or red top plain tube *on ice* (and 2 mL fluoride oxalate tube for concurrent glucose level) | 260–650 pmol/L (fasting) |
| Dehydro-epiandrosterone sulphate (DHEAS) | 5 mL blood gold top SST gel tube | Prepubertal children: <0.5 µmol/L Male: 0.4–13.4 µmol/L Female: 0.26–11.0 µmol/L |
| 7-Dehydrosterols | Random urine | |
| 11-Deoxycortisol | 5 mL blood gold top SST gel tube or red top plain tube | 7–13 nmol/L (09:00) |
| Dihydro-testosterone (DHT) | 5 mL blood red top plain tube | <0.27 nmol/L (6 months until puberty) From 9 years until 16 years depends on pubertal status Adult male: 0.32–1.64 nmol/L Adult female: <0.6 nmol/L |
| Follicle-stimulating hormone (FSH) | 5 mL blood gold top SST gel tube | <5 IU/L (prepubertal children) Male: 1.5–12.4 IU/L Female: 3.5–12.5 IU/L (follicular phase) 4.7–21.5 IU/L (mid cycle) 1.7–7.7 IU/L (luteal) 25.8–134.8 IU/L (postmenopausal) |
| Free $T_3$ | 5 mL blood gold top SST gel tube | 4.0–6.8 pmol/L |
| Free $T_4$ | 5 mL blood gold top SST gel tube | 12.0–22.0 pmol/L |
| Fructosamine | 5 mL blood gold top SST gel tube | 205–285 umol/L (non-diabetic) |

| | | |
|---|---|---|
| Gastrin (fasting essential) | 2 × 4 mL blood purple top EDTA *on ice* | <40 pmol/L |
| Gut hormones (fasting essential) | 2 × 4 mL blood purple top EDTA ON ICE | Vasoactive intestinal peptide <30 pmol/L |
| | | Pancreatic polypeptide <300 pmol/L |
| | | Gastrin <40 pmol/L |
| | | Somatostatin <150 pmol/L |
| | | Chromogranin A <60 pmol/L |
| | | Chromogranin B <150 pmol/L |
| Glucagon (fasting essential) | 2 × 4 mL blood purple top EDTA *on ice* | <50 pmol/L |
| Glucose | 3 mL blood light grey fluoride oxalate tube | 3.9–5.8 mmol/L |
| | or<br>0.5 mL cerebrospinal fluid fluoride light grey fluoride oxalate tube | 2.2–3.9 mmol/L |
| | or<br>5 mL fresh random urine | Not detected |
| Glucose (oral) tolerance test | 3 mL blood fluoride oxalate tube<br>Follow dynamic function test protocol | For interpretation see dynamic function test protocol |
| Glycated haemoglobin (HbA1c) | 4 mL blood purple top EDTA tube | 4.0–6.0% total Hb<br>20–42 mmol/mol (IFCC) |
| Growth hormone (GH) | 5 mL blood plain or SST gel gold top tube | <20 mU/L (fasting or random daytime)<br>Stimulation tests—see elsewhere in chapter |
| HCG, β subunit, as tumour marker | 5 mL blood gold top SST gel tube | 0–3 IU/L |
| Hydroxypro-gesterone (17α) | 5 mL blood gold top SST gel tube, redtop plain tube or green top lithium heparin tube | Male and female < 5 days: <3.0 nmol/L<br>Male and female <16 years: <4.0 nmol/L<br>Female >16 years: <5.0 nmol/L<br>Male >16 years: <5.0 nmol/L<br>Carriers for 21OHD may show higher values following Synacthen stimulation |

(Continued)

**Table 14.17** (*Contd.*)

| Insulin-like growth factor 1 (IGF-1) | 5 mL blood gold top SST gel tube | Age (years) | Female Male (nmol/L) |
|---|---|---|---|
| | | <1 | <17 <13 |
| | | 1–2 | <22 <19 |
| | | 3–5 | <33 <30 |
| | | 6–8 | 3–52 2–45 |
| | | 9–11 | 6.5–72 3–60 |
| | | 12–15 | 12–78 6.5–68 |
| | | 16–20 | 14–68 15.5–67 |
| | | 21–30 | 11–46 10.5–47 |
| | | 31–40 | 10–38 10.5–32 |
| | | 41–50 | 5.5–32 6.5–30 |
| | | 51–60 | 5.5–32 6.5–30 |
| | | 61–70 | 3.5–32 3.5–32 |
| | | 71–80 | 3–30 2.5–32 |
| | | >80 | 2–25 2–24 |
| IGFBP3 | 5 mL blood gold top SST gel tube or red top plain tube | 0–2 years: 0.5–2.9 mg/L 3–4 years: 0.8–3.4 mg/L 5–6 years: 1.0–3.8 mg/L 7–8 years: 1.1–4.3 mg/L 9–10 years: 1.3–4.6 mg/L 11–12 years: 1.6–5.0 mg/L 13–14 years: 2.1–5.3 mg/L 15–16 years: 2.5–5.4 mg/L 17–18 years: 2.4–5.4 mg/L 19–20 years: 2.3–5.3 mg/L 21–40 years: 1.7–5.2 mg/L 41–60 years: 1.3–4.8 mg/L 61–80 years: 0.7–4.4 mg/L >80 years: 0.5–4.3 mg/L | |
| Insulin | 5 mL blood gold top SST gel tube (and 2 mL fluoride oxalate tube for concurrent glucose level) | 2.6–24.9 mIU/L | |
| Inhibin B | 5 mL blood gold top SST gel tube | Male: 25–35 ng/L Female: day 3 <273 ng/dL Otherwise: <341 ng/dL Postmenopausal: <5 ng/L | |

| Luteinizing hormone (LH) | 5 mL blood gold top SST gel tube | Prepubertal children: <5 IU/L<br>Male: 1.7–8.6 IU/L<br>Female:<br>2.4–12.6 IU/L<br>(follicular phase)<br>14.0–95.6 IU/L (mid cycle)<br>1.0–11.4 IU/L (luteal)<br>7.7–58.5 IU/L<br>(postmenopausal) |
|---|---|---|
| Oestradiol | 5 mL blood gold top SST gel tube | Prepubertal children: 4–20 pmol/L<br>Male: 44–146 pmol/L<br>Female:<br>46–607 pmol/L (follicular)<br>315–1828 pmol/L<br>(mid cycle)<br>161–774 pmol/L (luteal)<br><201 pmol/L<br>(postmenopausal) |
| Osmolality | 5 mL blood gold top SST gel tube<br>5 mL random urine | 285–295 mOsmol/kg<br>300–900 mOsmol/kg |
| Phosphate | 5 mL blood gold top SST gel tube | 0–10 days: 1.45–2.91 mmol/L<br>10 days–2 years: 1.45–2.16 mmol/L<br>2–13 years: 1.45–1.78 mmol/L<br>>13 years: 0.87–1.45 mmol/L |
| Progesterone | 5 mL blood gold top SST gel tube | Male: 0.2–0.5 nmol/L<br>Female:<br>0.2–2.8 nmol/L (follicular)<br>0.4–38.1 nmol/L (ovulatory)<br>5.8–75.9 nmol/L (luteal)<br>0.2–0.4 nmol/L<br>(postmenopausal) |
| Prolactin | 5 mL blood gold top SST gel tube | Male: 86–324 mIU/L<br>Female: 102–496 mIU/L |

(Continued)

**Table 14.17** (Contd.)

| | | |
|---|---|---|
| PTH (parathyroid hormone) | 5 mL blood gold top SST gel tube TO LAB <2 hours | 1.6–6.9 pmol/L |
| Renin | 4 mL blood EDTA or lithium–heparin tube. Sample requires immediate transfer to laboratory. Routine transport not suitable. DO NOT send on ice. | 4–12 nmol/L/hour (1–3 months) 2–6 nmol/L/hour (3–12 months) 0.5–3.5 nmol/L/hour (>1 years) |
| Sex hormone-binding globulin (SHBG) | 5 mL blood gold top SST gel tube | Male <50 years: 16–55 nmol/L Male >50 years: 19–83 nmol/L Female <50 years: 27–146 nmol/L Female >50 years: 22–142 nmol/L |
| Sodium | 5 mL blood gold top SST gel tube | 135–145 mmol/L |
| Sodium, urine | 24-hour urine collected in plain or acid bottle or 10 mL random urine | 40–220 mmol/24 hours |
| Testosterone | 5 mL blood gold top SST gel tube | Male: 0–2 years: 0.4–0.7 nmol/L 2–7 years: 0.1–1.1 nmol/L 7–13 years: 0.1–2.3 nmol/L 13–18 years: 0.9–31.4 nmol/L >18 years: 7.6–31.4 nmol/L Female: 0–1.8 nmol/L |
| Thyroglobulin | 5 mL blood gold top SST gel tube | <0.9 mcg/L post thyroidectomy |
| Thyroid receptor Ab (TRAb) Thyroid peroxidase Ab (TPO) | 5 mL blood gold top SST gel tube | Index <20 is normal 0–34 mIU/L |

| | | |
|---|---|---|
| Thyroid-stimulating hormone | 5 mL blood gold top SST gel tube | 0.27–4.20 mIU/L |
| Thyroxine (free T₄) | 5 mL blood gold top SST gel tube | 12.0–22.0 pmol/L |
| Tri-iodothyronine (free T₃) | | 4.0–6.8 pmol/L |
| Vitamin D, 25-OH (cholecalciferol) | 5 mL blood gold top SST gel tube<br>or red top plain tube | Deficient <30 nmol/L<br>Insufficient 30–50 nmol/L<br>Sufficient >50 nmol/L<br>Excess/toxic >200 nmol/L |
| Vitamin D 1,25-(OH)₂ (calcitriol) | 5 mL blood gold top SST gel tube<br>or red top plain tube or green top heparin tube | 43–143 pmol/L |

# Patient support groups and other endocrine organizations

Androgen Insensitivity Syndrome Support Group
ℰ http://www.aissg.org

Australasian Paediatric Endocrine Group
ℰ https://apeg.org.au

British Society for Paediatric Endocrinology and Diabetes
(with many links to sites in paediatrics, endocrinology, and diabetes)
ℰ http://www.bsped.org.uk

CAH support group
ℰ http://www.livingwithcah.com

Child Growth Foundation
ℰ http://www.childgrowthfoundation.org

CLIMB (Children Living with Inherited Metabolic Diseases)
ℰ http://www.climb.org.uk

Diabetes UK
ℰ http://www.diabetes.org.uk

Endocrine Society (US)
ℰ https://www.endocrine.org

European Society for Paediatric Endocrinology
(with many links to sites in paediatrics, endocrinology, and diabetes)
ℰ http://www.eurospe.org

Gender Identity Development Service
ℰ http://www.gids.nhs.uk

Gender Identity Research and Education Society
ℰ http://www.gires.org.uk

International Society for Pediatric and Adolescent Diabetes
ℰ http://www.ispad.org

Juvenile Diabetes Research Forum
ℰ http://www.jdrf.org.uk

Klinefelter Organisation
ℰ http://www.klinefelter.org.uk

Klinefelter Syndrome Association
ℰ https://www.ksa-uk.net

Pediatric Endocrine Society (US)
https://www.pedsendo.org

Pituitary Foundation
⌕ http://www.pituitary.org.uk

Restricted Growth Association
⌕ http://www.restrictedgrowth.co.uk

Royal College of Paediatrics and Child Health growth charts
⌕ https://www.rcpch.ac.uk/resources/growth-charts

Society for Endocrinology (UK)
⌕ http://www.endocrinology.org

Turner Syndrome Society of the United States
⌕ https://www.turnersyndrome.org

Turner Syndrome Support Society
⌕ http://www.tss.org.uk

Unique (rare chromosomal disorders)
⌕ http://www.rarechromo.org

# Index

Tables, figures and boxes are indicated by *t*, *f* and *b* following the page number